THE GENETICS PROBLEM SOLVER®

**Staff of Research and Education Association,
Dr. M. Fogiel, Director**

Research and Education Association
61 Ethel Road West
Piscataway, New Jersey 08854

THE GENETICS PROBLEM SOLVER®

Printed in the United States of America

Library of Congress Catalog Card Number 85-62730

International Standard Book Number 0-87891-560-5

Revised Printing, 1989

PROBLEM SOLVER is a registered trademark of
Research and Education Association, New York, N.Y. 10018

WHAT THIS BOOK IS FOR

For as long as genetics has been taught in schools, students have found this subject difficult to understand and learn because of the broad scope of this subject and unusually large number of concepts involved. Despite the publications of hundreds of textbooks in this field, each one intended to provide an improvement over previous textbooks, genetics remains particularly perplexing and the subject is often taken in class only to meet school/department requirements for a selected course of study.

In a study of the problem, REA found the following basic reasons underlying students' difficulties with genetics taught in schools:

(a) No systematic rules of analysis have been developed which students may follow in a step-by-step manner to solve the usual problems encountered. This results from the fact that the numerous different conditions and principles which may be involved in a problem, lead to many possible different methods of solution. To prescribe a set of rules to be followed for each of the possible variations, would involve and enormous number of rules and steps to be searched through by students, and this task would perhaps be more burdensome than solving the problem directly with some accompanying trial and error to find the correct solution route.

(b) Textbooks currently available will usually explain a given principle in a few pages written by a professional who has an insight in the subject matter that is not shared by students. The explanations are often written in an abstract manner which leaves the students confused as to the application of the principle. The explanations given are not sufficiently detailed and extensive to make the student aware of the wide range of applications and different aspects of the principle being studied. The numerous possible variations of principles and their applications are usually not discussed, and it is left for the students to discover these for themselves while doing exercises.

Accordingly, the average student is expected to rediscover that which has been long known and practiced, but not published or explained extensively.

(c) The examples usually following the explanation of a topic are too few in number and too simple to enable the student to obtain a thorough grasp of the principles involved. The explanations do not provide sufficient basis to enable a student to solve problems that may be subsequently assigned for homework or given on examinations.

The examples are presented in abbreviated form which leaves out much material between steps, and requires that students derive the omitted material themselves. As a result, students find the examples difficult to understand--contrary to the purpose of the examples.

Examples are, furthermore, often worded in a confusing manner. They do not state the problem and then present the solution. Instead, they pass through a general discussion, never revealing what is to be solved for.

Examples, also, do not always include diagrams/graphs, wherever appropriate, and students do not obtain the training to draw diagrams or graphs to simplify and organize their thinking.

(d) Students can learn the subject only by doing the exercises themselves and reviewing them in class, to obtain experience in applying the principles with their different ramifications.

In doing the exercises by themselves, students find that they are required to devote considerably more time to genetics than to other subjects of comparable credits, because they are uncertain with regard to the selection and application of the theorems and principles involved. It is also often necessary for students to discover those "tricks" not revealed in their texts (or review books), that make it possible to solve problems easily. Students must usually resort to methods of trial-and-error to discover these "tricks", and as a result they find that they may sometimes spend several hours solving a single problem.

(e) When reviewing the exercises in classrooms, instructors

usually request students to take turns writing solutions on the board and explaining them to the class. Students often find it difficult to explain in a manner that holds the interest of the class, and enables the remaining students to follow the material written on the boards. The remaining students seated in the class are, furthermore, too occupied with copying the material from the boards, to listen to the oral explanations and concentrate on the methods of solution.

This book is intended to aid students in genetics in overcoming the difficulties described, by supplying detailed illustrations of the solution methods which are usually not apparent to students. The solution methods are illustrated by problems selected from those that are most often assigned for class work and given on examinations. The problems are arranged in order of complexity to enable students to learn and understand a particular topic by reviewing the problems in sequence. The problems are illustrated with detailed step-by-step explanations, to save the students the large amount of time that is often needed to fill in the gaps that are usually found between steps of illustrations in textbooks or review/outline books.

The staff of REA considers genetics a subject that is best learned by allowing students to view the methods of analysis and solution techniques themselves. This approach to learning the subject matter is similar to that practiced in various scientific laboratories, particularly in the medical fields.

In using this book, students may review and study the illustrated problems at their own pace; they are not limited to the time allowed for explaining problems on the board in class.

When students want to look up a particular type of problem and solution, they can readily locate it in the book by referring to the index which has been extensively prepared. It is also possible to locate a particular type of problem by glancing at just the material within the boxed portions. To facilitate rapid scanning of the problems, each problem has a heavy border around it. Furthermore, each problem is identified with a number immediately above the problem at the right-hand margin.

To obtain maximum benefit from the book, students should familiarize themselves with the section, "How To Use This Book," located in the front pages.

To meet the objectives of this book, staff members of REA have selected problems usually encountered in assignments and examinations, and have solved each problem meticulously to illustrate the steps which are difficult for students to comprehend. Special gratitude is expressed to them for their efforts in this area, as well as to the numerous contributors who devoted brief periods of time to this work.

Gratitude is also expressed to the many persons involved in the difficult task of typing the manuscript with its endless changes, and to the REA art staff who prepared the numerous detailed illustrations together with the layout and physical features of the book.

The difficult task of coordinating the efforts of all persons was carried out by Carl Fuchs. His conscientious work deserves much appreciation. He also trained and supervised art and production personnel in the preparation of the book for printing.

Finally, special thanks are due to Helen Kaufmann for her unique talents to render those difficult border-line decisions and constructive suggestions related to the design and organization of the book.

Max Fogiel, Ph.D.
Program Director

HOW TO USE THIS BOOK

This book can be an invaluable aid to students in genetics as a supplement to their textbooks. The book is subdivided into 15 chapters, each dealing with a separate topic. The subject matter is developed beginning with cell mechanics, chromosomes, Mendelian genetics, sex determination and linkage, mutation and alleles, genetic interactions and extending through linkage, recombination and mapping, population genetics, and bacterial and viral genetics. Extensive sections are also included on biochemistry, behavioral genetics, immunogenetics, and genetic engineering.

Each chapter of the book is accompanied by a series of short answer questions to help in reviewing the study material and preparation of exams.

TO LEARN AND UNDERSTAND
A TOPIC THOROUGHLY

1. Refer to your class text and read the section pertaining to the topic. You should become acquainted with the principles discussed there. These principles, however, may not be clear to you at that time.

2. Then locate the topic you are looking for by referring to the "Table of Contents" in front of this book, "The Genetics Problem Solver."

3. Turn to the page where the topic begins and review the problems under each topic, in the order given. For each topic, the problems are arranged in order of complexity, from the simplest to the most difficult. Some problems may appear similar to others, but each problem has been selected to illustrate a different point or solution method.

To learn and understand a topic thoroughly and retain its contents, it will be generally necessary for students to review the problems several times. Repeated review is essential in order to gain experience in recognizing the principles that should be applied, and in selecting the best solution technique.

TO FIND A PARTICULAR PROBLEM

To locate one or more problems related to a particular subject matter, refer to the index. In using the index, be certain to note that the numbers given there refer to problem numbers, not to page numbers. This arrangement of the index is intended to facilitate finding a problem more rapidly, since two or more problems may appear on a page.

If a particular type of problem cannot be found readily, it is recommended that the student refer to the "Table of Contents" in the front pages, and then turn to the chapter which is applicable to the problem being sought. By scanning or glancing at the material that is boxed, it will generally be possible to find problems related to the one being sought, without consuming considerable time. After the problems have been located, the solutions can be reviewed and studied in detail. For this purpose of locating problems rapidly, students should acquaint themselves with the organization of the book as found in the "Table of Contents."

In preparing for an exam, locate the topics to be covered on the exam in the "Table of Contents," and then review the problems under those topics several times. This should equip the student with what might be needed for the exam.

CONTENTS

CHAPTER 1

CELL MECHANICS

MITOSIS

● PROBLEM 1-1

What are the stages of mitosis?

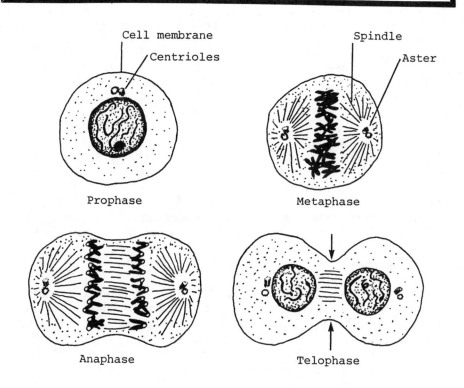

(a)   Animal cell

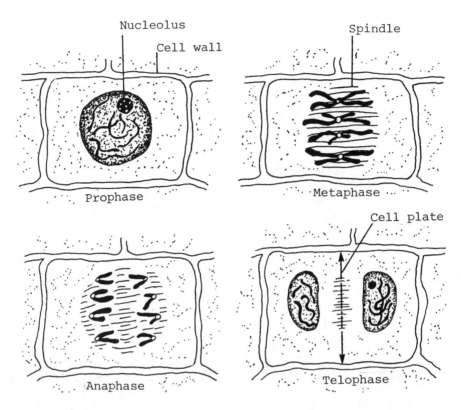

Nucleolus
Cell wall
Spindle
Prophase
Metaphase
Cell plate
Anaphase
Telophase

(b) Plant cell

Mitosis in (a) animal and (b) plant cells compared. Note the presense of centrioles in the animal cells, as well as division of the cytoplasm (cytokinesis) by constriction of the cell membrane (arrows). The cells of higher plants lack centrioles, and cytokinesis is effected by the formation of a cell plate which expands centrifugally (arrows).

Solution: Mitosis is the division of a cell in such a way that each new cell receives exactly the same number and kind of chromosomes that the parent cell had. Each mitotic division is a continuous process, but for descriptive purposes 5 separate stages have been defined: interphase, prophase, metaphase, anaphase and telophase.

I. Interphase

Interphase is the stage between mitotic divisions. Although the cell appears to be resting, it in fact is carrying out the processes of respiration, growth, differentiation and other functions necessary to the survival of the cell. It is during this stage that the genetic material is replicated.

II. Prophase

The next stage is prophase. During this stage, the cell prepares itself for the chromosomal separation necessary for cell division. The cell undergoes many changes that are visible through the use of dyes that react with RNA, DNA or protein. The chromosomes begin to appear as threads. As prophase proceeds the chromosomes condense, becoming shorter and thicker. This is probably due to an increase in the coiling of the structures. Meanwhile, the nucleolus becomes less distinct when viewed with a light microscope and the boundary between the nucleus and cytoplasm, the nuclear membrane, disintegrates. A system of fiber-like microtubules, the spindle, forms as the centrioles move to opposite sides of the nuclear area. Before continuing with the remaining mitotic stages, it would be helpful to describe a chromosome at this stage in detail. A chromosome in prophase is comprised of two separate strands, chromatids, which are genetically identical. Each chromatid has an area called a centromere. Identical chromatids are somehow bound to each other at their centromeres. The centromeres divide a chromosome into arms of characteristic lengths. A chromosome with its centromere equidistant from either end is metacentric, (in Greek meta = between). If the centromere is towards one end of the chromosome, it is called acrocentric. And if the centromere is at the very end of the chromosome, it is telocentric (in Greek telos = end).

Now, back to mitosis. It is in middle prophase when the chromosomes can be distinguished as being composed of two chromatids. During late prophase, the chromosomes begin to move to the middle (equator) of the spindle. We use the word equator since a cell is really spherical like a globe and not flat like our diagram. The end of prophase is marked by the complete disappearance of the nuclear membrane and the formation of the spindle to which the chromosomes are attached by their centromeres.

III. Metaphase

Metaphase is a brief stage when the chromosomes are arranged on the equatorial plane of the spindle. The diagram shows a cross-sectional view of an animal cell in this stage. Notice how the chromosomes appear to be lined up between the two centrioles. Metaphase ends when the chromatids of each chromosome separate. The chromatids are now considered to be independent daughter chromosomes. Therefore, the total number of chromosomes has actually doubled by this separation of chromatids.

IV. Anaphase

During anaphase the single-stranded daughter chromosomes move away from each other. The chromosomes, or more specifically, their centromeres, are attached to a microtubule of the spindle in a region of the centromere called the kinetochore. The spindle microtubules are involved in this chromosomal movement, since the drug colchicine, which disrupts microtubules, effectively inhibits the movement. Late anaphase is characterized by the approach of the chromosomes to the poles of the spindle.

V. Telophase

The final stage, telophase, finishes the mitotic process. Each set of chromosomes becomes enclosed in a new nuclear membrane and the spindle fibers disappear. The chromosomes uncoil, once again becoming indistinct, and the nucleoli reappear. Telophase is followed by cytokinesis, division of the cytoplasm. Both nuclei return to the interphase state.

There is an important difference between the beginning of interphase, directly after telophase, and the end of interphase when the cell enters prophase. The chromosomes are single-stranded in early interphase and double-stranded in late interphase. Replication of each chromosome must occur sometime during interphase. Thus, in the mitotic process, each daughter cell (the products of the mitotic division) receives a complete and exact copy of the genetic information of the parent cell.

● **PROBLEM** 1-2

Colchicine blocks mitosis. What does this reveal about the mitotic process?

Solution: The use of drugs with known biochemical targets reveals much about the chemical makeup of biological systems. Colchicine is a drug that causes the dissociation of microtubules into its component parts. Since colchicine effectively stops mitosis, microtubules must be involved in the mitotic process. Since microtubules are long fibrous molecules, it follows that they make up some long fibrous structure in the mitotic cell. Spindle fibers fit this description perfectly. Experiments using protein extraction techniques, in which fluorescent antibodies are sent to specific microtubule proteins, such as tubulin, and colchicine inhibition have confirmed that microtubules are the major component of spindle fibers.

● **PROBLEM** 1-3

> What is the importance of the centromere of a chromosome?

Appearance in
Anaphase

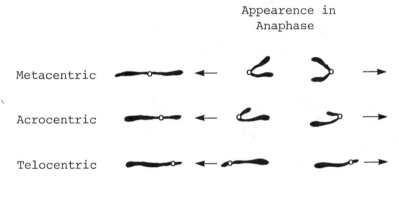

Figure 1.

Solution: Centromeres are regions on chromosomes that are most conspicuous during metaphase of mitosis. They are the areas that associate with homologous chromosomes and with the spindle fibers. A chromosome must contain a centromere if it is to behave properly on the spindle. Without a centromere, chromosome fragments may be lost from the spindle or left in the equatorial plane.

The kinetochore is the region of the centromere that attaches to the spindle. Nothing is known about the composition of this structure and how it is attached to the chromatin fibers. However, the attachments are firm: experiments have been done in which pressure from a needle tip was unable to break the connection.

Only the centromeres show active movement during anaphase. The rest of the chromosome seems to be pulled passively because of its attachment to the centromere. This active role has been used to characterize the shapes that individual chromosomes acquire as a result of the movement: metacentric, acrocentric and telocentric, see Fig. 2.

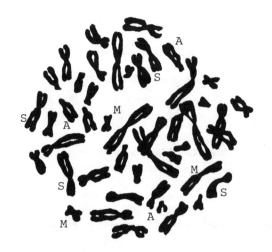

Fig. 2.

Human chromosomes (M = metacentric, S = submetacentric, A = acrocentric) of a metaphase cell.

Thus, the centromere is a necessary component for
the proper movement of chromosomes during meiosis and
mitosis. Its composition and precise structure has
remained enigmatic. However, its importance to future
generations of a cell line is apparent.

MEIOSIS

● PROBLEM 1-4

Differentiate between continuous fibers, kinetochore
(or chromosomal) fibers, neocentric fibers and astral
fibers.

Solution: All of these fibers make up the broad category
of spindle fibers. Figure 1 shows the various types.
Continuous fibers, A, run from pole to pole. These
fibers may cause elongation of the spindle during
anaphase. Kinetochore fibers, B, as their name
suggests, run from one pole to a kinetochore on a
chromosome. These fibers shorten and thus move the
chromosomes from the equatorial plane to the poles.

Neocentric fibers, C, attach to other parts of the chromosome. Astral fibers, D, radiate from the asters but do not run through the spindle. The differentiation among the various types of fibers indicates that microtubules can vary functionally even though the molecular structure is extremely similar, if not identical.

● **PROBLEM** 1-5

What are the stages of meiosis? How does meiosis differ from mitosis?

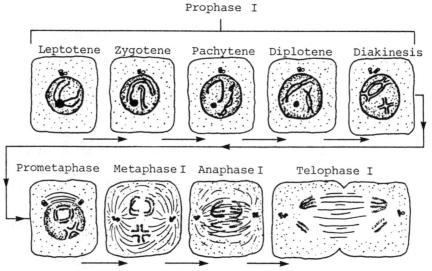

Fig. 1.   The stages of meiosis I in a schematicized animal cell

Solution: The stages of meiosis are basically the same as those described for mitosis, but there are important differences. Mitosis involves one division that produces two cells with identical genetic information. Meiosis involves two divisions that eventually produce four cells with half of the genetic information of the parent cell. In addition, meiosis involves genetic rearrangement so that great variability is introduced.

Meiosis takes days or weeks to complete, whereas mitosis is usually completed in a few hours. The same basic stages are used to characterize meiosis. But since there are two divisions, there are both a prophase I and a prophase II. The other stages are similarly numbered. Since prophase I of meiosis is so long, it is further divided into leptotene, zygotene, pachytene, diplotene and diakinesis. As in mitosis, none of these stages is distinct and the phases flow from one to the next.

I. Prophase

A. Leptotene - A cell at the leptotene stage has chromosomes identical to those in prophase of mitosis. The chromosomes appear as slender threads. Each thread is a pair of identical sister chromatids held together by a centromere.

B. Zygotene - In this stage, homologous sets of chromosomes join together, or synapse. Homologous chromosomes are similar chromosomes that contain genes for similar characters. In a meiotic cell, one homolog is maternal and the other is paternal. They contain similar genes but vary in their specific genetic sequence, hence the variability among traits. During synapsis the maternal chromosome finds its homologous chromosome from among the paternal chromosomes, or vice versa. Somehow the homologs find each other and synapse, gene for gene along their lengths. It is these synaptic complexes that mediate the exchange of genetic material via crossing over and recombination. This exchange is accomplished in such a way that information is neither gained nor lost. For instance, suppose two homologous chromosomes have the following makeup: ABCD and abcd. If crossing over between the homologs occurred, various new combinations could result: ABcd and abCD, or Abcd and aBCD are two possible results. Notice how, in both cases, no information has been lost or gained, but variability has been introduced.

C. Pachytene - The actual physical exchange of genetic material is believed to occur during this stage. This stage is characterized by the noticeably thicker and shorter strands (in Greek, pachynema means "thick strand").

D. Diplotene - In this stage, the pairs of chromosomes separate in a process called desynapsis. Sister chromatids continue to be held together by their centromeres. Desynapsis is not a complete dissociation of the homologous chromosomes: non-sister chromatids of the homologous chromosomes are connected by structures called chiasmata (chiasma - singular). The chiasmata are related to cross over events.

E. Diakinesis - The chromosomes are in their maximally condensed state in diakinesis. For some unknown reason, the chiasmata slide to the ends of the chromatids.

II. Metaphase I

As in mitosis, metaphase I involves the formation of the spindle and the disintegration of the nuclear membrane. The main differences between mitosis and meiosis at this stage are a smaller spindle diameter in meiosis due to the grouping of 4 chromatids per microtubule rather than 2, and no separation of chromatids.

III. Anaphase I

This phase involves the split of the homologous chromosomes so that the maternal goes to one pole and the paternal to the other. It does not matter which goes to which pole, resulting in a shuffling of the genetic material. Two complete sets of chromosomes are formed, but each has only half of the original amount of chromosomes. Variety has been introduced by recombination and reshuffling of the chromosomes.

IV. Telophase I

This stage is the same as in mitosis except that in mitosis the chromosomes are single-stranded and those of meiosis are double-stranded. Also, as mentioned earlier, in mitosis, the daughter cells have the same number of chromosomes as the parent while in meiosis, that number has become half.

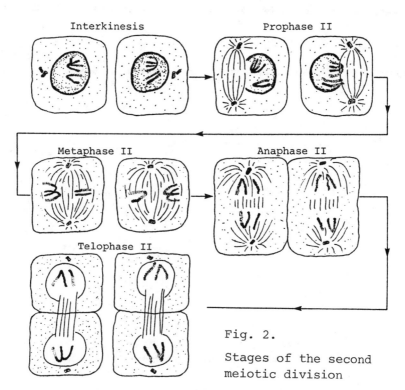

Fig. 2.

Stages of the second meiotic division

V. Interphase

This is the same as interphase of mitosis except that no DNA is replicated.

Following interphase is the second division of meiosis. This division is essentially mitotic. At metaphase II, the chromatids separate and move to opposite poles at anaphase II. Four daughter cells are produced in telophase II when a nuclear membrane forms in each cell.

Thus, after meiosis, the number of chromosomes is reduced to one half of the original number. In higher plants and animals each specific type of chromosome is present in the diploid state. Sex cell, or gamete formation, utilizes meiosis to produce haploid cells. When two haploid gametes fuse upon fertilization, the resulting zygote is diploid. Thus genetic information can come from two sources: a mother and a father, whereas in mitosis, the information comes from only one source: the parent cell. Therefore, meiosis provides genetic diversity due to recombination, reshuffling of maternal and paternal chromosomes and fusion of gametes upon fertilization.

● **PROBLEM** 1-6

What are the genetic consequences of meiosis?

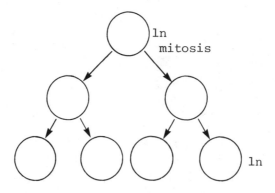

Fig. 1.

Haploid: all daughter cells
have identical genotypes

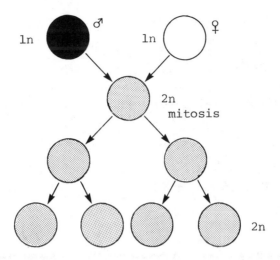

Fig. 2.

Diploid: fusion of two genetically different cells results
in daughter cells with a genotype different from that of
either parent

Solution: To answer this question, it is helpful to also examine the genetic consequences of mitosis. A comparison of these processes indicates certain advantages that reproduction involving meiosis has over reproduction involving mitosis.

An asexual organism reproduces mitotically. All of the progeny, therefore, have identical genotypes. The way that new genetic information is created is through mutation of existing genes.

Sexually reproducing parents produce haploid gametes by meiosis that combine upon fertilization. Thus, variability arises, not only through mutation, but as a consequence of the segregation of alleles and independent assortment of genes that occurs in meiosis. These reshuffling events are the basis of Mendel's Laws. Basically, segregation is the separation of alleles from a maternal and paternal source as a result of a segregation of homologous chromosomes during meiosis I. Although the original diploid set of chromosomes is reduced to a haploid set, each nuclei receives a full set of chromosomes. Since humans have 23 pairs of homologous chromosomes, the possible combinations due to segregation are enormous. Further variability arises because genes assort independently. This is another way of saying that recombination due to crossing over between homologous chromosomes can reshuffle alleles even further. A single chromosome can end up with alleles from both the mother and the father. Since in a species there are thousands of different genes, each with different alleles, the chance that any two gametes will have identical genotypes is very remote. Even further variability is introduced since a male gamete's nucleus must fuse with that of a female gamete. Statistically, the production of two individuals with identical genotypes is almost impossible, except in the case of identical twins. Thus meiotic gamete production and sexual reproduction guarantees genetic variety in each and every generation.

● **PROBLEM** 1-7

What are chiasmata? What important means of genetic exchange are they related to?

Solution: Chiasma (the singular form of chiasmata) means a cross. Chiasmata are areas of contact between nonsister chromatids of a meiotic diplonema nucleus which give the chromosomes a crosslike appearance under a light microscope.

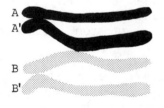

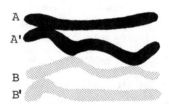

a) One A' - B chiasma   b) Two A' - B chiasmata

Fig. 1.

Two, three or all four chromatids can participate in chiasma formation and one chromatid can form numerous chiasmata. In normal meiosis, there is at least one chiasma per tetrad.

Chiasmata are almost certainly related to crossing over and recombination. There are two sets of experimental data that support this belief. One is that there is a correlation between physical exchange and the occurance of chiasmata. This was shown from studies of a strain of the plant Disporum sessile, which contains easily distinguishable homologous chromosomes called heteromorphic homologues. The other experiment shows a correlation between physical exchange and recombination. This was shown through studies on Drosophila strains with mutant X-chromosomes. Neither of these experiments prove that chiasma leads to genetic recombination, but they lend strong support to the hypothesis.

● PROBLEM 1-8

Meiosis proceeds systematically and precisely. How can individual genes be implicated as having specific effects on a process such as meiosis? Are there any aspects of meiosis that are under known genetic control?

Solution: The effects of individual genes can be studied indirectly through their mutant alleles. These mutations usually produce abnormal effects that can serve as a basis for the isolation of marked individuals. These mutations, or markers, can be followed through their phenotypic effects and enable investigators to infer what the normal function of the gene is.

Mutants have been found that influence meiosis in maize and Drosophila. These mutations affect either the genetic recombination event or chromosome segregation. They may affect the control of the events or the exchange process itself. Mutations have been found that specifically influence synapsis, crossing over, the centromere and the spindle.

Synapsis can be prevented or destroyed between all homologous loci in maize in the absence of a specific allele. Since there is no synapse between homologues, there is no exchange between them and the chromosome distribution during anaphase is irregular.

Normal (wild-type) crossing over in Drosophila differs in females and males. Females undergo normal meiosis and the resulting cross-over events. But in males there is no exchange between chromatids because leptotene, zygotene and pachytene stages are not apparent. These stages are those in which crossing over and exchange is thought to occur. Therefore, the homologous chromosomes stick together only in a localized heterochromatic region near the centromere during prophase I. Male mutants, Mr, have been found in which recombination does occasionally occur in the production of gametes.

The specific behavior of centromeres is also under some sort of genetic control. A mutant in Drosophila, nod, causes sister centromeres at metaphase II to separate early so that each goes to the poles independently. Sometimes both chromatids can orient to the same pole. This results in an unequal distribution of chromosomes.

The shape of the spindle is under some genetic influence. In maize and Drosophila there are mutations that change the shape of the spindle during meiosis but not during mitosis. These mutants have divergent, rather than convergent, spindle ends. The result of this may be the loss of some widely spread out chromosomes from the telophase nuclei. Abnormal chromosome contents could result. The orientation of the spindle is also under some genetic control. Usually both spindles of meiosis II are oriented in the same direction. When this direction is the same as that in meiosis I, a row of 4 nuclei or cells is the result. When the direction is opposite to that of meiosis I, a cluster of 4 nuclei or cells results. Different species or sexes orient the spindle according to one of these guidelines. However, no details are known.

Thus, several aspects of meiosis are under known genetic control. Many other are probably under similar control, but they may be hard to identify. Some types of mutants are difficult or impossible to isolate with existing techniques since they may make development of the organism impossible. At the present time, no system analogous to that of conditional mutants in bacteria exists for eukaryotes so the traits must be recessive. Regardless of these problems, meiotic mutants have been and continue to be discovered.

● **PROBLEM 1-9**

How does meiosis differ in males and females?

Solution: The actual stages of meiosis are the same in males and females. What differs is the time it takes to complete certain stages and the products of the meiotic divisions.

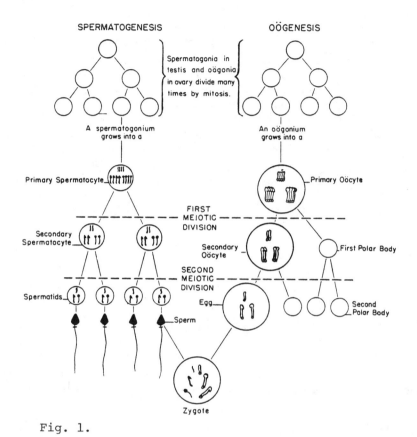

Fig. 1.

The production of sperm cells by the human male follows the normal meiotic scheme. For each complete round of meiosis, four haploid sperm cells are produced. This meiotic gamete production occurs only after puberty.

In the human female, things are very different. Meiosis begins very early, in the fetus. By birth, all of the potential female sex cells, oocytes, have begun meiosis I, but have stopped at the diplotene stage. They may remain in this state as long as fifty years. When the female reaches sexual maturity the meiosis process continues. Each month, one oocyte resumes meiosis. This meiosis is still dissimilar from that during sperm formation. After meiosis I, the cytoplasm divides unevenly to produce one small cell, a polar body, and one large cell, the oocyte. The polar body may undergo meiosis II to produce 2 such bodies. The oocyte, meanwhile, enters meiosis II, but it stops again about metaphase II and awaits sperm penetration. Once a sperm has penetrated, the oocyte finishes meiosis II and produces another polar body and a mature haploid egg. When the nuclei of the sperm fuses with that of the egg, the product is a diploid zygote. The polar bodies are usually discarded.

Thus, the meiotic products of male gametogenesis are four sperm cells and those of female gametogenesis are two or three polar bodies and one large oocyte. Since the oocyte must contain a lot of materials to form the initial cells of the developing embryo, it must be very large. The large size of the oocyte is a result of most of the cytoplasm from meiosis going towards the oocyte and very little going towards the remaining three meiotic products. Conversely, sperm don't need to be so large, since their purpose is only to reach the oocyte, to donate their genetic material and to stimulate the oocyte to mature. Thus, the form of meiosis that male and female sex cells undergo is very much determined by their cellular functions.

HAPLOID AND DIPLOID NUMBER

● **PROBLEM** 1-10

In an animal with a haploid number of 10, how many chromosomes are present in
a)   a spermatogonium?
b)   in the first polar body?
c)   in the second polar body?
d)   in the secondary oocyte?
Assume that the animal is diploid.

Solution: In solving this problem, one must keep in mind how meiosis is coordinated with spermatogenesis and oogenesis.

a) Spermatogonia are the male primordial germ cells. These are the cells that may undergo spermatogenesis to produce haploid gametes. But until spermatogenesis occurs, a spermatogonium is diploid just like any other body cell.

Since the haploid number is 10, the number of chromosomes in the diploid spermatogonium is 2 x 10 or 20 chromosomes.

b) It is essential to remember that while the polar body is formed as a result of unequal distribution of cytoplasm in meiosis, the chromosomes are still distributed equally between the polar body and the oocyte. Since the first polar body is a product of the first meiotic division, it contains only one of the chromosomes of each homologous pair; separation of homologous chromosomes has occurred. But daughter chromatids of each chromosome have not separated, so there are 2 identical members in each chromosome. Therefore there are 10 doubled chromosomes in the first polar body, or 20 chromatids.

c) The second polar body results from the second meiotic division. In this division, the duplicate copies of the haploid number of chromosomes separate, forming true haploid cells. Therefore the chromosome number is 10.

d) The secondary oocyte results from the first meiotic division, along with the first polar body. Since, as we have said, the chromosomes have segregated equally, the secondary oocyte has the same number of chromosomes as the first polar body, and for the same reasons. Therefore, it contains 10 doubled chromosomes or 20 chromatids.

● **PROBLEM 1-11**

An animal has a diploid number of 8. During meiosis, how many chromatids are present
a)   in the tetrad stage?
b)   in late telophase of the first meiotic division?
c)   in metaphase of the second meiotic division?

Solution: In doing this problem, one must remember that meiosis involves both the duplication of chromosomes and the separation of homologous pairs.

a) In the tetrad stage of meiosis, homologous chromosomes synapse, or pair. But prior to this, every chromosome had been duplicated. Synapsis therefore results in a tetrad, a bundle of 4 chromatids (2 copies of each one of the homologous chromosomes). The number of tetrads equals the number of haploid chromosomes. Therefore, there are $\frac{1}{2}$ x 8 or 4 tetrads. Since each tetrad has 4 chromatids, there are a total of 4 x 4 or 16 chromatids in the tetrad stage.

b) In late telophase of the first meiotic division, the homologous chromosomes of each pair have separated. But each chromosome is still double and composed of two daughter chromatids. So there are the haploid number (4) of doubled chromosomes, or a total of 8 chromatids.

c) In metaphase of the second meiotic division, the doubled chromosomes have lined up along the equator of the cell, but daughter chromatids have not yet separated. So the number of chromatids is still 4 x 2, or 8.

● **PROBLEM** 1-12

The toad, <u>Bufo americanus</u>, is a diploid organism whose haploid number of chromosomes is 11. How many sister chromatids are in its
a) mitotic metaphase nucleus?
b) meiotic metaphase I nucleus?
c) meiotic metaphase II nucleus?

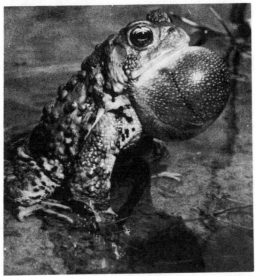

Fig. 1: Bufo americanus with expanded vocal sac

Solution: The important points to consider for this problem are:

1) mitosis produces daughter cells identical in chromosome number to the haploid parent cell;

2) meiosis I results in a split of the diploid (2n) nucleus to two haploid (n) nuclei;

3)   meiosis II is essentially mitotic;

4) meiosis II results in the production of four daughter cells, each with the haploid number of chromosomes;

5) metaphase, in both meiosis and mitosis, is the stage in which the chromosomes align along the equatorial plane in preparation for separation to the daughter cells' nuclei;

and 6) each chromosome in a metaphase nucleus is composed of two identical sister chromatids.

The toad has a haploid chromosome number (n) of 11. Therefore its diploid number (2n) is twice that, or 22. We now have all of the relevant information for this problem.

a) In mitotic metaphase, the haploid number of chromosomes are composed of twin sister chromatids and are aligned along the equatorial plane. In other words, the 11 chromosomes, or 22 chromatids, are preparing to split into separate haploid groups. Thus in the mitotic metaphase nuclei of <u>Bufo americanus</u> there are 22 sister chromatids.

b) The meiotic metaphase I nucleus contains a diploid chromosome content: 11 paternal chromosomes and 11 maternal chromosomes. Each of these chromosomes contains 2 chromatids. Thus:
$$2(11 + 11) = 44 \text{ chromatids.}$$

c) Meiotic metaphase II brings the cell back to a haploid state. There are $2(11 \text{ chromosomes}) = 22$ chromatids in a nucleus at this stage.

VARIATIONS IN MITOSIS AND MEIOSIS

● **PROBLEM** 1-13

The division of dinoflagellates, Syndinium, has an unusual variation in its mitotic process. What is the variation? What does it indicate about the evolution of mitosis?

Solution: Dinoflagellates are unicellular organisms that have two flagella attached laterally. They, along with diatoms, are the primary producers of organic matter in the sea. Their mitotic apparatus is slightly less complex than that of higher eukaryotes.

Throughout the entire cell cycle, the chromosomes remain attached to the microtubules. The microtubules run from the kinetochore to the centriole. The kinetochore is attached to the nuclear membrane, which does not disappear in metaphase. The spindle fibers do not elongate; they act like rigid rods rather than elastic fibers. Thus these organisms have not evolved a separate mechanism for moving their chromosomes via spindle fiber movement.

Figure 1 shows some of the mitotic steps. In A, the chromosomes are attached to both centrioles. When the chromosome appears as sister chromatids, B, each kinetochore is attached to one of the centrioles by a microtubule. Each daughter cell, C, receives one chromatid from the pair.

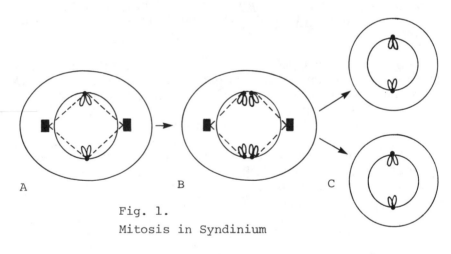

Fig. 1.
Mitosis in Syndinium

■   = centriole

•   = kinetochore

----   = spindle fiber

This form of mitosis may represent an earlier stage in the evolution of cell division. This is evolutionarily between direct attachment of chromosomes to the membrane and the evolution of the kinetochore as an active chromosome mover. In Syndiniumic mitosis, a separate mechanism for chromosome movement has not evolved.

Assume that the diploid number of chromosomes in a cell is 2n = 8. Suppose that in undergoing meiosis one pair of homologues fails to disjoin at the first meiotic division and both homologues of the pair proceed to the same pole.

(a) How many chromatids would be present in each daughter cell resulting from meiosis I?

(b) If the second meiotic division divides all the sister chromatids, how many chromatids would be present in each of the four resulting gametes?

Fig. 1.

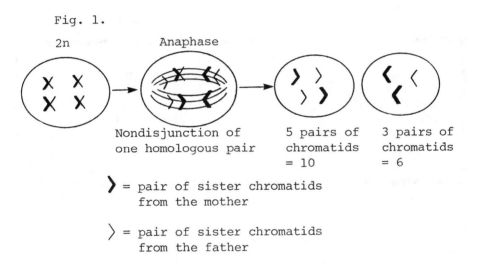

= pair of sister chromatids from the mother

= pair of sister chromatids from the father

Fig. 2.

Sister chromatids separate in meiosis II

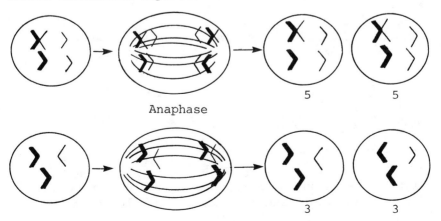

Solution: Nondisjunction is one way that cells can obtain an abnormal amount of chromosomes. Such diseases as Down's syndrome can be a result of nondisjunction. The problem gives a diploid number of 8. This tells us that the haploid number is one half of that, or 4. This information allows us to follow the events through diagrams.

a) If one pair of homologues fails to disjoin during the first meiotic division and both homologs of the pair proceed to the same pole there would be 10 chromatids in one daughter cell, and 6 in the other. See Figure 1.

b) If the second meiotic division proceeds correctly the number of chromatids present in the four resulting gametes would be 5, 5, 3, and 3 as shown in Figure 2.

● **PROBLEM** 1-15

Assuming 2n = 8, suppose the first meiotic division of a cell is normal, but in one of the two daughter cells nondisjunction of a pair of sister chromatids occurs during the second meiotic division. How many chromatids would be present in each of the four gametes?

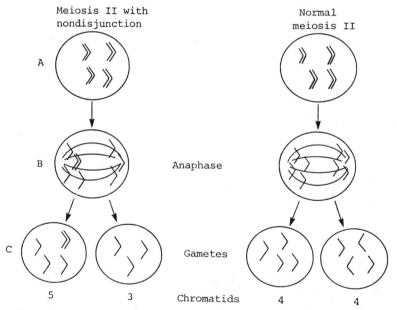

Fig. 1: Nondisjuntion in the second round of meiosis. Each bent line represents a single chromatid.

Solution: This problem is similar to the previous one except that the nondisjunction is occurring later, in the second meiotic division. This type of nondisjunction results in gametes with different numbers of chromosomes.

From the diagram, nondisjunction during meiosis II results in gametes with 5, 3, 4 and 4 chromatids, respectively.

SHORT ANSWER QUESTIONS FOR REVIEW

Choose the correct answer.

1. During mitosis the cell undergoes five
    different stages. In which stage does the
    cell replicate its DNA? (a) interphase (b)
    prophase (c) cytokinesis (d) metaphase
    (e) anaphase   a

2. In prophase the chromosomes condense and
    become shorter and thicker. This is due to
    (a) disintegration of the nuclear membrane.
    (b) increased coiling of the chromosomes. (c)
    microtubules pulling the chromosomes closer.
    (d) centrioles moving to opposite sides of
    nuclear area.   b

3. During mitotic metaphase the chromosomes (a)
    migrate toward the centrioles. (b) synapse
    with their homologous chromosomes. (c) line
    up on the equatorial plane of the cell. (d)
    uncoil and become less condense.   c

4. Which stage is arrested by the addition of
    colchicine to a cell undergoing mitosis? (a)
    metaphase (b) anaphase, at attachment of
    chromosomes to microtubules (c) telophase,
    at formation of spindle microtubules (d) both
    a and b   b

5. The main difference between mitosis and
    meiosis is (a) mitosis only occurs in plants.
    (b) mitosis produces two cells with different
    genetic information. (c) meiosis produces
    four daughter cells with exactly the same
    genetic information as the parent. (d) meiosis
    produces four daughter cells with half the
    genetic information of the parent.   d

6. During leptotene (a) the chromosomes appear
    as thin threads floating outside the nuclear
    membrane. (b) there are four pairs of
    chromatids for each chromosome. (c) chromo-
    somes line up on the equatorial plane. (d)
    both a and b (e) none of the above   e

7. One difference between metaphase in mitosis
    and meiosis is that in meiotic metaphase (a)
    the nuclear envelope is still present. (b) the

24

centromere breaks. (c) chromatids group in
sets of four. (d) spindle fibers form.

c

8. Which of the following characteristics does not
   apply to meiotic telophase I? (a) There are
   only two daughter cells. (b) Chromosomes are
   double stranded. (c) The daughter cells have
   the same number of chromosomes as the
   parent cell. (d) Recombination of genetic
   material has occured.

c

9. Genetic variability of individuals ensures a
   better chance of survival for the species as a
   whole. How does meiotic cell division provide
   individuals with a genetic make-up different
   from that of their parents? (a) Gametes are
   produced with only half of the genetic information of the parent cell. (b) Mutations are
   induced in some chromosomes. (c) During
   meiosis alleles are reshuffled through
   crossing over and recombination. (d) both a
   and c (e) all of the above

d

10. The process of meiosis is under genetic
    control just like any other living process,
    but only a few steps show evidence of this
    genetic control. Which specific steps in
    meiosis of Drosophila and maize have been
    found to be under direct genetic control?
    (a) synapsis (b) disintegration of the
    nuclear membrane (c) disintegration of
    centromeres (d) both a and b (e) both a
    and c

a

11. Female gametogenesis differs greatly from
    male gametogenesis in that the female's oocyte
    completes meiosis (a) during metaphase II
    only after sperm penetration. (b) during
    anaphase II only after penetration. (c)
    during diplotene only after sperm penetration
    (d) none of the above

a

12. The product of the fusion of the sperm and
    the ovum nucleus is (a) a haploid zygote.
    (b) a diploid zygote. (c) a triploid zygote.
    (d) a haploid zygote plus three extruded
    polar bodies.

b

SHORT ANSWER QUESTIONS FOR REVIEW

Fill in the blanks.

13. Essentially, the only difference between interphase II in meiosis and interphase in mitosis is that during meiotic interphase II _____ is not replicated.

    DNA

14. The two separate strands of a chromosome are called _____.

    chromatids

15. The region of the centromere which attaches to a microtubule is called the _____.

    kinetochore

16. Cytokinesis is the division of the _____.

    cytoplasm

17. The longest (most time consuming) phase of meiosis is _____ which is subdivided into _____ different stages.

    prophase I
    five

18. During the _____ stage of meiosis, the homologous sets of chromosomes join together.

    zygotene

19. Two chromosomes that contain identical loci for all traits are called _____.

    homologous

20. The formation of gametes in higher plants and animals occurs through _____ cell division.

    meiotic

21. Meiotic daughter cells are _____ because they contain only half the number of chromosomes than their _____ parents.

    haploid
    diploid

22. The complete genetic make-up of an individual is the _____.

    genotype

23. The complete expression of an individual's genotype is the _____.

    phenotype

24. Female oocytes become arrested at the _____ stage until after sexual maturity.

    diplotene

25. The _____ resulting from oogenesis are discarded at the completion of meiosis.

    polar
    bodies

Determine whether the following statements are true or false.

26. In a telocentric chromosome, the centromere

	is equidistant from both ends.	False
27.	The end of prophase is marked by the complete disappearance of the nuclear membrane.	True
28.	Chromosomes are single stranded during early interphase and double stranded during late interphase.	True
29.	After mitotic telophase, each daughter cell has an exact copy of the genetic make-up of the parent cell.	True
30.	Meiosis is completed in a few hours at the most.	False
31.	During diakinesis, the chromatids are maximally condensed and the chiasmata disappear completely.	False
32.	During meiotic anaphase, the homologous chromosomes migrate to the poles of the spindle so that the maternal chromosomes go to one pole and the paternal chromosomes to the other.	True
33.	Following meiotic telophase I, the two resulting daughter cells enter prophase II and continue to divide exactly as in mitosis.	False
34.	Meiotic sperm production results in two haploid sperm cells and two polar bodies.	False
35.	All the ova in a female have completed meiosis by puberty, and are ready for fertilization.	False
36.	After meiosis I, the cytoplasm of a parent oocyte divides evenly and produces two identical daughter cells.	False
37.	The large size of the daughter oocyte after meiosis II results from the uneven distribution of the cytoplasm which allows the zygote to divide mitotically before it begins growing.	True
38.	One function of the sperm is to bring the complementary genetic material to the oocyte.	True

In questions 39 through 42 match the terms in column A to their appropriate descriptions in column B.

	A		B	
39.	continous fibers	a)	chromosomal fibers- run from chromo- some to one pole	b
40.	kinetochore fibers	b)	run from pole to pole	a
41.	neocentric fibers	c)	radiate from aster but never pass through spindle	e
42.	astral fibers			c
		d)	runs from centriole to both poles	
		e)	runs from any chromosomal area except kinetochore	

In questions 43 through 47 match the appropriate events in column A to their descriptions in column B.

	A		B	
43.	pachytene	a)	normal breakage and exchange of parts between chromatids	c
44.	crossing over	b)	crossing over of non- sister chromosomes	d
45.	recombination	c)	physical exchange of genetic material	a
46.	diplotene	d)	interlocking of non- sister chromatids	f
47.	chiasmata	e)	separation of chromatids occurs	b
		f)	homologous chromo- somes separate	

CHAPTER 2

CHROMOSOMES

STRUCTURE

● **PROBLEM 2-1**

Describe the structure of a chromosome. What methods are used to study chromosomes?

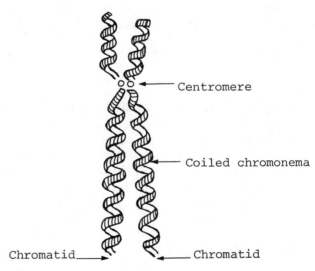

Fig. 1
Chromosome structure

Solution: Chromosomes contain DNA, histone proteins, a small amount of RNA and the enzymes necessary for DNA and RNA synthesis. These chromosomes reside in the nucleus of cells in numbers and morphologies that are characteristic of each species. Humans have 23 pairs of chromosomes: two of these chromosomes determine the sex of the individual and are hence called sex chromosomes. The remaining 44 (or 22 pairs) are called autosomes. The structures of the chromosomes have been studied by various techniques including chemical analysis, X-ray diffraction, electron microscopy, and autoradiography. Individual chromosomes have also been studied by karyotype and banding techniques.

Chromosomes owe their linear structure to the linear nature of DNA. Each eukaryotic chromosome contains one DNA duplex molecule. This molecule twists and coils to produce the compact shape of the chromosomes seen during mitosis and meiosis. A chromosome also contains histone proteins. The DNA complexes to a group of eight histone proteins (an octamer). The DNA winds around this bundle of protein to form a structure called a nucleosome. Electron micrographs have been produced that show these repeating structures to look like a string of beads if the chromosome is artificially stretched out. These protein complexes help to protect the DNA from degradation by nucleases in the nuclei.

The centromere region, described in a previous question, is the area of spindle fiber attachment (and possibly formation). See Figure 1. The centromere is necessary for chromosome transport towards a pole during nuclear division. Little is known about the chemical composition of the centromere since no method exists which is sensitive to the centromere region alone.

Further characteristics of chromosomal structure can be described through cytogenetic analysis. Chromosomes can be studied by karyotype technique and through various staining techniques. The karyotype technique permits the study of the complete chromosome set of a cell. Figure 2 shows this technique. Blood cells are first placed in a solution that stimulates mitosis. Colchicine is then added to stop mitosis at metaphase (colchicine disrupts the microtubules of the mitotic spindle). The white blood cells are separated and collected from the culture medium by centrifugation. A hypotonic solution (distilled water) is added to disperse the chromosomes and the cells are then fixed and spread on a slide. The slide is stained with various dyes and a selected cell is photographed through a microscope. Each chromosome is then cut out and arranged by size, shape and banding pattern. Karyotypes can be used to analyze abnormal chromosomal patterns and to correlate these patterns with clinical symptoms.

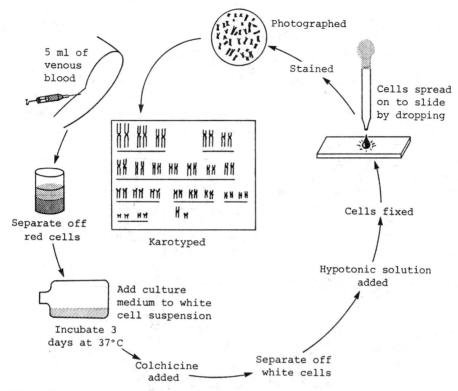

Fig. 2.

Preparation of a karotype

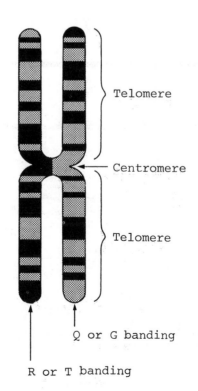

Fig. 3.

Chromosome banding

31

Karyotype analysis usually involves staining or banding techniques. Each chromosome produces a unique pattern of dark and light bands when stained with certain reagents. One reagent is Giemsa reagent. Giemsa stain reveals G-bands. G-bands have patterns almost identical to Q-bands which are a result of staining with quinacridine. Quinacridine inserts itself into the DNA duplex and produces fluorescent bands when excited by ultraviolet light. R- and T-banding techniques produce bands where G- and Q-banding techniques do not, see Figure 3. Thus, since G- and Q-bands do not form at the ends of chromosomes, R- and T-banding techniques can be used to detect terminal deletions. Through these banding techniques abnormal chromosomes of an individual can be detected. These banding techniques have also been used to study chromosomes comparatively. Differences between chromosomes of related species can be determined to aid in studies of an evolutionary nature.

Chromosomes have been analyzed in ways that reveal structural differences. In addition, the DNA of the chromosomes is being studied in detail. Eventually a correlation between DNA sequences and chromosome structure may be established. But there is much more research that has to be done before anything conclusive is accomplished.

● PROBLEM 2-2

What are histones?

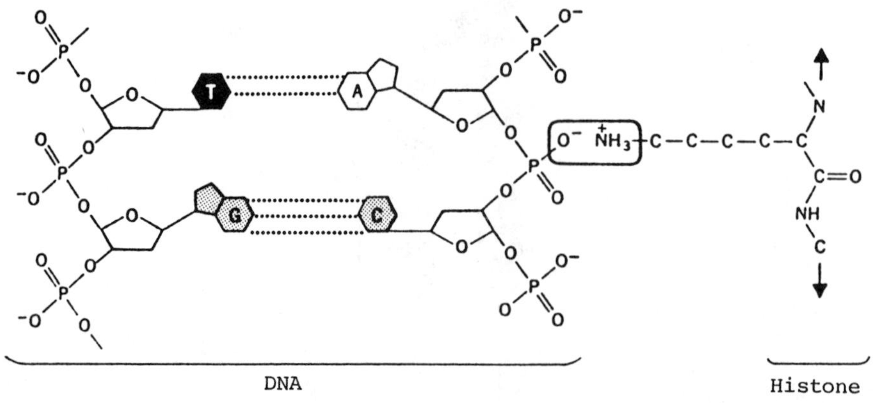

DNA   Histone

Fig. 1

32

Solution: Histones are small, basic proteins which bind tightly to the DNA of eukaryotes. The DNA-histone complex is called chromatin. Histones have a high content of positively charged side chains, especially lysine and arginine residues. A possible mechanism of binding is shown in Figure 1. Half of the mass of chromosomes is due to the presence of histones, the remaining mass is from the DNA. Thus, histones are a major component of eukaryotic chromosomes.

There are five types of histones: H1, H2A, H2B, H3 and H4. Each of these types of histones can be modified by methylation, ADP-ribosylation or phosphorylation. These posttranslational modifications may be important in regulating the availability of DNA for replication and transcription by changing the charge or hydrogen bonding capabilities.

● **PROBLEM 2-3**

Can a metacentric chromosome be derived from two acrocentric chromosomes?

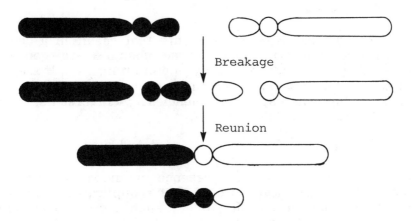

Fig. 1.
Formation of metacentric chromosomes from reunion of acrocentric types

Solution: Metacentric chromosomes are chromosomes that have their centromeres at or near the middle of their length. Acrocentric chromosomes have their centromeres towards the end of their length. If the acrocentric chromosomes break and rejoin properly, metacentric chromosomes may be formed.

● **PROBLEM 2-4**

What are the effects, if any, of changes in chromosomal structure? What are the various structural changes that can occur?

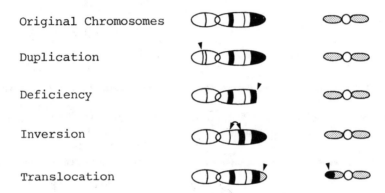

Original Chromosomes

Duplication

Deficiency

Inversion

Translocation

Solution: There are several events that result in a change in chromosomal structure. These changes are generally harmful and result in many debilitating syndromes in humans. The various structural changes that can occur are: duplications, deficiencies, inversions and translocations.

I. Duplication

A duplication is the presence of an extra copy of a piece of chromosomal material. The duplication may be a result of unequal crossing over; such a cross-over would result in one chromosome with a duplication and one with a deficiency. Down's syndrome manifests itself only if one band of chromosome 21 is present in triplicate. Down's syndrome results in mongolism and a low resistance to disease.

II. Deficiency

A deficiency (or deletion) is the loss of a piece of genetic information. As mentioned earlier, deficiencies

34

most commonly arise from unequal crossing over (see Figure 1). If there is a deficiency in the short arm of chromosome 5 in humans, cri-du-chat syndrome results. This syndrome includes severe mental retardation and a very cat-like cry in young infants.

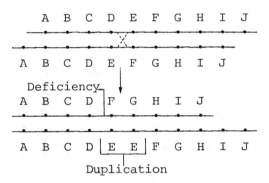

Deficiency for "E"
Duplication for "E

Fig. 1

III.   Inversions

In inversions, the arrangement of the chromosomal material is changed, rather than the amount, as in duplications and deficiencies. Inversions occur when a chromosome is broken and the broken piece is reversed and reinserted. (See Figure 2.) Paracentric inversions are those which do not involve the centromere. Pericentric inversions do involve the centromere, and thus alter the morphology of the chromosome with respect to the location of the centromere. The karyotype has presumably evolved by such chromosomal changes.

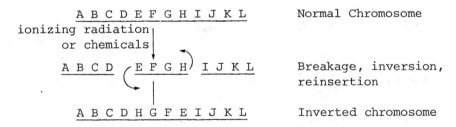

A B C D E F G H I J K L   Normal Chromosome

ionizing radiation
    or chemicals

A B C D E F G H I J K L   Breakage, inversion,
                              reinsertion

A B C D H G F E I J K L   Inverted chromosome

Fig. 2

IV.   Translocations

Translocations involve the rearrangement of genetic material between nonhomologous chromosomes. Such exchanges are usually reciprocal, meaning that each chromosome both donates and receives a piece of chromosome. A person who carries a translocation could have one normal chromosome 14 and one normal chromosome 21 but also a chromosome that is a result of a fusion between chromosomes 14 and 21. This translocated chromosome is designated t(14;21). This person may be phenotypically normal since he carries the full diploid set of chromosomes. When meiosis occurs however, some gametes will contain 14 but not 21 or 21 and t(14;21). Translocation Down's syndrome can appear in one of this person's offspring if a gamete 21 + t(14;21) fuses with a normal gamete containing 14 and 21 since there will be 3 copies of chromosome 21.

These chromosomal aberrations are not always deleterious. For instance, small duplications may become advantageous. Resistance to pesticides and antibiotics may arise by duplications of the genes that produce the gene products that are susceptible to the substance. Duplications are also important substrates through which mutations can occur. Since the cell contains a complete genetic complement plus a duplication, a mutation in the duplication will not adversely affect the organism's survival. Mutations of these types are a means through which evolution can occur.

● **PROBLEM 2-5**

The order of the genes on a chromosome is:

$$\underset{O}{\bullet} \quad \text{A} \quad \text{B} \quad \text{C} \quad \text{D} \quad \text{E} \quad \text{F} \quad \text{G} \quad \text{H} \quad \text{I}$$

where O represents the centromere. If a shift in the homologous chromosome resulted in the insertion of the genes C, D, and E between genes G and H, how could a chromosome containing a duplication and one containing a deficiency be formed?

Solution: To answer this problem, diagrams should be drawn. This will enable one to understand the question and to visualize possible events. The question describes an event that results in a chromosome that differs from the original. When genes C, D, and E are inserted between "G" and "H", our two homologous chromosomes look like this:

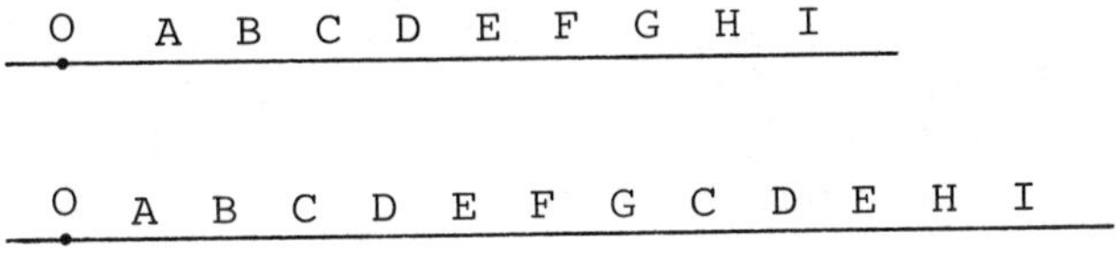

```
O   A   B   C   D   E   F   G   H   I
```

```
O   A   B   C   D   E   F   G   C   D   E   H   I
```

Notice how the chromosomes do not line up completely. Since molecules tend to be in the state of lowest energy, the homologues may line up so as to reduce their energy state by binding at areas of homology. In order to do this loops must form. This is possible since DNA is relatively flexible. One such loop formation is:

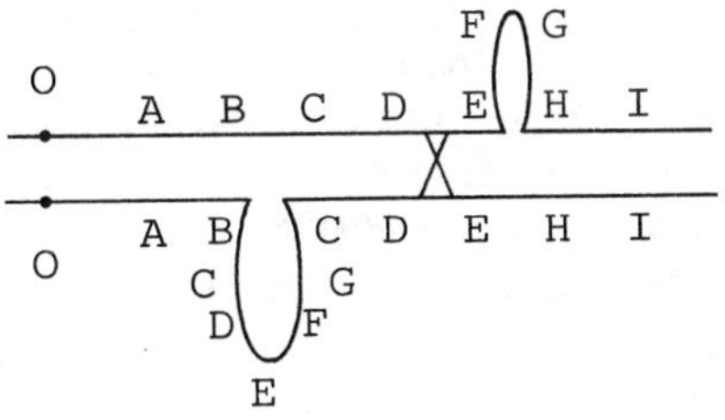

If, during pachytene of meiosis I, crossing over were to occur where indicated in the diagram, one chromosome would gain information and the other would lose information. In other words, one chromosome would have a duplication and the other would have a deficiency. The final gene sequences would be:

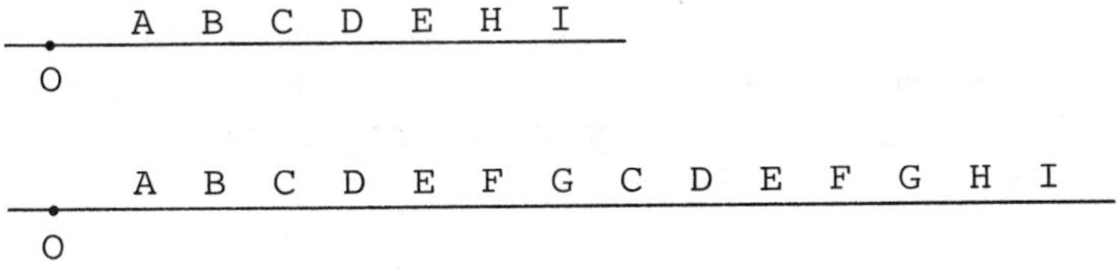

```
        A   B   C   D   E   H   I
    O
```

```
        A   B   C   D   E   F   G   C   D   E   F   G   H   I
    O
```

● **PROBLEM 2-6**

How are chromosomal breaks produced? What factors modify these breaks?

Solution: Energy is required to disrupt the relatively stable chromosome. Any form of high energy radiation can

37

provide sufficient energy to break a chromosome. Factors such as radiation frequency, ion density, length of exposure, and chromosome state can determine how effectively a chromosome is broken.

The effective power depends on the frequency of the radiation. Higher frequency radiation, such as ultraviolet light, is more effective than the lower frequency visible light. X-rays and gamma rays, having even higher frequencies than ultraviolet rays, are much more effective chromosome breakers.

Another factor that influences the breakage is the length and density of the ion track which varies according to the type of ionizing radiation. Ions break the chromosome by breaking bonds between atoms. Molecules are formed by shared atomic electrons. Ionizing radiation knocks out the electrons, thus ionizing the affected atom. If the electrons that are knocked out are those that are shared in a molecule, then the molecule will no longer hold together. Thus, the more concentrated the track of ions, the more harmful the radiation is to chromosomal molecules. Ion clusters can also produce more than one break in a chromosome by attacking it in separate, independent tracks. Such rearrangements show a breakage frequency that is faster than the dosage; these are non-linear relationships. These rearrangements also show a threshold dose.

When chromosomes are broken by radiation, "sticky" ends are produced. These ends are capable of rejoining. If the rejoining of ends can take place so that normal chromosomes are reformed (this is known as restitutional union), prolonging the delivery of the radiation will reduce the frequency of such rejoinings. Thus, when irradiated for longer stretches of time, the chromosomes are unable to rejoin properly resulting in more abnormal chromosomes.

The physio-chemical state of the chromosomes and other cellular structures also modifies the frequency of breakage. The type of structural change depends on the mass of chromosomal material present in the nucleus and upon the numbers and sizes of the chromosomes.

● **PROBLEM 2-7**

Can chromosome instability cause cancer?

Solution: There are a number of diseases that result in a high incidence of cancer. Many of these diseases are also associated with an increased frequency of chromosomal instability. This instability causes gaps, breaks, exchanges in, and rearrangement of chromosomal structure. Chromosomal instability may not "cause" cancer but it may create an environment that is highly susceptible to certain forms of cancer.

Xeroderma pigmentosum is a disease in which the mechanism that repairs ultraviolet induced damage in DNA is defective. In cell culture, clones of affected cells with chromosomal rearrangements have been found. Various skin cancers have been reported in patients with this disorder.

Bloom's syndrome is characterized by dwarfism. Individuals who are homozygous for this recessive trait show a high frequency of spontaneous chromosome breaks in their cells. Individuals with Bloom's syndrome have a high incidence of leukemia and malignant neoplasms.

Individuals who are homozygous or heterozygous for Fanconi's anemia are also cancer-prone. This disorder is characterized by chromosomal aberrations, anatomical defects, and mental retardation.

Victims of these diseases show an instability in their chromosomal structures. They also show a heightened susceptibility to cancer. Since the chromosomes of individuals with these afflications are easily and effectively disrupted, they must have various defects in the repair pathways that normally protect chromosomes. Thus, chromosomal instability is not necessarily a cause of cancer — cancer is one result of chromosomal instability.

● **PROBLEM 2-8**

A chromosomal sequence is A↑BCDEF↑G•HIJ. The arrows indicate breaks induced by radiation. The centromere is located between G and H. What are the consequences of these breaks?

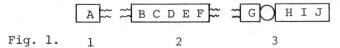

Fig. 1.   1   2   3

Solution: When a chromosome is broken by radiation, "sticky" ends are produced. These ends have unsaturated nucleotide sequences that can rejoin to other such "sticky" ends. Thus, when radiation breaks chromosomes, the pieces are free to bind to each other in ways that allow the original chromosomes to be produced - restitutional union - or in ways that create chromosomes with new gene sequences - nonrestitutional union. These reunions usually occur during interphase when the chromosomes are in the dispersed chromatin state.

Restitutional union is more likely to occur when the chromosome breaks in a single place on one chromatid. In this case, the other unbroken chromatid of the pair can act as a support for the broken chromatid piece. The pieces can be brought close to each other and rejoin, recreating the original gene sequence. This rejoining becomes more difficult when there are two or more breaks along a length of chromosome.

The most likely result of the breaks outlined in this problem is that some kind of nonrestitutional union will take place. Since rejoining can only occur at "sticky" ends, we should draw them to help us see the possible reunions, see Figure 1.

The wavy lines on each fragment represent the "sticky" ends left by the radiation. These are the only areas that can rejoin.

There are several ways that these fragments can rejoin. Fragments 1 and 3 can bind, leaving fragment 2 to its own fate, see Figure 2. Fragment 2 can produce a circular chromosome by binding its own sticky ends, or it may be left out of any binding completely.

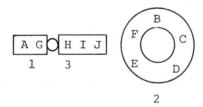

Fig. 2

These deficient chromosome fragments are usually lost before the next nuclear division is completed. Occasionally, however, these chromosomes may survive if the deleted segment is not terribly essential for the survival of the cell. This genetic loss is termed "hypoploid" with respect to the normal genetic complement (in Greek, hypo means under). Thus, a hypoploid nucleus contains less genetic information than a normal nucleus.

Another rearrangement results in a euploid nucleus. A euploid nucleus has the same amount of genetic material as a normal nucleus, but a paracentric inversion is involved. A paracentric inversion does not involve the centromere. (An inversion which does is termed a pericentric inversion.) If fragment 2 is inverted and, consequently, joined backwards between fragments 1 and 3, the following chromosome is formed:

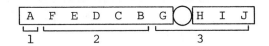

Fig. 3

This type of rearrangement usually has no detectable phenotypic effect since all genes are present. Only when the gene order is important (in an operon, for instance), is there a noticable affect.

A hyperploid nucleus - one which has more genetic information than the normal nucleus - can also be created by these chromosomal breaks. If the rejoining is delayed until the chromosomes replicate, duplication of fragment 2 can occur. This process is diagrammed in Figure 4. A duplication is produced in one chromatid and a deletion is caused in the other. Thus, when the chromatids separate in metaphase II of meiosis, one daughter cell will have a hyperploid nucleus and the other will have a hypoploid nucleus.

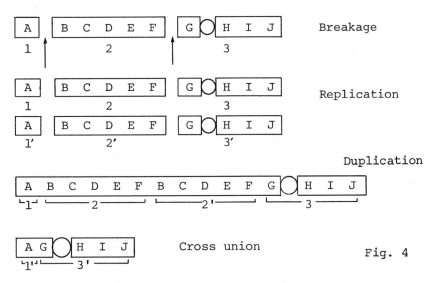

Fig. 4

The chromosomal breaks induced by radiation can result in several new gene sequences. The affect that such breaks have depend on the functions of the genes and their gene products.

POLYPLOIDY AND ANEUPLOIDY

What are the terms that describe variations in the number of chromosomes?

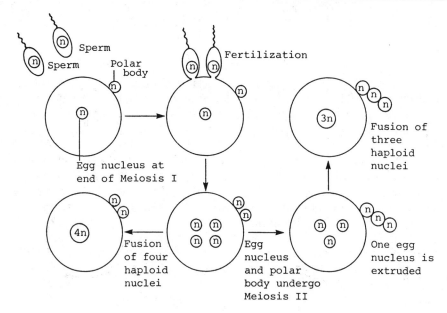

Fig. 1(a)

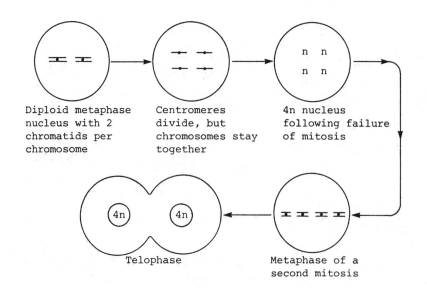

Fig. 1(b)

Solution: Variations in chromosome number are described by the terms euploidy and aneuploidy. Euploidy describes the existence of the entire set of chromosomes in multiples. Aneuploidy describes additions and deletions of only parts of the chromosomal set.

I. Euploidy

The following is a list of the different types of euploidy:

Euploidy type	Chromosome sets
1. Haploid	One (n)
2. Diploid	Two (2n)
3. Polyploid	More than two
a. Triploid	Three (3n)
b. Tetraploid	Four (4n)
c. Pentaploid	Five (5n)
d. Hexaploid	Six (6n)

Haploidy is the normal state of gametes. Diploidy is the state of zygotes, higher plants, and animals. Polyploidy is of agricultural importance since polyploid plants have greater vigor, larger flowers and larger fruits than diploid plants. Polyploidy in animals usually results in sterility since animals contain differentiated sex chromosomes. Fertility seems to depend on a delicate balance between the numbers of sex chromosomes and the numbers of autosomes - polyploidy upsets this balance.

There are two types of polyploidy: autopolyploidy and allopolyploidy. Autopolyploidy refers to polyploidy when all of the chromosome sets are homologous. Allopolyploidy refers to nonhomologous chromosome sets that arise from different species. Figure 1 shows two ways that autopolyploidy is produced: the first case is when two or more sperm fertilize an egg; the second case is when mitosis fails to separate chromosomes.

Allopolyploidy describes nonhomologous chromosome sets that are contributed by different species. Since the chromosomes of different species are essentially nonhomologous, chromosome pairing in meiosis is absent. The chromosomes are distributed randomly to the gametes. This leads to sterility. But, if a mitotic failure producing tetraploidy (4n) occurs, meiosis will proceed normally since each chromosome has something to pair with. Figure 2 shows a summary of allopolyploidy.

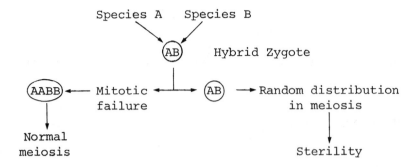

Fig. 2

II. Aneuploidy

Another type of variance in chromosome number involves only parts of the chromosome set. This is called aneuploidy. In aneuploidy some chromosomes are copied while others are deleted. There are several types of aneuploidy: monosomic, trisomic, tetrasomic, double trisomic and nullosomic. These names refer to the number of the affected chromosome. Monosomics are diploids missing one chromosome of a pair (2n-1). Two types of gametes are formed by monosomics: (n) and (n-1). The abnormal (n-1) gametes usually do not function in plants.

In animals (n-1) gametes result in a genetic imbalance which shows itself through reduced fertility or high mortality.

Trisomics are designated (2n+1). They contain an extra copy of one chromosome. They can create (n) and (n+1) gametes. The (n+1) gametes have various phenotypic effects depending on the chromosome that is in triplicate. In humans, this may be deleterious; Down's syndrome is a result of an extra copy of chromosome 21.

Tetrasomics have two extra copies of one chromosome (2n+2). Double trisomics (2n+1+1) have two extra different chromosomes. Nullosomics (2n-2) have completely lost a pair of chromosomes and this is usually lethal in diploids; however, polyploid organisms may survive, with reduced vitality, when nullosomic. Their survival is due to their additional chromosome copies.

Variance in chromosome number is a way in which organisms can evolve genetic and, therefore, phenotypic changes. Thus, these changes can result in increased adaptability of the organism.

Monoploid lines of many species exist. Plant breeders often convert these to diploids or polyploids through colchicine treatment. Can you see any advantages to this?

Solution: Polyploid and diploid nuclei can be made through the use of colchicine. Colchicine blocks microtubule formation. If added during cell division, the spindle will not form. The chromosomes will not be able to separate and migrate to separate poles. When the nuclear membrane reforms, a polyploid nucleus is the result.

By manipulating their plants in this way, plant breeders can control the euploidy of their nuclei. There are several advantages to this procedure. First, by doubling the chromosomes of a monoploid nucleus a diploid, homozygous for all of its gene pairs, is produced. The production of such a genetically pure organism by inbreeding is extremely time consuming. Secondly, some polyploids have phenotypes that are more desirable than their corresponding diploids. As a result, many disease-resistant strains of plants have been developed. Nicotiana tobacum is resistant to the tobacco mosaic virus which produces lesions on the leaves of the plant. Polyploid individuals also can produce larger fruits and flowers. The tetraploid watermelon, with 44 chromosomes, is larger than the normal watermelon.

This colchicine treatment can also convert a sterile species hybrid into a fertile "double diploid". The hybrid, which contains a set of nonhomologous chromosomes, will not be able to produce gametes with complete sets of chromosomes. The "double diploid" that results from the colchicine treatment has two copies of each chromosome so that balanced chromosome sets will be produced in the gametes. The once sterile hybrid will now be fertile.

There are ways to manipulate the chromosome complement of plants to obtain desirable traits. The treatment with colchicine is an effective method to obtain polyploids and diploids from monoploids. This manipulation has proven to be time-saving and economically advantageous to plant breeders.

What is the genetic basis of Down's syndrome?

Solution: Down's syndrome occurs in approximately one of every 600 live births, and the syndrome increases in frequency as the age of the mother at parturition increases. Usually, the syndrome is a result of trisomy of chromosome 21. The relationship between maternal age and incidence of Down's syndrome suggests that nondisjunction occurs more often in older egg cells. Recall that the human egg cell remains in a diplotene state from the fetal stage onward. It is possible that egg cells in older women are simply more prone to mechanical difficulties.

About 10% of the cases of Down's syndrome are caused by a translocation. The translocation chromosome arises as a fusion between chromosomes 14 and 21. A woman who has such a translocation has a normal chromosome 14 and a normal chromosome 21. She also has the translocated chromosome which is designated t(14;21). She will be phenotypically normal since she has a full diploid set of chromosomes. However, in meiosis, synaptic pairing is asymmetric and hence the orientation of the spindle can become abnormal. Such a woman may produce eggs that have chromosome 14 but not chromosome 21, 21 but not 14, 21 and t(14;21) or 14 and t(14;21). If an egg with the constitution 21 and t(14;21) is fertilized by a normal sperm containing both chromosomes 14 and 21, Down's syndrome will be the result. The child will have the 3 copies of chromosome 21 necessary to display Down's syndrome.

Translocation has occurred in a wild-type male Drosophila between chromosomes 2 and 3 in 1% of the sperm. Each male of the testing population is crossed with a female that is homozygous for the traits bw and st. The allele bw is located at the end of chromosome 3 and st is located near the centromere on chromosome 2. Flies homozygous for this gene cannot form colored pigment in their eyes and hence have white eyes. How can you detect the translocation?

Fig. 1.

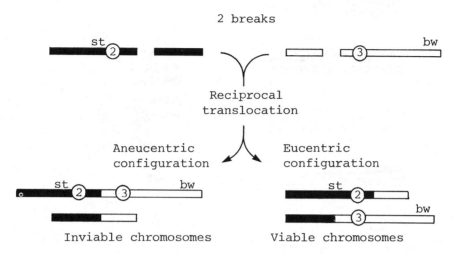

2 breaks

Reciprocal
translocation

Aneucentric
configuration

Eucentric
configuration

Inviable chromosomes   Viable chromosomes

Solution: To detect the translocation, we must first know how the translocation affects the chromosomes. Figure 1 shows two types of reciprocal translocations.

To detect a translocation the phenotypes of the progeny of various crosses must be compared. The offspring from a union of a sperm containing the translocation and the homozygous egg will be different from the union of the egg with a normal sperm. If an F_1 male has a normal sperm, he will produce 4 types of gametes in equal frequency: ++, bw+, +st, and bw st. A test cross of these gametes with the bw st gametes of the homozygous female yields:

Female gamete

bwst

Male gametes		Female gamete bwst	
	++	bwst ++	wild type
	bw+	bwst bw+	brown-eyed
	+st	bwst +st	scarlet-eyed
	bwst	bwst bwst	white-eyed

The phenotypic ratio is 1:1:1:1.

If the sperm contains a translocation, the situation is different. A cross-shaped double tetrad segregates differently at the first meiotic anaphase,

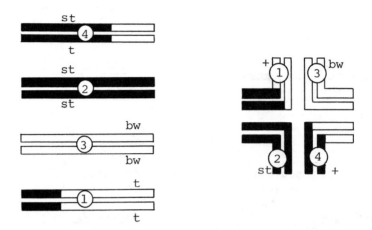

chromatids 2 and 3 go towards one pole and chromatids 1 and 4 go towards the other pole. This will produce the following gametes in the affected male:

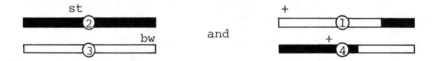

and

When these gametes are fused with the homozygous eggs, only white-eyed and wild-type offspring are produced:

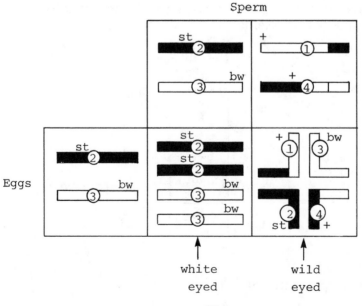

Therefore, the offspring that are produced by a test cross of a male with a translocation and a homozygous female are all white-eyed or wild-type. Of the cultures produced in these crosses, 1% will have only white-eyed or wild-type flies and 99% will have all four phenotypes since we began with a translocation in 1% of the sperm.

● **PROBLEM** 2-13

The chromosomes in a translocation heterozygote consist of two original chromosomes: ABCDEF and GHIJKL, and two translocated chromosomes: ABCJKL and GHIDEF. Diagram and explain the viable and lethal chromosome combinations.

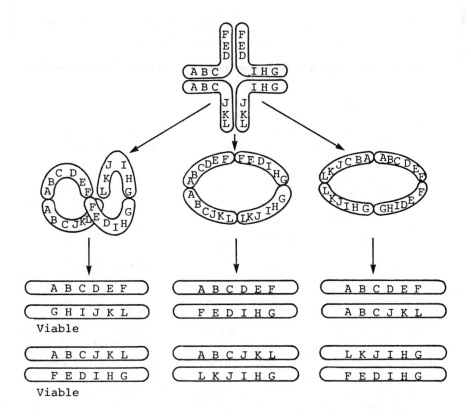

Fig. 1.

Diagram of viable and lethal chromosome combinations in a translocation heterozygote.

Solution: The homologous parts of a chromosome will associate with each other. As shown in Figure 1, such an association gives the gene sequence a definite order in a ring-shaped structure. At anaphase I of meiosis the ring is broken and two chromosomes move to each pole of the spindle. If the chromosomes were distributed at random, six different types of gametes would form. The only sets of gametes that would be viable would be the ones that had the complete genetic sequences: ABCDEF, GHIJKL and ABCJKL, FEDIHG. The other types of gametes would be unbalanced and hence nonviablesince they do not have a complete set of the genetic information. For instance, in the gamete set ABCDEF, ABCJKL, the sequence ABC occurs twice while the sequence GHI is missing entirely. The other gamete types are lethal for similar reasons.

● PROBLEM 2-14

What is the genotypic ratio produced by the self-fertilization of a duplex autotetraploid?

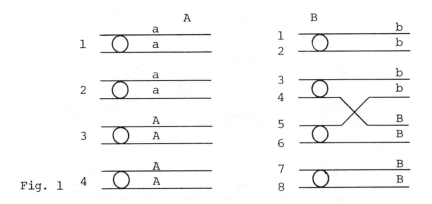

Fig. 1

Solution: Three points have to be considered in order to answer this question. First, we must know what a duplex autotetraploid is. Second, we must know what gametes such a species will produce. Third, we must answer the question in terms of centromere position, since differences in centromere position affect the genotypic ratios.

To begin with, an autotetraploid nucleus has four homologous sets of chromosomes. The genetics of such a species is therefore more complicated than that of a diploid species which has only two homologous sets of chromosomes.

If, in a diploid nucleus, there are two allelic forms of a gene, B and b, there are three possible combinations: BB, Bb and bb. If B is dominant to b, then the recessive trait b will only be expressed in the bb genotype.

The autotetraploid nucleus can be considered in a similar manner. Again, if we have two alleles, B and b, we can get the genotypic combinations: BBBB(quadruplex), BBBb(triplex), BBbb(duplex), Bbbb(simplex) and bbbb(nulliplex). If B is dominant to b, then the recessive trait will only manifest in the nulliplex, bbbb.

The position of the centromere is another important consideration in this problem. If the locus under consideration is close to the centromere it can be considered linked to the centromere. Chiasmata will not be able to form between the locus and the centromere, so crossing over will rarely occur. The assortment of genes into gametes can be determined by considering all of the ways that each of the 4 chromosomes can separate into pairs. If, on the other hand, the locus is far enough from the centromere to allow chiasmata and cross-over to occur, then each chromatid of the pair must be considered separately.

We now have enough information to solve this problem. Next, we must determine what gametes are formed when crossing over occurs and when it does not affect the locus that we are interested in. Figure 1 shows both types of duplex autotetraploids.

Let us consider the case where the gene is close to the centromere. A list of all of the gametes produced is obtained by recognizing all of the combinations of chromosomes:

1-2	aa	1	
1-3	aA		
1-4	aA	4	The gametic ratio is 1:4:1.
2-3	aA		
2-4	aA		
3-4	AA	1	

The genotypic and phenotypic ratios can be obtained through an examination of the self-fertilizing cross where the male gametes and the female gametes are the same:

Female gametes

		AA	4Aa	aa
Male gametes	AA	AAAA 1	AAAa 4	AAaa 1
	4Aa	AAAa 4	AAaa 16	Aaaa 4
	aa	AAaa 1	Aaaa 4	aaaa 1

Fig. 2

The genotypic ratio will be: 1 quadruplex:8 triplex:18 duplex:8 simplex:1 nulliplex. The phenotypic ratio will be 35 dominant:1 recessive.

A list of gametes that are a result of the type of locus which may change chromatids on account of recombination is a bit more lengthy than when crossing over does not occur. The list is more lengthy because each chromatid must be combined with another separately. Refer to Figure 1 to find which chromatid is represented by which number.

1-2	bb								
1-3	bb	2-3	bb						
1-4	bB	2-4	bB	3-4	bB				
1-5	bb	2-5	bb	3-5	bb	4-5	bB		
1-6	bB	2-6	bB	3-6	bB	4-6	BB	5-6	bB
1-7	bB	2-7	bB	3-7	bB	4-7	BB	5-7	bB
1-8	bB	2-8	bB	3-8	bB	4-8	BB	5-8	bB
	6-7	BB							
	6-8	BB	7-8	BB					

By adding all of the similar types, bb:Bb:BB, gametes are produced in the ratio 6:16:6 or 3:8:3. The BBbb x BBbb cross will yield the following progeny:

Female gametes

		3BB	8Bb	3bb
Male gametes	3BB	BBBB 9	BBBb 24	BBbb 9
	8Bb	BBBb 24	BBbb 64	Bbbb 24
	3bb	BBbb 9	Bbbb 24	bbbb 9

Fig. 3

The results of this cross are a genotypic ratio of 9 quadruplex: 48 triplex: 82 duplex: 48 simplex: 9 nulliplex and a phenotypic ratio of 187 dominant: 9 recessive or 21:1.

A regular diploid cross of Bb x Bb will yield a phenotypic ratio of 3:1. Thus, autotetraploids produce the recessive phenotype much less frequently. Working with genetics of this type requires much larger populations and much greater patience.

● **PROBLEM** 2-15

In Drosophila, when females homozygous for the X-linked gene for white eyes are crossed to red-eyed males, they normally yield red-eyed females and white-eyed males. However, white-eyed females are occasionally seen. Explain.

Solution: This problem describes the first sex-linked trait that was discovered by Thomas Hunt Morgan in 1910. Sex-linkage occurs when a gene is present on the X-chromosome but not on the Y. Thus, a female (XX in Drosophila as well as humans) can be homozygous and can express a recessive trait. A male (XY) is considered hemizygous since he can only possess one set of such genes. Males can thus express a recessive trait more often than females since the recessive trait in a male cannot be masked.

In the case of eye color in Drosophila, red eyes are dominant to white. Since a dominant trait is seen most often in normal populations of organisms, the trait is called wild-type and is denoted by (+). Thus, (+) can represent the gene for red eyes and (w) can represent the gene for white eyes.

Now we can take the information given to us in the problem and study the results of the cross. The female is homozygous for the gene for white eyes. The genotype on her X-chromosomes are therefore (ww); her phenotype shows white eyes. The male is red-eyed. His X-chromosome contains the wild-type gene. His Y-chromosome does not have a locus for this gene and is therefore silent. A cross between two flies of this kind should yield the results shown in Figure 1.

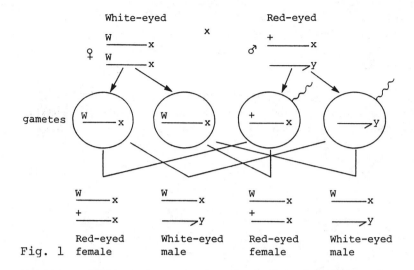

Fig. 1

The progeny of such a cross are either red-eyed females or white-eyed males. No white-eyed females are produced in a normal cross. In order to produce a white-eyed female, two X-chromosomes that contain the recessive trait are needed. The reason that no white-eyed females are produced in a normal cross is that the alleles segregate to separate gametes. To get a white-eyed female, both X-chromosomes have to come from the mother. But how is this possible? It is only possible if the X-chromosomes do not segregate properly during meiosis in the mother. This abnormality is termed nondisjunction and results in both X-chromosomes going to the same pole of the meiotic spindle. This faulty meiosis creates two eggs with two X-chromosomes and two eggs without any sex chromosome. The fertilization of these eggs creates exceptional types of offspring:

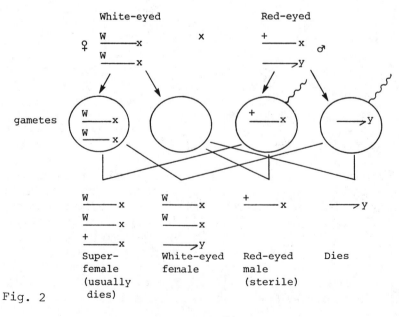

Fig. 2

54

This cross produces the white-eyed female that we were looking for.

What is the F_1 phenotypic ratio in the jimson weed, Datura stramonium, when a purple female (PPp) is crossed with a purple male (PPp)?

PPp ♀ x PPp ♂

gametes: P, P, Pp, Pp, PP, p   P, P, p

Female gametes

		2P	2Pp	PP	P
Male gametes	2P	PP 4	PPp 4	PPP 2	Pp 2
	p	Pp 2	Ppp 2	PPp 1	pp 1

Fig. 1

Solution: This problem involves a cross between two individuals that have three alleles for the color of their flowers. Since they have three alleles, they probably have the rest of the chromosomes to go with them. They are, therefore, trisomic. Jimson weed plants that are trisomic in their flower color allele have an extra copy of chromosome 9. In this gene purple is dominant over white. But since these are trisomics, the alleles will not segregate in the usual 3:1 Mendelian ratio, as will be seen.

The female plant produces P, Pp, PP, and p megaspores. The male, on the other hand, only produces functional P and p pollen; pollen with more or less than the normal 12 chromosomes will be nonfunctional.

The cross is shown in the diagram.

By counting the numbers of similar progeny, a genotypic ratio of 4PP:4Pp:5PPp:2Ppp:2PPP:1pp is obtained. The presence of one or more P alleles is expressed phenotypically as purple flowers. White flowers are only expressed in plants homozygous for the recessive p allele. Thus, the phenotypic ratio is 17 purple:1 white.

SHORT ANSWER QUESTIONS FOR REVIEW

Choose the correct answer.

1. Chromosomes lack which one of the following items? (a) DNA (b) centrioles (c) histones (d) RNA

   b

2. Of the 23 pairs of chromosomes present in humans, what is the number of autosomal pairs? (a) 20 (b) 21 (c) 22 (d) 23

   c

3. Histones make up approximately_____ of the mass of the chromosomes. (a) 75% (b) 50% (c) 33% (d) 25%

   b

4. Ions break chromosomes by (a) causing them to fracture during replication. (b) allowing disjunction of certain genes. (c) adding electrons to the chromosomes to increase the charge. (d) breaking bonds between atoms.

   d

5. The types of structural changes that can occur on chromosomes depend on the _____ of chromosomal material present in the nucleus and upon the _____ and sizes of the chromosomes. (a) mass, shapes (b) charge, number (c) charge, shapes (d) none of the above

   d

6. Which of the following diseases have been linked to some form of cancer? (a) Xeroderma pigmentosum (b) Bloom's syndrome (c) Fanconi's anemia (d) all of the above

   d

7. Which of the following term represents the euploidy state of gametes? (a) diploid (b) haploid (c) polyploid (d) tetraploid

   b

8. Autopolyploidy refers to (a) polyploidy when all chromosomes are homologous. (b) polyploidy with non-homologous chromosomes from different species. (c) the normal state of human gametes. (d) none of the above

   a

9. An advantage to creating polyploid and diploid nuclei in plants is (a) creating sterile hybrids (b) producing a larger quantity of less desirable mutations. (c) producing more desirable phenotypes. (d) decreasing the economic value of products grown on these plants.

   c

10. Down's syndrome is usually the result of
(a) nullosomy of chromosome 14. (b)
tetrasomy of chromosome 21. (c) double
trisomy of chromosomes 14 and 21. (d)
trisomy of chromosome 21.   d

11. To detect a translocation, the _____ of
the progeny of various crosses must be
compared. (a) phenotypes (b) genotypes
(c) gametes (d) none of the above   a

12. The chromosomes in a translocation
heterozygote consist of two original chromosomes: ABCDEF and GHIJKL, and two
translocated chromosomes: ABCJKL and
GHIDEF. Which of the following choices is
a viable chromosome combination? (a)
ABCDEF, FEDIHG (b) ABCJKL, LKJIHG
(c) ABCJKL, FEDIHG (d) LKJIHG, FEDIHG.   c

13. The number of possible genotypic combinations from an autotetraploid nucleus is (a)
4. (b) 5. (c) 6, (d) 8.   b

14. White eyes are a recessive trait in
Drosophila and the gene for white eyes is
only present on the X chromosome. In order
to produce a white eyed female (a) the male
parent must be recessive for this trait. (b)
the female must have the geneotype XYXX.
(c) both X chromosomes must come from the
female parent, caused by nondisjunction of
these X chromosomes. (d) it is impossible
to produce a white eyed female.   c

15. In the jimson weed, purple flower color is
dominant over white. If a purple male of
genotype PP_p is crossed with a female of the
same genotype, what would be the phenotypic
ratio of the progeny? (a) 3 purple:1 white
(b) 1 purple:3 white (c) 17 purple:1 white
(d) 1 purple:17 white   c

In questions 16 through 19 match the appropriate
terms to their corresponding definitions.

57

16. Duplication   (a) the amount of chromo-   d
                                  somal material remains

17. Deficiency   unchanged, while the   c
                                  arrangement of this

18. Inversion   material is altered   a

                     (b) genetic material is

19. Translocation   rearranged between   b
                                  non-homologous
                                  chromosomes

                     (c) involves the loss of a
                                  piece of genetic infor-
                                  mation

                     (d) an extra copy of a
                                  piece of chromosomal
                                  material is present

In questions 20 - 22 match the type of aneuploidy to its correct genetic designation. Use 2n to represent a diploid nucleus.

20. Trisomic   (a) (2n - 2)   b

21. Tetrasomic   (b) (2n + 1)   c

22. Nullosomic   (c) (2n + 2)   a

The following set of questions, #23 through #26, refers to a cell with a hyperploid nucleus due to a break and then a nonrestitutional union. Match the appropriate terms to the diagrams they best describe.

23. Breakage   (a) [A] [BCDEF] [G◯HIJ]   c
                            1 ↑   2   ↑   3

24. Replication   [A] [BCDEF] [G◯HIJ]   a
                            1' ↑   2'   ↑   3'

25. Duplication   (b) [A BCDEFBCDEF   G◯HIJ]   b
                            1   2   2'   3

26. Cross union   (c) [A][BCDEF] [G◯HIJ]   d
                            1 ↑   2   ↑   3

                     (d) [AG◯HIJ]
                            1'   3'

Fill in the blanks.

27. Using the _____ technique, the complete set
of chromosomes of a cell can be studied.   karyotype

28. Histones are_____,_____ _____ which, in
the chromosomes of eukaryotes, bind tightly
to DNA.

small basic
proteins

29. Metacentric chromosomes have their centromeres near the _____ of their length, while
acrocentric chromosomes have their centromeres toward the _____ of their length.

middle,
end

30. Inversions and deficiencies are two examples
of _____ _____ that can occur in
chromosomes.

structural
changes

31. In the accompanying diagram of two once-
homologous chromosomes, Chromosome A
contains a _____ while chromosome B
contains a _____ .

duplication,
deletion

Chromosome A . ABCDEFGHFGH _____

Chromosome B / . ABCDGH _____

centromeres

32. _____ is required to cause a break in the
structure of the relatively stable chromosome.

Energy

33. Many times when a chromosome is broken
by radiation, a _____ _____ occurs, and
the original gene is recreated.

restitutional
union

34. Plant breeders produce polyploid and diploid
nuclei in their plants by using the chemical
_____ .

colchicine

35. An autotetraploid has _____ _____ _____
of chromosomes.

four
homologous
sets

36. In Drosophila, red eyes occur more
frequently in normal populations than white
eyes. They are, therfore, the _____ trait
and are also called the _____ _____ of
the species.

dominant,
wild type

Determine whether the following statements are
True or False.

To be covered
when testing
yourself

37. Higher frequency radiation, such as x-ray, is less effective than radiation of a lower frequency in disrupting the structure of the chromosome.

False

38. When a chromosome is broken, the ends are incapable of rejoining.

False

39. Though chromosomal instability may not be the sole cause of cancer, it may create an environment that is highly susceptible to certain forms of cancer.

True

40. A nonrestitutional union - one in which the original chromosome is not recreated - is the more likely union to occur.

True

41. If a normal sperm containing both chromosomes 14 and 21 fertilizes an egg with the constitution 21 and t(14;21), Down's Syndrome will not occur.

False

CHAPTER 3

MENDELIAN GENETICS

MENDEL'S LAWS

● **PROBLEM 3-1**

What are Mendel's Laws and how did he formulate his hypothesis?

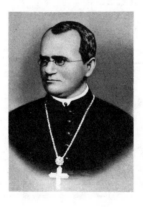

Fig. 1.
Gregor Johann Mendel

Solution: Gregor Mendel was able to formulate his laws on the basis of his work with the garden pea. He chose to work with garden peas because they were readily hybridized and had well defined traits. Mendel studied seven garden pea traits that appeared in one form or another without blending to produce intermediate traits, see Figure 1. The traits he studied included round vs. wrinkled seeds, yellow vs. green seeds, and tall vs. dwarf plants.

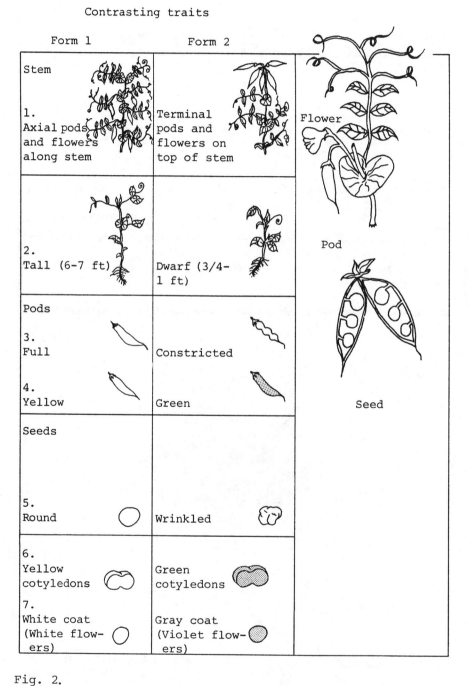

Contrasting traits

Form 1	Form 2	
Stem 1. Axial pods and flowers along stem	Terminal pods and flowers on top of stem	Flower
2. Tall (6-7 ft)	Dwarf (3/4-1 ft)	Pod
Pods 3. Full	Constricted	
4. Yellow	Green	Seed
Seeds 5. Round	Wrinkled	
6. Yellow cotyledons	Green cotyledons	
7. White coat (White flowers)	Gray coat (Violet flowers)	

Fig. 2.

Seven traits of the garden pea

After many crosses, Mendel was able to demonstrate that the seven traits each behaved in mathematically precise and predictable ways. When tall plants that had come from a line of tall parents were self-fertilized, they produced only tall offspring. The same held true for dwarf plants, which produced only dwarf offspring. Mendel also found that when the tall plants were crossed with dwarf plants, the first generation plants, the F_1 generation, were all tall. However, when these tall hybrids were allowed to self-fertilize, the next (F_2) generation was composed of 787 tall plants and 277 short plants, roughly a 3:1 ratio. When the F_2 generation was self-fertilized, Mendel found that all of the short plants produced only short offspring. On the other hand, 1/3 of the F_2 tall plants produced only tall offspring while the other 2/3 produced both tall and short plants in, roughly, a 3:1 ratio.

From these results Mendel was able to theorize that the determinants of heredity (called "factors" by Mendel, but now known as genes) occur in pairs, and that they segregate in the formation of gametes, allowing only one of each pair to be transmitted to a gamete. The double number is restored when the gametes come together to form the zygote. This principle is known as the Law of Segregation.

Mendel also noted that the pattern of inheritance in his peas featured a dominant and recessive relationship between alternate forms of each trait. For example, the tall trait is shown to be dominant over the dwarfness trait because hybrids between tall and short strains produce only tall plants, even though the hybrid contains genes for both tallness and dwarfness. Mendel designated dominant factors with capital letters and recessive ones with corresponding lower case letters. Thus, a pure tall plant would be designated DD, and a dwarf plant dd. A hybrid tall would be designated Dd.

In addition to the single factor crosses, Mendel made several hybridizations in which he studied two or three pairs of factors simultaneously. For example, one cross involved plants producing round yellow seeds with those producing wrinkled green seeds. The seeds from the first generation were all round and yellow, since these are the dominant traits. When these plants were self-fertilized, 4 types of seeds resulted in the F_2 generation. They were found in proportions of 9/16 round and yellow, 3/16 wrinkled and yellow, 3/16 round and green, and 1/16 wrinkled and green, a 9:3:3:1 ratio. Mendel recognized that this 9:3:3:1 ratio resulted from the independent assortment of 2 single factor crosses. The segregation of both factors was occurring independently for both factors. The ratio resulting from this cross could be predicted from results for each pair when crossed individually. When only looking at seed color, a 3:1 yellow to green ratio occurred. A 3:1 round to wrinkled ratio is seen when shape is considered individually. Multiplying these together:

$$3(\text{yellow}) + 1(\text{green})$$
$$\underline{x \quad 3(\text{round}) + 1(\text{wrinkled})}$$
$$9(\text{yellow, round}) + 3(\text{yellow, wrinkled}) +$$
$$3(\text{green, round}) + 1(\text{green, wrinkled})$$

yields the ratio expected, based on what Mendel found in his cross involving two simultaneous factors. This is called the Law of Independent Assortment. Each factor in the cross segregates independently of the other factors involved. The principle makes it easy to predict the results of crosses involving multiple pairs of factors by merely multiplying together the results for each pair considered individually.

● **PROBLEM 3-2**

Suppose pure line lima bean plants having green pods were crossed with pure line plants having yellow pods. If all the F_1 plants had green pods and were allowed to interbreed, 580 F_2 plants, 435 with green pods and 145 with yellow pods would be obtained. Which characteristic is dominant and which is recessive? Of the F_2 plants, how many are homozygous recessive, homozygous dominant and heterozygous? Using G to represent the dominant gene and g to represent the recessive gene, write out a plan showing the segregation of genes from the parents to the F_2 plants.

Solution: This example is used to illustrate the basic concepts of genetics and the methods of solving genetic problems. First, some definitions:

a) chromosomes - filamentous or rod-shaped bodies in the cell nucleus which contain the hereditary units, the genes.

b) gene - the part of a chromosome which codes for

a certain hereditary trait.

c) genotype - the genetic makeup of an organism, or the set of genes which it possesses.

d) phenotype - the outward, visible expression of the hereditary constitution of an organism.

e) homologous chromosomes - chromosomes bearing genes for the same characters.

f) homozygote - an organism possessing an identical pair of alleles on homologous chromosomes for a given character or for all given characters.

g) heterozygote - an organism possessing different alleles on homologous chromosomes for a given character or for all given characters.

In solving genetic problems, one uses letters to represent the genotype of the organism. For example, "a" represents the gene for blue color and "A" represents the gene for red color. A capital letter is used for a dominant gene; that is, the phenotype of that gene will be expressed in a heterozygous state. For example, if the genotype Aa is expressed as red, then A is the dominant gene. Small letter a represents the recessive gene; that is, one whose phenotype will be expressed only in the homozygous state. Therefore, aa would be expressed as blue.

To solve a genetic problem, one writes down the genotypes of the two parents in the cross. Mendel's First Law tells us what to do. This law, also known as the Law of Independent Segregation, states that genes, the units of heredity, exist in individuals in pairs. In the formation of sex cells or gametes, the two genes separate and pass independent of one another into different gametes, so that each gamete has one, and only one, member of each pair. During fertilization, the gamete of one parent fuses with that of the other parent. Fusion brings the genes from each parent together, giving rise to offspring with paired genes. Now we will illustrate the Law of Segregation as it applies to the problem given. Let G represent the gene for green pod color and g represent the gene for yellow pod color. Since the parents come from pure lines, meaning that the two members of each gene pair are identical, we write the genotype of the parent plant with green pods as GG, and that of the parent plant with yellow pods as gg. Each gamete from the first parent will have one G and each gamete from the second will have one g. (Recall the Law of Independent Segregation.) Writing out a schematic cross, we have:

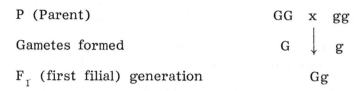

P (Parent)   GG x gg

Gametes formed   G ↓ g

F₁ (first filial) generation   Gg

The genotype of the F_1 generation is written as Gg because it results from the fusion of the two gametes.

We are told that all the F_1 generation from the above cross are green, and we observe that they are all heterozygous. Therefore G, which stands for the gene with green pods, must be dominant (by definition), and g, which stands for the gene with yellow pods, must be recessive.

To determine the possible genotypes of the F_1 plants, or the second generation offspring, we mate two F_2 plants. The possible gametes derived from the parents are again obtained using Mendel's First Law. But now we obtain two types of gametes, G and g, from each parent, because either gene can come from the parental genotype of Gg.

Schematically, then:

P   Gg x Gg

gametes G_1 g ↓ G_1 g

It is easier to determine the F_2 generation using the Punnet square. The square is constructed as follows:

	G	g
G	GG	Gg
g	Gg	gg

possible gametes from male parent

possible gametes from female parent ——→

It gives all possible combinations of the parental gametes, so in F_2 we have genotypically:

1 GG : 2 Gg : 1 gg

Phenotypically:

GG is homozygous dominant and green because G is dominant;

Gg is heterozygous and green because G is dominant; and

gg is homozygous recessive and yellow because g is recessive.

It is important to note that we cannot observe the genotype itself because it lies in the constitution of the gene. Our observations come only from what we actually see, that is, the phenotypic differences.

We know from the Punnet square that in the F_2 generation the ratio of homozygous dominant to the entire progeny is $\frac{1}{4}$; the ratio of heterozygous is 2/4 or $\frac{1}{2}$, and the ratio of homozygous recessive is $\frac{1}{4}$. Therefore, the number of homozygous dominant (GG) plants is

$$1/4 \times 580 \quad \text{or} \quad 145,$$

the number of heterozygote (Gg) plants is

$$1/2 \times 580 \quad \text{or} \quad 290$$

and the number of homozygous recessive (gg) plants is

$$1/4 \times 580 \quad \text{or} \quad 145.$$

When added together, they total 580, the number of F_2 plants.

● **PROBLEM 3-3**

(a) In garden peas, yellow seed color is determined by the dominant allele G and green by the recessive allele g. Diagram a cross between a pea plant homozygous for yellow seeds (GG) with one that produces green seeds (gg). Do this for the F_1 and F_2 generations. In addition to the use of Punnett squares, also give the possible phenotypes, the possible genotypes, the genotypic frequency, and the phenotypic ratio for the F_2 generation.

(b) When Mendel did this cross, from a total of 8023 F_2 seeds obtained, he classified 6022 yellow seeds and 2001 green seeds. Using a chart with the headings phenotypes, observed (Mendel's results), calculated, and deviations, compare the expected results calculated in (a) with Mendel's results.

67

<u>Solution</u>: This problem can be solved by applying Mendel's Law of Segregation, which states that hereditary characteristics are determined by particulate factors (now called genes), that these factors occur in pairs, and that these factors are segregated in the formation of gametes so that only one member of the pair is given to each gamete. According to the Mendelian hypothesis, the gametes are combined according to chance, following certain fixed probabilities. The following Punnett square shows the resulting F_1 generation combinations:

G - Yellow seeds
g - Green seeds
GG - Yellow homozygous
Gg - Yellow heterozygous
gg - Green homozygous

F_1 generation:

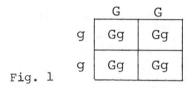

Fig. 1

As seen in the Punnett square, every member of the F_1 generation is heterozygous yellow.

When a member of the F_1 generation is self-pollinated, the following F_2 generation results:

F_2 generation:

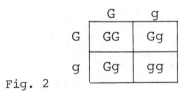

Fig. 2

Below is a summary of the expected F_2 generation, showing expected phenotypic and genotypic ratios:

Phenotypes	Genotypes	Genotypic Frequency	Phenotypic Frequency
Yellow	GG	1	3
	Gg	2	
Green	gg	1	1

(b) The ratio of yellow to green seeds is 3:1 according to the calculated F_2 generation. This means that for every 4 seeds, 3 are yellow and 1 is green. This theoretical relationship can be compared to the experimental values that Mendel obtained. By comparing the theoretical total of 4 seeds to the given total of 8023 seeds, the expected number of each type of seed can be obtained. These values can then be compared to the values that Mendel got (6022 yellow and 2001 green) to find the deviation from the theoretical values.

To do this the expected number of each type of seed must first be found. The following relationship is used:

$$\frac{4(\text{total expected})}{3(\text{yellow expected})} = \frac{8023(\text{total obtained})}{X(\text{yellow obtained})}$$

where X is the number of yellow seeds that should be produced if Mendel's ratio is correct. By cross-multiplying and then dividing, X is found to equal 6017. Thus of a total of 8023 seeds, 6017 should be yellow.

Similarly, the relationship for green seeds to the total is:

$$\frac{4(\text{total expected})}{1(\text{green expected})} = \frac{8023(\text{total obtained})}{X(\text{yellow obtained})}$$

Here, X = 2006 green seeds.

Now, these theoretical values (6017 yellow and 2006 green) can be compared to the given values in order to calculate the deviation.

Phenotypes	Observed (given)	Calculated	Deviation
Yellow	6022	6017	5
Green	2001	2006	5

The deviation values show that there were 5 more yellow seeds than expected and 5 fewer green seeds than expected. Of a total of 8023 seeds, only 10 behaved differently than Mendel's theoretical calculations predicted. Finding the deviation in terms of percentages will help to illustrate how minimal this discrepancy really is:

$$\frac{10 \text{ deviates}}{8023 \text{ total}} \times 100\% = 0.12\%$$

This deviation of less than 1% could be expected to decrease even further if a larger number of seeds were classified.

MONOHYBRID CROSS

Two long-winged flies were mated. The offspring consisted of 77 with long wings and 24 with short wings. Is the short-winged condition dominant or recessive? What are the genotypes of the parents?

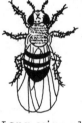 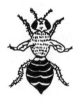

Long-winged   Short-winged
  (male)   (female)

Fruit flies (enlarged)

Solution: When we are not told which of the characteristics is dominant and which is recessive, we can deduce it from the ratio of phenotypes in the progeny. We know that 77 flies have long wings and 24 have short wings. This gives us an approximate ratio of 3 long-winged flies to every 1 short-winged fly.

$$\frac{77}{24} \sim \frac{3}{1}$$

As previously noted, the three-to-one ratio signifies that dominant and recessive characteristics are most likely involved. Moreover, because there are three long-winged flies to every short-winged one, it suggests that short-wingedness is the recessive characteristic, and long-wingedness is dominant.

We cannot immediately conclude that both the long-winged parents are homozygous. In fact they are not, because if they were, no short-winged offspring could have resulted in the cross. So the presence of short-winged flies (homozygous recessive) in the progeny suggests that both parents carry the recessive gene and are thus heterozygotes.

Let L be the gene for long wings in flies and ℓ be the gene for short wings in flies. In the cross between two long-winged heterozygous parents:

P   Lℓ   x   Lℓ

Gametes   L;ℓ ↓   L;ℓ

F_1 1 LL: 2Lℓ: 1 ℓℓ

               long wing   short wing

The phenotypes of the F_1 show the three-to-one ratio of long-winged flies to short-winged flies, which concurs with the data given. Therefore, the genotypes of the parents are the same, both being heterozygous (Lℓ).

● PROBLEM 3-5

Predict the genotypic and phenotypic results from each of the following crosses in garden peas:
(a) a tall (homozygous dominant) plant crossed with a dwarf plant;
(b) the progeny of (a) when self-pollinated;
(c) the progeny of (a) crossed with a homozygous tall plant;
(d) the progeny of (a) crossed with a dwarf plant.

Solution: (a) D - tall
              d - dwarf

              DD - homozygous tall
              Dd - heterozygous tall
              dd - homozygous dwarf

```
        D   D
    ┌────┬────┐
  d │ Dd │ Dd │
    ├────┼────┤
  d │ Dd │ Dd │
    └────┴────┘
```

Genotypic results: All Dd.
Phenotypic results: All tall.

(b) This part asks for a cross between two F_1 individuals: Dd x Dd

```
        D    d
    ┌────┬────┐
  D │ DD │ Dd │
    ├────┼────┤
  d │ Dd │ dd │
    └────┴────┘
```

There are 4 different progeny. Of these 4, 1 is homozygous dominant, or DD; hence the fraction 1/4. The remaining fractions were obtained in a similar fashion.

Genotypic results: 1/4 DD; 1/2 Dd; 1/4 dd.
Phenotypic results: 3/4 tall; 1/4 dwarf.

(c) This part of the problem asks for the following cross: Dd x DD.

```
        D    d
    ┌────┬────┐
  D │ DD │ Dd │
    ├────┼────┤
  D │ DD │ Dd │
    └────┴────┘
```

Genotypic results: 1/2 DD; 1/2 Dd.
Phenotypic results: All tall.

(d) This final part asks for a Dd x dd cross.

```
        D    d
    ┌────┬────┐
  d │ Dd │ dd │
    ├────┼────┤
  d │ Dd │ dd │
    └────┴────┘
```

Genotypic results: 1/2 Dd; 1/2 dd.
Phenotypic results: 1/2 tall; 1/2 dwarf.

From these results it can be seen that in order for a dwarf variety to be produced, both of the parents must carry the recessive allele, d.

● **PROBLEM 3-6**

Consider the trait, body color in the flour beetle, Tribolium castaneum, to be controlled by a pair of genes exhibiting complete dominance. The pair of contrasting alleles are E for red body which is dominant to e for ebony body color. In a cross between a red-bodied female and an ebony-bodied male, 32 progeny are recovered, of which 18 are red-bodies and 14 are ebony-bodied. What are the genotypes of the parents and progeny?

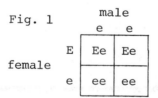

Fig. 1

Solution: Since the gene for ebony body color is recessive to that for red body color, we can determine the genotypes of both the ebony male parent and ebony progeny to be ee homozygotes. The occurence of ebony progeny dictates that the genotype of the female parent must be Ee, since ebony progeny were observed. Similarly, the genotypes of the red progeny must be Ee since both parents contribute a gene for body color, E, from the female parent and e, from the male parent.

The cross can be illustrated by a Punnett square, as shown in Figure 1.

Consider that in horses a single pair of genes controls gait. Some horses can only exhibit a trotting gait, while others exhibit only a pacing gait. In an attempt to determine the pattern of inheritance displayed by this trait, a horse breeder crossed a stallion (σ) that came from a long line of pacers to several mares ($\varphi\varphi$) that were trotters. All of the foals were trotters.

Which gait is under the control of the dominant gene?

Using the letters $\underline{T}$ and $\underline{t}$ to represent the dominant and recessive genes, respectively, identify the genotypes of the stallion, the mares and the foals.

Solution: Since all of the foals were trotters, and since both the stallion and the mares came from long lines showing their respective gaits, we can say that the trotting gait is controlled by the dominant gene, $\underline{T}$.

Thus, the genotype of the stallion is $\underline{tt}$, that of the mares is $\underline{TT}$, and the genotypes of the foals is $\underline{Tt}$.

Given: two strains of snapdragons which differ by a single character; position of the flowers. Strain A has flowers that are positioned axially on the plant stem, while Strain B has terminal flowers. Both strains are considered to be pure breeding for their respective form of the character.

When plants from the two strains are reciprocally crossed (i.e., A φ x B σ and B φ x A σ), the first progeny generation gives only axially positioned flowers. Second generation progeny exhibited the following:

Phenotype	Number
axial	716

a) How is this trait inherited?

b) Using A and a for gene symbols, determine the genotypes for the parent strains, the F_1 generation and F_2 generation progenies.

Solution: a) Since both strains were pure bred, we can assume that they were homozygous. Therefore, on the basis of the results observed (a 3:1 axial to terminal ratio), the trait appears to be inherited as controlled by a single gene pair. The gene for axially-placed flowers is dominant to its counterpart for terminally-placed flowers, since only axial flowers were observed in the F_1 progeny. Terminal flowers did not reappear until the F_2 generation.

b)

Plant	Phenotype	Genotype
Strain A parent	axial	AA
Strain B parent	terminal	aa
F_1 progeny	axial	Aa
F_2 progeny	axial	AA or Aa
	terminal	aa

● **PROBLEM 3-9**

A homozygous tall pea plant was crossed with a homozygous dwarf pea plant. The gene for tall is dominant to its allele for dwarf. What will be the expected phenotypic and genotypic results in the F_1 and F_2 generations?

Solution: D-tall, d-dwarf.   homozygous   homozygous
                                      tall   X   dwarf
              Genotype   DD   dd
         Types of gamete   D   D   d   d

	D	D
d	Dd	Dd
d	Dd	Dd

F$_1$ progeny all Dd and tall

To obtain the F$_2$ progeny two F$_1$ Dd individuals are mated

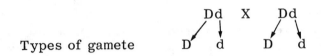

Types of gamete   Dd   X   Dd

	D	d
D	DD	Dd
d	Dd	dd

F$_2$ Genotypic results   Phenotypic results

1/4 DD
1/2 Dd   } 3/4 tall

1/4 dd   1/4 dwarf

● **PROBLEM 3-10**

If two fruit flies, heterozygous for genes of one allelic pair, were bred together and had 200 offspring
a) about how many would have the dominant phenotype?
b) of these offspring, some will be homozygous dominant and some heterozygous. How is it possible to establish which is which?

Solution: Let A be the dominant gene and a be the recessive gene. Since the flies are heterozygous, each must therefore be Aa.

a) In the cross, we have:

P   Aa   x   Aa

Gametes   A; a   A; a

76

F₁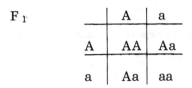

1 AA : 2 Aa : 1 aa

homozygous   hetero-   homozygous
dominant   zygous   recessive

The proportion of offspring expressing the dominant phenotype is $1/4 + 2/4 = 3/4$. Therefore, the expected number with the dominant phenotype is $3/4 \times 200$ or 150.

b) To establish which of the dominant phenotypes are homozygous and which are heterozygous, we have to perform a test cross; i.e., crossing one fly whose genotype is to be determined with a homozygous recessive fly. If the test fly is homozygous dominant:

P_2 AA   x   aa

Gamete   A ↓ a

F_2 100% Aa

All the progeny will show the dominant phenotype. This implies that the test fly is homozygous dominant.

If the test fly is heterozygous, then in the back cross:

P_2 Aa   x   aa

Gamete   A, a ↓ a

F_2 Aa ;   aa

So half the progeny will show dominant phenotype and the other half will show recessive phenotype. This indicates that the test fly was heterozygous.

Therefore, by performing a test cross between a fly whose genotype we do not know and homozygous recessive fly, we can determine if the fly is homozygous or heterozygous by looking at the phenotypes of the progeny.

The ability to roll the tongue into almost a complete circle is conferred by a dominant gene, while its recessive allele fails to confer this ability. A man and his wife can both roll their tongues and are surprised to find that their son cannot. Explain this by showing the genotypes of all three persons.

Solution: Let us represent the dominant allele for the trait of tongue-rolling by R, and the recessive allele by r. We know that if a gene is dominant for a trait, it will always be expressed if it is present. Since the son cannot roll his tongue, he cannot possess the dominant gene for this trait, and his genotype must be rr. This means that each parent must have at least one recessive allele to donate to their son. Also, each parent must have a dominant allele for this trait because they have the ability to roll their tongues. Thus, the genotype of parents for this trait must be Rr.

We can illustrate this by looking at the mating of two such parents,

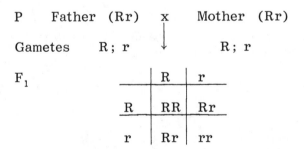

P   Father (Rr)   x   Mother (Rr)

Gametes   R; r   R; r

The offspring will be obtained in the following ratio:

F   1/4 RR,   Homozygous dominant; tongue roller.
        1/2 Rr,   Heterozygous; tongue roller.
        1/4 rr, Homozygous recessive;
                              non-tongue roller

We see then that there is a one-in-four chance that two parents who are heterozygous for a dominant trait will produce offspring without that trait. It is not unlikely, then, that the parents in this problem could have had a son who does not have the ability to roll his tongue.

A man and a woman are heterozygous for tongue rolling, and have three sons. The three sons marry women who are not tongue rollers. Assuming that each of the three sons has a different genotype, show by diagram what proportion of their children might have the ability to roll their tongues.

Solution: Let us again use the letter R to represent the dominant tongue rolling allele, and r to represent the recessive allele. Only three possible genotypes could result from the cross of the heterozygous parents. These alleles are: RR, Rr and rr. Let one of the sons be RR and therefore a tongue roller, the second son Rr and also a tongue roller, and the third son rr (homozygous recessive) and thus unable to roll his tongue. All three sons have married women who are not tongue rollers and who are therefore rr.

Let us now determine the proportion of the offspring who will be able to roll their tongues.

Case 1

	Son 1 x Woman 1	
P$_1$	RR x	rr
Gametes	R ↓	r
F$_1$	Rr	100% Rr: tongue rollers

Case 2

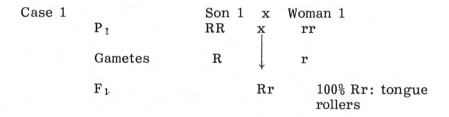

	Son 2 x Woman 2	
P$_1$	Rr	rr
Gametes	R;r ↓	4
		50% Rr: tongue rollers
		50% rr: non-
F$_1$	Rr; rr	tongue rollers

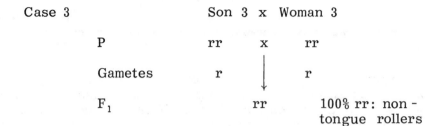

Case 3   Son 3 x Woman 3

    P   rr   x   rr

    Gametes   r   │   r
                            ↓
    F₁   rr   100% rr: non -
                                    tongue rollers

As a result of the three crosses, we can see that of the total offspring from the three marriages, half will be tongue rollers and half will be non-tongue rollers. The tongue rollers consist of all the children of the first son plus half the children of the second son. The non-tongue rolling children consist of all the offspring of the third son's marriage plus half the offspring from the second son's marriage.

● PROBLEM 3-13

The ability to roll the tongue is conferred by a dominant gene, while its recessive allele fails to confer this ability. If 16% of the students in a school cannot roll their tongues, what percentage of students are heterozygous?

Solution: The 16 percent of the students that cannot roll their tongues must have a homozygous recessive genotype because the trait is determined by a dominant allele. The homozygous dominant or heterozygous condition will give one the ability to roll his tongue. If we represent the dominant allele by R and the recessive allele by r, then the three possible genotypes will be RR, Rr, and rr.

We are told that the non-tongue rolling phenotype and thus the homozygous recessive genotype (rr) occurs with a frequency of 16% or .16. To find the frequency of the recessive allele r we take the square root of .16

$$\sqrt{.16}, = .40$$

Thus, .4 is the frequency of the non-roller allele. Knowing that the frequencies of the two alleles must add to 1 (i.e., R+r = 1) we can calculate the frequency of the roller allele (R) to be .60 (i.e., R + .40 = 1; R = 1 - .40; R = .60). Squaring .60 will give us the frequency of the homozygous dominant rollers (RR). It is .36 ($.60^2$ = .36).

The total homozygous proportion of the student population can be obtained by adding the homozygous recessive's frequency (rr) with the homozygous dominant's frequency (RR). 0.36 + 0.16 = 0.52. To obtain the heterozygous proportion of the population we can use the fact that total population = homozygous population + heterozygous population. Thus, 1 = .52 + heterozygous population or, heterozygous population = 1 - .52 = .48. Therefore, 48 percent of the students are heterozygotes and have the ability to roll their tongues.

DIHYBRID CROSS

● PROBLEM 3-14

The checkered pattern of pigeons is controlled by a dominant gene C; plain color is determined by the recessive allele c. Red color is controlled by a dominant gene B, and brown color by the recessive allele b. Complete a Punnett square for a dihybrid cross involving a homozygous checkered red bird and a plain brown bird. For this cross, show the expected phenotypes, genotypes, genotypic frequencies and phenotypic ratios for the F_2 generation.

CCBB × ccbb   P

(CB)   (cb)   gametes

CcBb × CcBb F_1 × F_1

Gametes	(CB)	(Cb)	(cB)	(cb)
(CB)	CCBB	CCBb	CcBB	CcBb
(Cb)	CCBb	CCbb	CcBb	Ccbb
(cB)	CcBB	CcBb	ccBB	ccBb
(cb)	CcBb	Ccbb	ccBb	ccbb

Solution: This problem involves the Law of Independent Assortment - Mendel's Second Law. The law states that any pair of genes will segretate independently of all other pairs. Because of this, the results of an experiment involving several sets of characters may be obtained by multiplying the proportions expected for each factor when considered individually. The cross would result in the following:

Summary of F_2:

Phenotypes	Genotypes	Genotypic frequency	Phenotypic ratio
checkered red	CCBB	1	9
	CCBb	2	
	CcBB	2	
	CcBb	4	
checkered brown	CCbb	1	3
	Ccbb	2	
plain red	ccBB	1	3
	ccBb	2	
plain brown	ccbb	1	1

● **PROBLEM 3-15**

In peas, tall (D) is dominant to dwarf (d) and yellow cotyledons (G) is dominant to green (g). If a tall, homozygous, yellow pea plant is crossed with a dwarf, green pea plant, what will be the phenotypic results in the F_1 and F_2?

Solution: Homozygous tall, yellow × Homozygous dwarf, green

$$DDGG \qquad\qquad ddgg$$

F_1 individuals have 1 gene from each parent in each pair. Hence, DdGg are tall and yellow.

The F_2 generation is obtained by mating F_1 individuals.

$$\underline{DdGg} \quad \times \quad \underline{DdGg}$$

This problem can be solved by first determining the results for each individual gene pair.

Dd   x   Dd   Gg   x   Gg

	D	d
D	DD	Dd
d	Dd	dd

	G	g
G	GG	Gg
g	Gg	gg

3/4 (D_) tall   3/4 (G_) yellow

1/4 (dd) dwarf   1/4 (gg) green

Then apply the rule of probability for independent events. The probability of independent events occuring together is the product of their individual probabilities.

The P of tall and yellow = 3/4 tall x 3/4 yellow = 9/16

The P of tall and green = 3/4 tall x 1/4 green = 3/16

The P of dwarf and yellow = 1/4 dwarf x 3/4 yellow = 3/16

The P of dwarf and green = 1/4 dwarf x 1/4 green = 1/16

These calculations are readily done by multiplying each P for height in the first column times each P for color in the second column.

● PROBLEM 3-16

In peas, tall (D) is dominant to dwarf (d) and yellow cotyledons (G) is dominant to green (g). If a tall, heterozygous pea plant with green cotyledons is crossed with a dwarf pea plant heterozygous for yellow cotyledons, what will be the phenotypic results in the progeny?

83

Solution:

Phenotypes of parents:	heterozygous tall, green	X	dwarf, heterozygous yellow	

Genotypes
of parents: Ddgg   ddGg

This problem can be solved by using the rule of probability for independent events. The probability of independent events occurring together is the product of their individual probabilities.

First, determine the results for each gene pair separately. Then put the results together using the rules of probability by multiplying each P for size times each P for color.

	D	d
d	Dd	dd
d	Dd	dd

	g	g
G	Gg	Gg
g	gg	gg

1/2 tall   1/2 yellow

1/2 dwarf   1/2 green

Phenotypic results:

1/2 tall x 1/2 yellow = 1/4 tall, yellow

1/2 tall x 1/2 green = 1/4 tall, green

1/2 dwarf x 1/2 yellow = 1/4 dwarf, yellow

1/2 dwarf x 1/2 green = 1/4 dwarf, green

● **PROBLEM 3-17**

In peas, tall (D) is dominant to dwarf (d) and yellow cotyledons (G) is dominant to green (g). A tall pea plant with yellow cotyledons was crossed with a tall pea plant with green cotyledons. These were the results in the progeny:

    6 tall, green
    5 tall, yellow
    2 dwarf, yellow

2 dwarf, green

What are the genotypes of the parents?

Solution: First, fill in as much of the genotype as possible from the phenotypic description of the parents. If a parent shows a dominant trait it must possess at least one dominant gene. If it shows a recessive trait, it must be homozygous recessive in the gene pair controlling that trait.

$$\text{Tall, yellow} \quad \text{X} \quad \text{Tall, green}$$
$$\text{D\_G\_} \qquad\qquad \text{D\_gg}$$

The rest of the genotype is determined by looking at the progeny. If recessive traits appear in the progeny, both parents must have contributed a recessive gene. Dwarf offspring occur, so both parents must have a d gene. Green offspring occur, so the first parent must be heterozygous Gg.

$$\text{DdGg} \quad \text{X} \quad \text{Ddgg}$$

● **PROBLEM 3-18**

Normal-length fur in rabbits is controlled by the dominant allele R, and a short type of fur, called "rex", is determined by the recessive allele r. The dominant allele B controls black fur color; the recessive allele b controls brown.

(a) Diagram a dihybrid cross between a homozygous rabbit with normal-length black fur and a rex rabbit with brown fur. What are the phenotypic ratios resulting from this cross?

(b) What proportion of the normal, black rabbits in the F_2 generation of this cross can be expected to be homozygous for both pairs of genes?

(c) What would be the expected phenotypic and genotypic results of a backcross between a member of the F_1 generation and a fully recessive rex, brown parent?

```
BBRR × bbrr        P

(BR)   (br)        gametes

BbRr               F₁

BbRr × BbRr        F₁ × F₁
```

Gametes	(BR)	(Br)	(bR)	(br)
(BR)	BBRR	BBRr	BbRR	BbRr
(Br)	BBRr	BBrr	BbRr	Bbrr
(bR)	BbRR	BbRr	bbRR	bbRr
(br)	BbRr	Bbrr	bbRr	bbrr

Summary of F_2 phenotypes: 9 black, long: 3 black, rex: 3 brown, long: 1 brown, rex.

<u>Solution</u>: (a) This is an example of a typical dihybrid cross. Assuming the genotype of the homozygous black rabbit with normal length fur is BBRR and that the genotype of the homozygous brown rex rabbit is bbrr, the results of the cross are shown in Figure 1. This 9:3:3:1 ratio is expected from all dihybrid crosses involving simple dominance.

(b) By scanning the above diagram, one counts 9 normal-furred black F_2 rabbits (either BB or Bb for fur color, and either RR or Rr for fur length, since normal-length fur and black color are dominant traits); of these, only one is homozygous for both traits - BBRR.

Total number of normal, black F_2 rabbits expected = 9

Number of these expected to be homozygous for both traits = 1

Ratio = 1/9

The proportion of normal, black rabbits that can be expected to be double homozygous is thus 1/9.

(c) Genotype of F_1 member - BbRr
Genotype of brown, rex parent - bbrr

The genotypic and phenotypic results of this back cross are:

86

BbRr × bbrr

Gametes	(BR)	(Br)	(bR)	(br)
(br)	BbRr	Bbrr	bbRr	bbrr

Summary of back cross results: 1 black, long:
1 black, rex: 1 brown, long: 1 brown rex.

● **PROBLEM** 3-19

Consider the following two traits in domestic rabbits, each controlled by a single pair of contrasting alleles exhibiting complete dominance:

hair color

black hair = B
(dominant)

white hair = b

hair texture

straight hair = K
(dominant)

kinky hair = k

Assume that each pair of genes is located in a different pair of chromosomes (i.e., independent gene pairs). For each of the crosses, below, predict what phenotypes will occur, and in what proportions they will occur, for progeny produced by each:

a) Bb Kk ♀ X   BB Kk ♂

b) Bb kk ♀ X   Bb Kk ♂

Solution: There are two approaches we can use in determining the answer to the problem. We will use one for cross (a) and the second to solve cross (b).

(a) Using the method of construction of the Punnett square, we first must determine the gametes produced by each parent. The female parent is heterozygous for both gene pairs and thus will produce one of four possible kinds of gametes in respect to gene content: BK, Bk, bK and bk. The male parent is heterozygous for only one gene pair and will produce one of two possible kinds of gametes, Bk and Bk. Now we can construct the Punnett square as follows:

♀ \ ♂	(BK)		(Bk)	
(BK)	$\underline{BB}$ $\underline{KK}$ black, straight		$\underline{BB}$ $\underline{Kk}$ black, straight	
(Bk)	$\underline{BB}$ $\underline{Kk}$ black, straight		$\underline{BB}$ $\underline{kk}$ black, kinky	
(bK)	$\underline{Bb}$ $\underline{KK}$ black, straight		$\underline{Bb}$ $\underline{Kk}$ black, straight	
(bK)	$\underline{Bb}$ $\underline{Kk}$ black, straight		$\underline{Bb}$ $\underline{kk}$ black, kinky	

Summarizing the phenotyes we see that we get 6 that are black and straight, and 2 that are black and kinky. We must reduce this phenotypic ratio to its lowest whole number, which will be 3 that are black and straight, and 1 that is black and kinky. This gives us a 3:1 ratio.

(b) For the second cross, we will use the expansion of the binomial, $(aX + bY)^n$, where X and Y represent the dominant and recessive phenotypes of a given trait, a and b represent the coefficients of each phenotype expected, respectively, based on the type of cross involved, and n represents the number of traits involved.

Thus, the expansion of the binomial for this can be represented as follows:

(3 black + 1 white)(1 straight + 1 kinky)
which will give an expected phenotypic ratio of 3 black and straight; 3 black and kinky; 1 white and straight; 1 white and kinky.

TRIHYBRID CROSS

● PROBLEM 3-20

In the common garden pea, <u>Pisum</u> <u>sativuum</u>, the alleles for tall plants, yellow seeds and round seeds -

D, G, and W, respectively - are all dominant over the alleles for dwarf plants, green seeds, and wrinkled seeds - d, g, and w.

(a) A homozygous tall, yellow round plant and a dwarf, green, wrinkled plant are mated. Show all possible gametes from each parent and the F_1 generation.

(b) Using the forked line method, show a cross between two F_1 plants.

(c) Show the results of a cross between an F_1 plant and a dwarf, green, wrinkled parent by using the forked line method again. Give results for the phenotypes, the genotypes, the genotypic frequency, and the phenotypic ratio.

Solution: Virtually no two cross-fertilizing plants have the exact same combination of alleles. These plants usually differ in more than one or two pairs of alleles, and mating in natural breeding populations usually involves new combinations of many genes. Crosses between parents that differ at three gene loci - trihybrid crosses - are a combination of three monohybrid crosses operating together:

    Tall - D; Dwarf - d
    Yellow seed - G; Green seed - g
    Round seed - w; Wrinkled seed - w

genotype of homozygous tall, yellow, round parent:

DDGGWW

genotype of dwarf, green, wrinkled parent:

ddggww

(a) A cross between a tall, yellow, round-seeded parent and a dwarf, green wrinkle-seeded parent is shown in Figure 1.

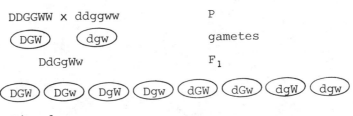

Fig. 1

(b) The forked-line method is used here to visualize the segregation of alleles. All combinations are obtained by starting with one trait. For instance, by starting with the trait Dd, a cross of these parents would be Dd x Dd. The result of this could be DD, Dd or dd. Looking at only the next trait, the cross is Gg x Gg. This results in the genotypes GG, Gg, and gg in a 1:2:1 ratio. As shown in the diagram, each of these is connected to the first allele by a line, hence the name forked-line method. Each of the succeeding traits work in a similar manner until all are completed. This can be done for any number of traits.

By following a line from one set of alleles out to the end, the entire genotype can be determined. For example, starting at DD follow the line to GG and then to WW. The genotype of this pea plant would be DDGGWW. By following a different line from GG, we could get the genotype DDGGww. All the possible genotype combinations can then be found.

DdGgWw x DdGgWw   F$_1$ gametes

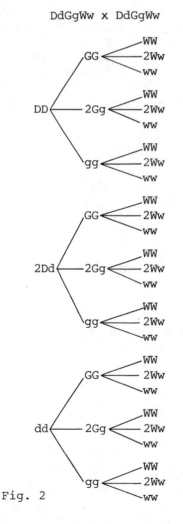

Summary of F$_2$ phenotypes:

27 tall, yellow, round
 9 tall, yellow, wrinkled
 9 tall, green, round
 9 dwarf, yellow, round
 3 tall, green, wrinkled
 3 dwarf, yellow, wrinkled
 3 dwarf, green, round
 1 dwarf, green, wrinkled

Fig. 2

(c)

DdGgWw x ddggww
Summary of backcross results:

Phenotypes		Genotypes	Genotypic frequency	Phenotypic ratio
Dd — **Gg** Ww	tall, yellow, round	DdGgWw	1	1
Gg ww	tall, yellow, wrinkled	DdGgww	1	1
gg Ww	tall, green, round	DdggWw	1	1
gg ww	tall, green, wrinkled	Ddggww	1	1
dd — Gg Ww	dwarf, yellow, round	ddGgWw	1	1
Gg ww	dwarf, yellow, wrinkled	ddGgww	1	1
gg Ww	dwarf, green, round	ddggWw	1	1
gg ww	dwarf, green, wrinkled	ddggww	1	1

Fig. 3

● **PROBLEM 3-21**

In peas, Tall (D) is dominant to dwarf (d), Yellow (G) is dominant to green (g), and Round (W) is dominant to wrinkled (w). What fraction of the offspring of this cross would be homozygous recessive in all gene pairs? GgDdww X GgddWw

Solution: This problem can be solved using the rule of probability for independent events. The probability of independent events occurring together is the product of their individual probabilities.

First determine the expected frequency of homozygous recessive offspring for each gene pair.

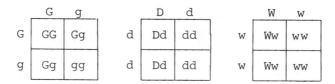

Then, multiply the expected homozygous recessive frequencies together to find the fraction of offspring with all the homozygous recessive gene pairs.

$$1/4 \text{ gg} \quad X \quad 1/2 \text{ dd} \quad X \quad 1/2 \text{ ww} = 1/16 \text{ ggddww}$$

MULTIGENE CROSS

● **PROBLEM 3-22**

There are two highly inbred strains of laboratory mice whose adult body weights are very different. Assume that the mouse's body weight is under the control of three pairs of contrasting genes: A vs. a, B vs. b and D vs. d. Assume further that each capital letter gene is responsible for contributing 5.0 grams to the total body weight, and that lower case letters contribute 2.5 grams to total body weight. The average weight of mice in Strain I is 30 grams, while that of Strain II mice is 15 grams.

a) What are the most likely genotypes of these two strains?

b) Suppose Strain I and Strain II are crossed. What will be the phenotype of the F_1 progeny?

Solution: a) Since there are three pairs of genes that control body weight, there will be a total of six genes present. Because the strains are highly inbred, we can assume them to be homozygous. Strain I exhibits a total weight of 30 grams. Since each capital letter gene contributes 5.0 grams, there must be six capital letter genes present. Thus, the genotype of Strain I will be <u>AA BB DD</u>. Strain II weights 15 grams and since each lower case letter gene contributes 2.5 grams to the body weight, the genotype for this strain will be <u>aa bb dd</u>.

b) Crossing Strains I and II will give an F_1 with a genotype of <u>Aa Bb Dd</u>. Thus, with three capital letter genes, each contributing 5.0g, and three lower case letter genes, each contributing 2.5g, the phenotype of the F_1 will be 22.5g.

● **PROBLEM** 3-23

What are the possible gametes that can be formed from the following genotypes, assuming all the gene pairs segregate independently? What are the gamete frequencies?

(a) AaBBCc
(b) DdEEffGg
(c) MmNnOo

Solution: Mendel recognized quite early that the segregation of one pair of alleles is independent of the segregation of other pairs of alleles. Using the Law of Independent Assortment discussed in previous problems, let us consider an example: Let AaBb be a diploid double hybrid parent. Aa and Bb are separate pairs of alleles that will segregate to separate gametes independently of each other. Each gamete will get one allele for each trait, making it haploid. Four combinations are possible, see Figure 1.

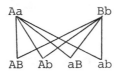

Fig. 1

These gametes occur in the following frequencies:

1/4 AB : 1/4 Ab : 1/4 aB : 1/4 ab

The gamete frequencies of all the genotypes given in the problem can be obtained similarly.

(a) The parental genotype is AaBBCc. If only the A and B loci are examined, AB and aB are possible in equal frequencies. One half the gametes will contain AB and one half will contain aB. Since the third locus also contains two different alleles, C and c, they will segregate so that 1/2 the gametes will have C and the other 1/2 c. There is a 50% change that any one gamete will contain C, and a 50% chance that it will contain c. Both types of gametes can combine with either AB or aB. The gamete frequencies for all three loci can be calculated by multiplying the chances of each individual frequency:

$$1/2 \text{ AB} \times 1/2 \text{ C} \rightarrow 1/4 \text{ ABC}$$

$$1/2 \text{ AB} \times 1/2 \text{ c} \rightarrow 1/4 \text{ ABc}$$

$$1/2 \text{ aB} \times 1/2 \text{ C} \rightarrow 1/4 \text{ aBC}$$

$$1/2 \text{ aB} \times 1/2 \text{ c} \rightarrow 1/4 \text{ aBc}$$

Each of the gamete types occurs 1/4 of the time, so there is a 25% chance of one gamete containing one of the four combinations of alleles.

(b) Since the parent contains homozygous genotypes of both EE and ff, the Dd trait is the only one that varies in segregation. There is a 50% chance of D segregating with Ef and a 50% chance of d segregating with Ef. But E has to segregate with f in both instances since both traits are homozygous. With this information, the following results are obtained:

Parent - DdEEffGg

$$1/2 \text{ DEf} \left\langle \begin{array}{l} 1/2 \text{ G} \rightarrow 1/4 \text{ DEfG} \\ 1/2 \text{ g} \rightarrow 1/4 \text{ DEfg} \end{array} \right.$$

$$1/2 \text{ dEf} \left\langle \begin{array}{l} 1/2 \text{ G} \rightarrow 1/4 \text{ dEfG} \\ 1/2 \text{ g} \rightarrow 1/4 \text{ dEfg} \end{array} \right.$$

The various gametes and frequencies would be:

$$1/4 \text{ DEfG} : 1/4 \text{ DEfg} : 1/4 \text{ dEfG} : 1/4 \text{ dEfg}$$

(c) This problem is slightly different since all three traits have heterozygous genotypes. Because of this there are more possible allele combinations. By drawing a diagram similar to that used in previous parts of this problem,

94

but incorporating the third varying trait into it, we obtain the following:

Parent - MnNnOo

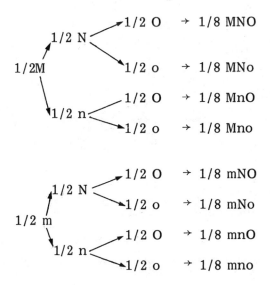

1/2 N
1/2 O → 1/8 MNO
1/2 o → 1/8 MNo

1/2M

1/2 n
1/2 O → 1/8 MnO
1/2 o → 1/8 Mno

1/2 N
1/2 O → 1/8 mNO
1/2 o → 1/8 mNo

1/2 m

1/2 n
1/2 O → 1/8 mnO
1/2 o → 1/8 mno

the following frequencies occur:

1/8 MNO; 1/8 MNo; 1/8 MnO; 1/8 Mno; 1/8 MNO; 1/8 mNo; 1/8 mnO; 1/8 mno.

● **PROBLEM 3-24**

Given the following genotype for an individual organism that has six pairs of independent genes:

<u>Aa</u>   Bb   <u>DD</u>   ee   <u>Ff</u>   <u>Gg</u>

a) How many different gametes, with respect to gene content, can this individual produce?

b) List all of the possible gametes that can be produced.

Solution: a) The number of different kinds of gametes that can be produced is dependent upon the number of loci for which the individual is heterozygous. There will be 2^n gametes produced, where n = the number of loci that are heterozygous. This individual is heterozygous for four (4) loci; thus, there will be 2^4 or 16, different gametes that can possibly be produced.

b)

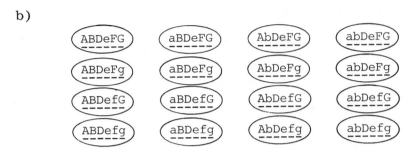

Assume there is an organism in which there are five (5) contrasting independent gene pairs, A vs. a, B vs. b, D vs. d, E vs. e and F vs. f, for which the organism is heterozygous. If the organism were able to undergo self-fertilization,

a) what is the probability that the first progeny will have a genotype identical to that of the parent?

b) what proportion of the total progeny will be homozygous?

c) assuming complete dominance for each gene pair, what proportion of the total progeny will phenotypically exhibit the dominant form for the five characters?

Solution: a) In a cross between two individuals that are heterozygous for a single pair of genes (eg. Aa X Aa), the probability of a progeny being heterozygous is 1/2. Since each of the gene pairs in question are independent, then the probability of the first progeny being identical to that of its parent(s), (i.e., Aa Bb Dd Ee Ff), is:

$P=(1/2)^5 =1/32$.

b) For a single pair of genes, a cross between two heterozygotes will yield 1/2 of the progeny that are homozygous, either $\underline{AA}$ or $\underline{aa}$. Thus, for five independent pairs, the proportion of the total progeny that are homozygous will be $(1/2)^5 = 1/32$.

c) A cross between two heterozygotes for a single gene pair with complete dominance will yield 3/4 of the progeny exhibiting the dominant phenotype. Thus, the proportion of the total progeny exhibiting the dominant form for all five characters will be $(3/4)^5 = 243/1,024$.

SHORT ANSWER QUESTIONS FOR REVIEW

Choose the correct answer.

1. Two mice with long tails were mated. The
    offspring consisted of 32 mice with long tails
    and 9 mice with short tails. We can determine
    that _____ is the dominant trait, and given
    that L represents long tail and 1 represents
    short tails the genotype of each parent was
    _____. (a) short tails, LL (b) long tails,
    LL (c) short tails, L1 (d) long tails, L1   d

2. A cross between a homozygous dominant tall
    pea plant and a homozygous recessive dwarf
    pea plant would yield (a) 4DD. (b) 1DD,
    2Dd, 1dd. (c) 4Dd. (d) 3Dd, 1DD.   c

3. A phenotypic ratio of 9:3:3:1 can be expected
    when crossing (a) any parental strains.(b)
    F_1 x F_1 heterozygotes with two pairs of
    factors being determined. (c) F_2 x F_1
    heterozygotes with two pairs of factors being
    determined. (d) P x F_2 with three pairs of
    factors being determined.   b

4. In lima beans, green color is dominant over
    yellow color. A cross between a pure green
    bean and a pure yellow bean yields 40 hybrid
    beans. A cross between two of these hybrid
    beans yielded 80 F_2 beans. How many of these
    F_2 beans should be green? (a) 40 (b) 50
    (c) 60 (d) 80   c

5. A cross between a homozygous tall pea plant
    (DD) and a heterozygous tall pea plant (Dd)
    should yield (a) one homozygous tall, two
    heterozygous tall, one homozygous dwarf. (b)
    two homozygous tall, two heterozygous tall.(c)
    one homozygous tall, three heterozygous tall.
    (d) four heterozygous tall.   b

6. In horses, a trotting gait is dominant over a
    pacing gait. A stallion that was a heterozygous
    trotter was mated repeatedly with a mare over
    a number of years. The offspring produced
    were all trotters. What was the genotype of
    the mare? (a) heterozygous trotter (b)
    homozygous pacer (c) heterzygous pacer
    (d) homozygous trotter   d

98

SHORT ANSWER QUESTIONS FOR REVIEW

7. Tongue rolling in humans is a dominant trait, while the inability to roll the tongue is recessive. Out of 60 people, 15 cannot roll their tongues. How many of these people are homozygous dominant for tongue rolling? (a) 15 (b) 30 (c) 45 (d) 60

b

8. In garden peas, yellow seed color is dominant over green seed color. A total of 4092 off-spring resulted from a cross between a hetero-zygous yellow and a homozygous green. How many of these seeds are homozygous green? (a) 4092 (b) 3069 (c) 2046 (d) 1023

c

9. A homozygous tall pea plant was crossed with a homozygous dwarf pea plant. What would be the predicted genotypic ratio for the F_2 generation? (a) 1 heterozygous tall : 2 homozygous tall : 1 homozygous dwarf (b) 4 heterozygous tall (c) 3 homozygous tall : 1 homozygous dwarf (d) 1 homozygous tall : 2 heterozygous tall : 1 homozygous dwarf

d

10. As mentioned before, tongue rolling is dominant in humans. If a man can roll his tongue but his wife cannot, what is the largest percentage of their children that would be able to roll their tongues? (a) 50% (b) 66% (c) 75% (d) 100%

a

11. In rabbits, a special type of short fur, called "rex", is determined by a recessive allele, while long hair is its dominant trait. Brown fur color is recessive and black fur color is dominant. Multiple crosses between a hetero-zygous black rex rabbit and a brown rabbit heterozygous for long hair yield 28 offspring. Approximately how many would be expected to be brown with long hair? (a) 0 (b) 7 (c) 14 (d) 28

b

12. A 9:3:3:1 genotypic ratio usually yields a _____ phenotypic ratio. (a) two dominant : two recessive (b) one dominant : one recessive (c) one homozygous dominant : two heterozygous dominant : one homozygous recessive (d) three dominant : one recessive

d

SHORT ANSWER QUESTIONS FOR REVIEW

13. In order to determine whether an organism is homozygous or heterozygous for a trait, it must be crossed with a _____ and the results checked. (a) homozygous recessive (b) homozygous dominant (c) heterozygous recessive (d) heterozygous dominant

a

14. An organism has these 10 pairs of independent genes: Aa BB cc Dd Ee Ff Gg HH ii Jj How many gametes, with respect to gene content, can this individual produce? (a) 16 (b) 32 (c) 64 (d) 128

c

Fill in the blanks.

15. Mendel's first law, The _____, stated that there were paired heredity factors which separate, and only one from each pair was transmitted to the _____ from each parent.

Law of
Segregation
gamete

16. In the flour beetle, Tribolium castaneum, red body color (E) is dominant over ebony color (e). A cross between an ebony male and a red female yielded 16 offspring - nine red and seven ebony. The predicted genotype of the male parent is _____, and that of the female is _____.

ee,
Ee

17. A checkered pattern on pigeons is dominant over a plain color and red feather color is dominant over brown. A cross between a heterozygous red checked pigeon and a homozygous plain brown pigeon yields 16 offspring. The predicted number of heterozygous red checked pigeons out of these offspring is _____.

4

18. A man and woman who can both roll their tongues have two sons. Is it possible for for both sons to be unable to roll their tongues?

No

Questions 19 through 22 deal with the following Purnett Square.

SHORT ANSWER QUESTIONS FOR REVIEW

	AB	Ab	AB	Ab	Female
AB	AABB	AABb	AABB	AABb	
Ab	AABb	1	AABb	AAbb	
Male					
aB	AaBB	AaBb	2	AaBb	
ab	AaBb	Aabb	AaBb	Aabb	

KEY: A and B are Dominant
a and b are recessive

19. The genotype of the male parent is _____

AaBb

20. The genotype of the organism in box 1 is
_____.

AAbb

21. The organism in box 2 is _____ for
trait "A".

heterozygous

22. This organism exhibits _____ genetic traits.
(number)

2

In questions 23 through 26 match each word to
the term that best defines it.

23. Genes   (a) outwardly visible
characteristics of an

d

24. Phenotype   organism

a

25. Chromosomes   (b) different alleles for
specific traits on
homologous chromosomes

c

26. Heterozygote   (c) contain hereditary units
(d) once called the
inheritance "factors" by
Mendel

b

27. Mendel theorized that gametes were combined
according to _____.

chance

28. _____ are to genotype as characteristics
are to phenotype.

Genes

29. In the following cross there are _____
different gametes that can be made:

SHORT ANSWER QUESTIONS FOR REVIEW

AABB x AaBb   4

30. A cross between a homozygous dominant male and a heterozygous dominant female would have _____% homozygous recessive   0

Determine whether the following statements are true or false

31 Mendel crossed different types of pea plants to blend their characteristics.   False

32. Homozygotes have identical alleles for a given trait on homologous chromosomes.   True

33. An organism having the genotype Gg contains one gamete.   False

34. All organisms with identical phenotypes will have identical genotypes.   False

35. The phenotype is dependent upon the geno-genotype.   True

36. A test cross is positive if a heterozygous recessive trait is present in the offspring.   False

37. Phenotype determines whether an organism is heterozygous or homozygous.   False

38. Any organism displaying a recessive trait must be homozygous for that trait.   True

39. Mendel's Law of Independent Assortment prevents genetic variance.   False

40. Crossing two heterozygotes represented genotypically as Qq yields 50% of the offspring being phenotypically dominant.   False

41 A cross between a homozygous dominant tall pea plant and a heterozygous tall pea plant yields 100% tall pea plants.   True

42. The inability for a human to roll his tongue represents a complete absence of the dominant gene (assuming tongue rolling is the dominant trait).   True

CHAPTER 4

SEX DETERMINATION AND SEX LINKAGE

SEX DETERMINATION

Explain the mechanism of the genetic determination of sex in man.

Solution: The sex chromosomes are an exception to the general rule that the members of a pair of chromosomes are identical in size and shape and carry allelic pairs. The sex chromosomes are not homologous chromosomes. In man, the cells of females contain two identical sex chromosomes, or X chromosomes. In males there is only one X chromosome and a smaller Y chromosome with which the X pairs during meiotic synapsis. Men have 22 pairs of ordinary chromosomes (autosomes), plus one X and one Y chromosome, and women have 22 pairs of autosomes plus two X chromosomes.

Thus, it is the presence of the Y chromosome which determines that an individual will be male. Although the mechanism is quite complex, we know that the presence of the Y chromosome stimulates the gonadal medulla, or sex organ, forming a portion of the egg to develop into male gonads, or sex organs. In the absence of the Y chromosome, and in the presence of two X chromosomes, the medulla develops into female gametes. [Note: a full complement of two X chromosomes is needed for normal female development.]

In man, since the male has one X and one Y

chromosome, two types of sperm, or male gametes, are produced during spermatogenesis (the process of sperm formation, which includes meiosis). One half of the sperm population contains an X chromosome and the other half contains a Y chromosome. Each egg, or female gamete, contains a single X chromosome. This is because a female has only X chromosomes, and meiosis produces only gametes with X chromosomes. Fertilization of the X-bearing egg by an X-bearing sperm results in an XX, or female offspring. The fertilization of an X-bearing egg by a Y-bearing sperm results in an XY, or male offspring. Since there are approximately equal numbers of X- and Y-bearing sperm, the numbers of boys and girls born in a population are nearly equal.

● **PROBLEM** 4-2

Sex can be determined by staining for Barr bodies of cells. Explain what a Barr body is. How reliable is the method?

Interphase nuclei from a buccal smear

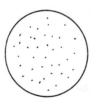

Male cell

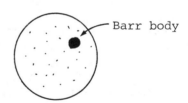

Barr body

Female cell

Solution: In the 1940s Barr and Bertram discovered the presence of a dark-staining body in the cells of female cats, but no such body could be observed in male cat cells. It was later suggested that this body, now called a Barr body, was formed during mammalian development as a result of inactivation of one of the female's X chromosomes. The body is found in the nucleus of all female tissues, characteristically situated close to the nuclear membrane, as in the figure.

The inactivation of the X chromosome results in what is called dosage compensation. The female cells are compensating for genes that are present in two doses;

only one dose is needed, as exists in the male. The process of inactivation is random. Some cells of one individual will have one X chromosome inactivated, while other cells will have the other X chromosome inactivated.

Because of the various sex chromosome anomalies that exist, the presence of Barr bodies is not completely reliable. The process works in a way such that all but one of the X chromosomes present are inactivated. When an individual, male or female, does not have the normal number of sex chromosomes, the result of Barr body staining may not reflect the person's phenotypic sex. For example, individuals with Turner's syndrome, who have only one X chromosome and no Y chromosomes, are phenotypically female. However, they have no Barr bodies. Individuals with Klinefelter's syndrome are phenotypically male, but have Barr bodies in their cells because they have two X chromosomes along with a Y. In cases such as these, one cannot rely on the presence of Barr bodies to classify males and females.

The following table shows that the number of Barr bodies detected is not always an accurate indicator of sex.

● **PROBLEM** 4-3

Chromosomal sex in mammals has been shown to be strongly Y chromosome determined. How was this shown to be true?

Individual designation	Sex chromosome constitution	Sex
Normal male	XY	Male
Normal female	XX	Female
Turner female	X	Female
Triplo-X female	XXX	Female
Tetra-X female	XXXX	Female
Penta-X female	XXXXX	Female
Klinefelter males	XXY	Male
	XXXY	Male
	XXXXY	Male
	XXYY	Male
	XXXYY	Male
XYY male	XYY	Male

Fig. 1: Sex chromosome anomalies and sex determination in humans

Solution: From various cytogenetic and chromosomal studies it was found that the presence of a Y chromosome usually determines maleness in mammals. Evidence for this can be seen in the table below. Organisms with an XO set of sex chromosomes were shown to be male in Drosophila, but female in mammals. In addition, mammals with an XXY set of chromosomes were shown to be male. The theory was consistently supported by the discovery that males always had at least one Y chromosome while females had at least one X but no Y chromosome.

● PROBLEM 4-4

How do chromosomal variations influence sex determination in humans?

Solution: Chromosomal variations in humans result in intermediate sex individuals. Most of the variants are associated with chromosomal abnormalities involving either an excess or a deficiency of sex chromosomes. With modern techniques it is possible to observe and count human chromosomes accurately. Numbers above and below the usual 46 can be detected. One in every 200 newborns has been shown to have a numerical chromosome irregularity.

The most common sex chromosome anomalies are Turner's syndrome and Klinefelter's syndrome. Turner's syndrome occurs in one out of every 2,000 births. These individuals have 45 chromosomes, and are monosomic for the X chromosome; they are XO. They are short in stature and usually have webbed necks. They are sexually infantile, and often have primary amenorrhea in addition to a failure to develop signs of puberty. Plasma concentrations of follicle stimulating hormone (FSH) and luteinizing hormone (LH) are elevated. The patients lack ovaries, accounting for the failure to develop sexually. Since they have only one X chromosome, buccal smears show no Barr bodies. Therefore, they cannot be distinguished from the cell preparation of a male.

A person with Klinefelter's syndrome has an XXY karyotype and shows male characteristics even though his cells contain Barr bodies. It is sometimes difficult to distinguish these individuals from normal males, although they usually have small testes and are below normal in intelligence. Pubic hair and fat distribution may also follow a female pattern. They are usually sterile.

Other chromosomal variations influencing sex determination have been reported. Males with XXXY, XXYY, and XXXXXY chromosomes are known to exist, as are females with XXX, XXXX, and XXXXX chromosomes. The presence of a Y chromosome is usually linked with "maleness"; the absence of it will lead to an individual with female characteristics.

● **PROBLEM** 4-5

Chromosomes in which one arm has been deleted and replaced by a piece identical to the remaining arm are called isochromosomes.

(a) Explain how this might occur.

(b) What are the consequences of carrying one normal X chromosome and either the long-arm isochromosome of X($X^L.X^L$) or the short-arm isochromosome of X ($X^S.X^S$)?

(c) What are the consequences of carrying one normal X and the isochromosome $Y^L.Y^L$ or $Y^S.Y^S$?

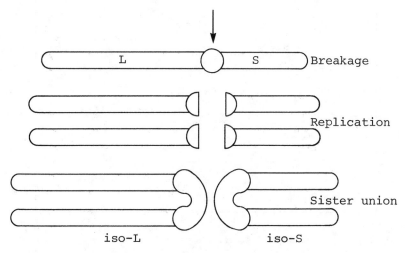

Fig. 1.   Formation of isochromosomes following centromeric breakage and chromosome replication

Solution: (a) Chromosomes can undergo any one of several types of breakage rearrangement. If breakage occurs near or within the centromere, and sister ends fuse after replication, isochromosomes (chromosomes made up of identical lengthwise halves) are made. This process is shown in Figure 1.

(b) Persons who carry either $X^L.X^L$ or $X^S.X^S$ isochromosomes (Fig. 2) along with a normal X chromosome are sterile females. X^LX^L individuals appear to have typical Turner's syndrome, while X^SX^S women do not have the nonsexual features of Turner's syndrome, such as the neck webbing and short stature. Because of this, the nonsexual features of Turner's syndrome have been attributed to the loss of genetic material in X^S.

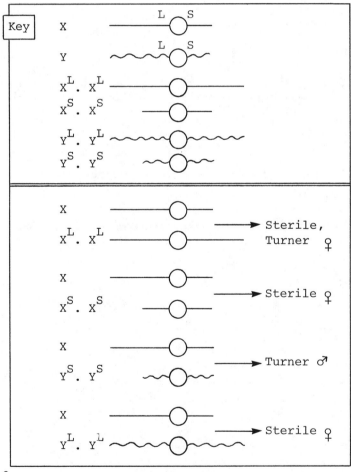

Fig. 2

(c) Phenotypic females result when the $Y^L.Y^L$ isochromosome is accompanied by a normal X. Because no nonsexual features of Turner's syndrome are present, it is thought that the genes for male sex determination are mainly in the short-arm of the Y chromosome. Individuals having $XY^S.Y^S$ are phenotypic males with many of the nonsexual features found in Turner's syndrome. This is possibly because Y^L and X^S may have homologous regions.

● **PROBLEM** 4-6

Even though sex determination does not appear to be controlled by the chromosomal method in some dioecious organisms, it is still gene determined. Explain.

Solution: The chromosomal method of sex determination implies that the presence or absence of a particular "accessory" chromosome determines what type of gametes an organism will produce. Most dioecious organisms, such as those that produce only a single kind of gamete, reproduce in this way. For those organisms in which sex is not determined by the chromosomal method, some form of genetic control is still instrumental.

The following examples will illustrate some variations of chromosomal method. The asparagus plant is normally dioecious, with some plants producing only staminate flowers and others only pistillate. In the asparagus plant maleness (staminate flowers) is controlled by a dominant gene and femaleness (pistillate flowers) is controlled by its recessive allele. Sometimes, pistillate flowers are found with non-functional stamens, and some staminate flowers may be found to have immature pistils, but sex determination seems to come from this single gene.

In the case of honeybees the process of sex differentiation seems to be dependent on outside factors. Male bees, known as drones, develop from unfertilized eggs and thus are haploid, possessing only 16 chromosomes. Female workers and queen bees both develop from fertilized eggs and are diploid, possessing 32 chromosomes. The queen bee determines which eggs will be fertilized and which will not, and so she determines the number of males. The type and amount of food given to the fertilized eggs determines which will becomes fertile females (queen bees), and which will become sterile female workers.

L. Powers has found that three pairs of genes control the breeding behavior of the guayule plant, Partheniun argentatum. The recessive gene a, when homozygous, leads to the formation of unreduced eggs; gene b, when homozygous, prevents fertilization; and unfertilized eggs will undergo embryogenesis when gene c is present in the homozygous form. Because of this, guayule plants of the genotypes aaBBCC or aaBBcc will reproduce sexually and produce polyploid offspring, while those of genotypes AABBCC or AABBcc will form diploids through sexual reproduction. AAbbcc and aabbCC plants are sterile, and aabbcc ones are apomictic. If 2 plants with the genotype AaBbCc are crossed, what phenotype ratios can be expected?

Solution: This problem deals with three segregating gene pairs - a trihybrid cross. The genotype and phenotype ratios from this cross will follow Mendelian principles. One approaches this problem like any other trihybrid cross. Using the forked-lines method, the cross would look like this:

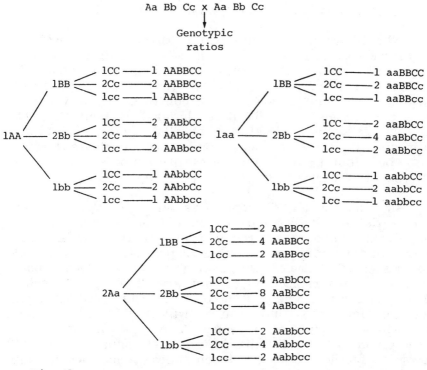

Fig. 1.

The phenotypic ratios can be summarized as follows:

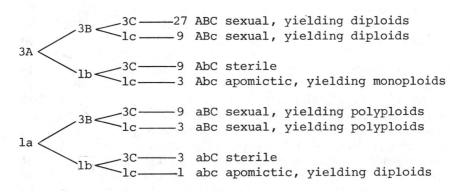

Phenotypic
ratios

3A

  3B
    3C——27 ABC sexual, yielding diploids
    1c—— 9 ABc sexual, yielding diploids

  1b
    3C—— 9 AbC sterile
    1c—— 3 Abc apomictic, yielding monoploids

1a

  3B
    3C—— 9 aBC sexual, yielding polyploids
    1c—— 3 aBc sexual, yielding polyploids

  1b
    3C—— 3 abC sterile
    1c—— 1 abc apomictic, yielding diploids

Total ratios:

36 sexual, yielding diploids
12 sterile
12 sexual, yielding polyploids
3 apomictic, yielding monoploids
1 apomictic, yielding diploids

● **PROBLEM 4-8**

How is sex determination in the parasitic wasp
Habrobracon junglandis different from the method
characteristic of the insect order Hymenopteca?

P: S^1S^2♀ x S^3♂

F_1: S^1S^3♀ S^2S^3♀ S^1♂ S^2♂

Mate F_1 x F_1; for example:

S^1S^3♀ x S^1♂

F_2: S^1S^3♀   (S^1S^1♂) S^1♂ S^3♂

A diploid ♂ homozygous for one of the sex alleles
Fig. 1.

111

Solution: This wasp is know to produce males by homozygosity as well as parthenogenesis. Parthenogenesis is the development of organisms from unfertilized eggs. In the Hymenoptera insect order, these haploid organisms result in male insects. Usually this is the only way for males to develop, but in the parasitic wasp diploid males are also produced by homozygosity at a single gene locus. The diagram shows a cross which results in one of these males.

At least nine sex alleles are known to exist at this gene locus, and the alleles may be represented as $s^1, s^2, s^3, \ldots, s^9$. Haploid males carry only one of the alleles at this locus. Diploid females are heterozygous at the locus; examples are the alleles $s^1 s^2$, $s^1 s^4$, or $s^3 s^4$. Any insect that is homozygous for an allele, $s^1 s^1$ or $s^8 s^8$, for example, will develop into a diploid male. Thus, if any allele at this locus, whether present in single or double condition, has no complement with which to interact, it will produce a male insect.

SEX LINKED TRAITS

Some sex-linked traits are expressed more often in girls than in boys, while others are expressed more often in boys than in girls. How is this possible?

Solution: The X chromosome carries not only the genes for sex, but also many other genes not related to sex, such as the gene for color blindness and the gene for hemophilia. Such genes are called sex-linked, because they are located on the sex chromosome. The Y chromosome does not carry any genes that we know of other than those which are related to the expression of the male sex.

Girls have two X chromosomes. Boys have one X chromosome and one Y chromosome. Each individual inherits one sex chromosome from each parent; thus, a girl gets one X chromosome from her mother and one X chromosome from her father. A boy receives an X chromosome from his mother and a Y chromosome from his father. (His mother cannot give him a Y chromosome since she only has X chromosomes to give.)

Since the genes for sex-linked traits are carried only in the X chromosome, it follows that a girl would have twice the chance of receiving a sex-linked gene than would a boy, because she receives two X chromosomes, while a boy receives only one. Thus, a girl has a chance to receive a sex-linked gene if either of her parents carry that gene. A boy, however, could only receive such a gene from his mother, even if his father carried that gene on his X chromosome.

Although a girl has a greater chance than a boy of receiving a sex-linked gene, the chance that either of them will express the trait coded for by that gene varies according to the dominant, or recessive, nature of the gene.

For example, if the gene for sex-linked trait is dominant, that trait would be more commonly expressed in girls than in boys. Because it is dominant, only one copy of the gene is necessary for its expression. Since girls have a greater chance of receiving a copy of a sex-linked gene, they have a greater chance of expressing its trait.

If a sex-linked trait is recessive, a boy would have a greater chance of expressing the trait. In order for a girl to express that trait, she would have to have two copies of the recessive gene, because its expression would be masked by the presence of a normal X chromosome or one with a dominant allele. Thus, both her parents would have to carry the gene. A boy, however, need only have one copy of the gene in order to express its trait, because his Y chromosome does not carry any genes that would mask the recessive gene. So only his mother need carry the gene. The chances of this happening are much greater than the chance that two people carrying the gene will mate and have a girl, so the trait is more commonly expressed in boys.

It is important to note that girls still have a greater chance of receiving a single copy of a recessive gene, although they may not express it. Such individuals are called carriers, and their frequency in the population is greater than that of individuals expressing the trait, be they male or female.

● **PROBLEM** 4-10

Vitamin D-resistant rickets is produced by an X-linked dominant allele. Two recessive alleles together will lead to normal bone development. What

113

are the expected results from the following crosses?

(a) A normal woman and a man with Vitamin D-resistant rickets.

(b) A normal man and a woman with the condition who has a normal father.

Solution: The common form of rickets usually occurs in infants or children because of low levels of Vitamin D. Vitamin D-resistant rickets, caused by a mutant X-linked dominant allele, is resistant to normal treatment. Exceptionally large amounts of calcium and Vitamin D must be given to treat it.

Mutant X-linked traits which are dominant are seen in both males and females whenever they carry the mutant allele. Affected females will transmit the allele to 1/2 of all their offspring while affected males can only give the alleles to their daughters.

(a) Letting "R" represent the mutant allele and "r" the recessive normal allele, the following would result:

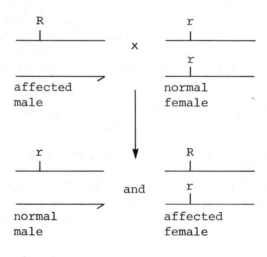

Fig. 1.

In this type of problem, _____ represents a Y chromosome. __R__ stands for X chromosome with the rickets disorder and ___r___ stands for an X chromosome with a normal allele. All of the males from this cross would be normal, and all of the females would have the disorder.

(b) Similarly, the solution for question (b) is:

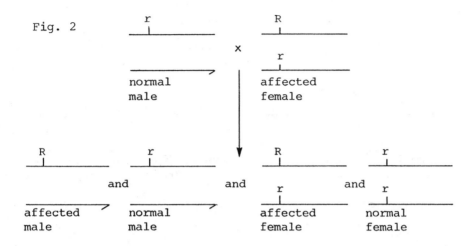

Fig. 2

Fifty percent of the males and fifty percent of the females will be affected.

• **PROBLEM** 4-11

A sex-linked recessive allele "d" determines the presence of pseudohypertrophic (Duchenne) muscular dystrophy in humans. A person requires the allele "D" for muscles to be normal. What would be the result of the following crosses?

(a) A man with the dystrophy and a woman heterozygous for it.

(b) A man with normal muscles and a woman with the disorder.

(c) A woman homozygous for the "D" allele and a man with the dystrophy.

Solution: This problem can be solved in the same way as the preceding one.

(a)
Half of the sons will have the dystrophy and half will have normal muscles. Half of the daughters will be carriers and half will have the dystrophy.

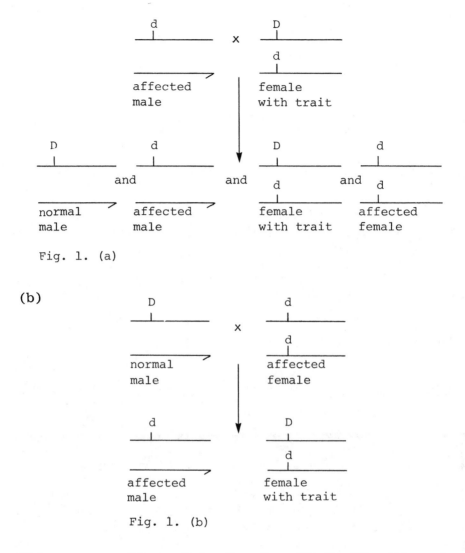

Fig. 1. (a)

(b)

Fig. 1. (b)

This cross would result in all males with the disorder and carrier females.

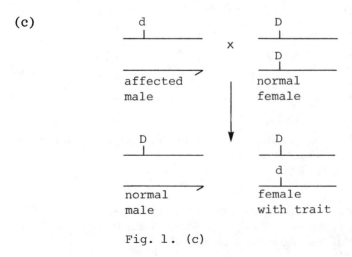

Fig. 1. (c)

All the males from this cross would be normal. All the females will be carriers with normal muscles.

Explain the mode of inheritance for color blindness.

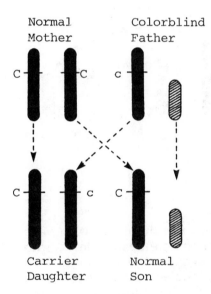

Fig. 1.

Normal woman × color-blind man

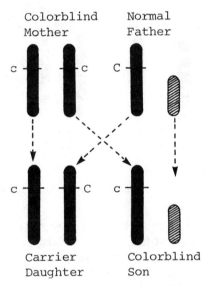

Fig. 2.

Colorblind woman × normal man

Solution: Color blindness is one of the most common genetic disorders that occurs in the human race. About 8% of males in the U.S. are red-green color defective. The trait for color blindness is caused by a recessive gene located on the X chromosome. Since the Y chromosome does not contain an allele for this gene, men are hemizygous for either the normal allele or the color-defective one. Because of this, the usual "dominant" and "recessive" terms do not apply in males. Whichever allele is present is expressed. The terms can be used in females since they have 2 X chromosomes. Because it is a recessive gene, a woman heterozygous for the trait will be phenotypically normal.

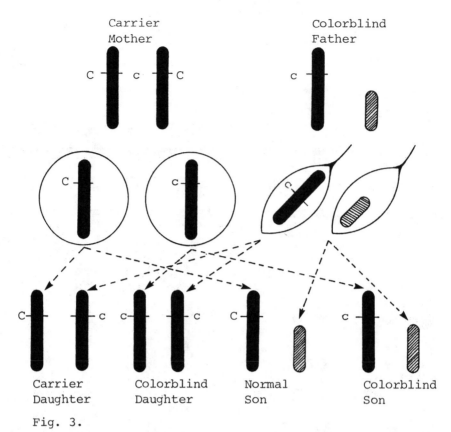

Fig. 3.

Carrier woman x colorblind man

Females heterozygous for color blindness will pass the mutant gene on to 1/2 of their children. Males who get this allele will be color blind because, possessing only 1 X chromosome, this is the only allele they have. Female children with the mutant allele will be heterozygous like their mother as long as the father has normal vision. Females homozygous for the trait are rare, since both parents would have to possess the defective allele.

The daughters of normal females and color blind males will all be carriers with normal vision. They will all inherit the defective X gene from their father and a normal X gene from their mother. Because males do not inherit X chromosomes from their fathers, all sons of color blind males and normal females will have normal vision. The transmission of color blindness is illustrated in figures 1, 2, and 3.

● **PROBLEM 4-13**

Hemophilia, a genetic blood disorder, is caused by a

recessive sex-linked gene. A phenotypically normal couple had a son with hemophilia. What is the probability that their next child, if a girl, would also have hemophilia?

Solution: The following cross is occuring:

	X^C	Y
X^C	$X^C X^C$	$X^C Y$
X^c	$X^C X^c$	$X^c Y$

There is no chance that a daughter will have hemophilia.

A daughter would have to be homozygous $X^c X^c$ to have hemophilia. A phenotypically normal father could not pass a gene for hemophilia to any children.

● **PROBLEM 4-14**

A girl is a hemophiliac.

a) What are the possible genotypes and phenotypes of her parents?

b) Assuming that her mother is normal, what were this girl's chances of being born with the disease?

c) Several cases of hemophilia in girls have been reported within a small region in England where there is often close intermarriage. Explain this high frequency of hemophilia in girls.

Solution: a) Hemophilia is a sex-linked trait carried on the X chromosome. It is also a recessive trait and will not be expressed in the presence of a normal X chromosome. It will be expressed, however, in the presence of a normal Y chromosome, because that chromosome does not carry any genes that would mask its expression. In order for a boy to be a hemophiliac, he need only have a mother who carries the gene, since this is who he gets his X chromosome from. Because he only gets a Y chromosome from his father, he will not inherit any alleles from his father's X chromosome. A girl, however, would have to have both parents carry the gene, since she receives one X chromosome from each parent.

Let ^+X represent the chromosome carrying the gene for hemophilia, and X and Y represent the normal sex chromosomes. The father of a hemophiliac girl, in order to be able to give his daughter the gene for hemophilia, must be ^+X Y, and therefore a hemophiliac himself. The mother could be either $^+X^+X$, (a hemophiliac), or ^+XX, (a carrier), in order to pass the hemophilia gene to her daughter.

b) If the mother is normal, her genotype must be ^+XX. Let us look at the cross that produced the hemophiliac girl.

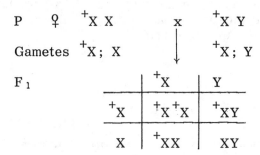

P   ♀ ^+X X   x ^+X Y

Gametes ^+X; X ^+X; Y

F_1

	^+X	Y
^+X	$^+X^+X$	^+XY
X	^+XX	XY

The offspring will be as follows:

1/2 normal
      1/4 female carrier (X^+X)
      1/4 normal male ($^+X^+X$)

1/2 hemo-
  philiac
      1/4 hemophiliac male (^+X Y)
      1/4 hemophiliac female ($^+X^+X$)

Since half the possible offspring are hemophiliac, the girl had a 50% chance of being born with the disease.

c) As a member of the family above, a female has the same chance as a male of being a hemophiliac; this is not the case in the population as a whole. Because a father must be a hemophiliac and a mother be at least a carrier in order to produce a hemophiliac girl, there are only rare cases of girls being born with hemophilia. The hemophilia gene has a lower frequency than the normal gene in the population, and the chances that both parents will have this gene are very low.

However, within the particular region in question, there is much intermarriage. If a gene is carried by a family member, its frequency among other family members will be much higher than in the population as a whole. If an individual carries a particular gene, in this case the gene for hemophilia, and marries within the family, there is a good chance that their spouse will also carry the gene. There is thus, an increased probability that it will be carried by offspring in the homozygous state, resulting in hemophiliac girls.

● **PROBLEM** 4-15

In humans, the disease known as the "bleeder's disease", or hemophilia, is inherited as an X-linked recessive trait.

Sally and Sam, both of whom are normal, marry, and they have three children: (1) Saul, a bleeder, who marries a normal woman and has a daughter, Sarah, who is normal; (2) a normal daughter, Sheryl, who marries a normal man and has a son, Solomon, who is a bleeder; and (3) Shirley, also normal, who marries and has six normal sons.

Using the letters H and h for the normal and hemophilia genes, respectively, and /\ to represent the Y chromosome, determine the genotypes of Sally, Sam, Saul, Sarah, Sheryl, Solomon and Shirley.

Solution: Sally must be heterozygous Hh since her son Saul is a bleeder. Sam's genotype is H/\ since he is normal, and Saul's must be h/\ since he is a bleeder. Sarah, who is normal, receives the hemophilia gene from Saul, and therefore is Hh. Since Sheryl has a son who is a bleeder she must also be Hh. Her son, Solomon, must be h/\ . Since Shirley had six sons, none of whom was affected, she most likely is homozygous normal, HH.

● **PROBLEM** 4-16

Red-green colorblindness is caused by a recessive sex-linked gene. If a red-green colorblind man marries a woman with normal vision whose father was red-green colorblind, what will be the expected phenotypic results in their children?

Solution: Always write out the genotypes of the parents with the sex chromosomes. Remember the Y chromosome carries essentially no genes except those for "maleness".

Red-green colorblind man and	X	Heterozygous woman
X^cY		X^cX^C

Then solve the problem in the usual way for single gene pairs, but carry along the sex chromosomes.

Results in progeny

	X^C	Y
X^C	X^CX^c	X^CY
X^c	X^cX^c	X^cY

1/4 female, normal vision

1/4 male, normal vision

1/4 female, colorblind

1/4 male, colorblind

● PROBLEM 4-17

In the fruit fly, Drosophila melanogaster, the gene for white eyes is sex-linked recessive, w. Its wild-type allele, w^+, gives dull red eyes. The gene for black body, b, is an autosomal recessive and contrasts its wild-type allele, b^+, which gives a gray body. For a cross between females who are heterozygous for both genes, and white-eyed, black-bodied males, determine the phenotypes of the progeny, and in what proportions they occur.

Solution: We use the Punnett square to solve this problem. First, we determine what gametes are produced by each parent. The genotypes of the parents are ww bb for the females and w bb for the males.

♀ \ ♂	$\underline{wb}$	$\underline{b}$
$\underline{w}^+\,\underline{b}^+$	$\underline{w}^+\underline{w}\ \underline{b}^+\underline{b}$ red,gray ♀	$\underline{w}^+\!/\ \underline{b}^+\underline{b}$ red, gray ♂
$\underline{w}^+\,\underline{b}$	$\underline{w}^+\,\underline{wbb}$ red, black ♀	$\underline{w}^+\!/\ \underline{bb}$ red, black ♂
$\underline{wb}^+$	$\underline{wwb}^+\underline{b}$ white, gray ♀	$\underline{w}\!/\ \underline{b}^+\underline{b}$ white, gray ♂
$\underline{w}\ \underline{b}$	$\underline{ww}\ \underline{bb}$ white, black ♀	$\underline{w}\!/\ \underline{bb}$ white, black ♂

Summarizing the progeny, we see that the phenotypic distribution of the progeny is the same for both females and males: 1 red-eyed, gray-bodied: 1 red-eyed, black-bodied: 1 white-eyed, gray-bodied: 1 white-eyed, black-bodied.

● PROBLEM 4-18

Consider the gene for vermilion eye color (v) in the fruit fly, Drosophila melanogaster, to be X-linked and recessive to its wild-type allele ($\underline{v}^+$), which produces dull red eye color. The heterogametic sex (XY) in the fruit fly is the male. A female with wild-type eyes is crossed with an unknown male and the following progeny are observed:

Females	Males
64 wild-type	42 wild-type
57 vermilion	59 vermilion

a) What is the genotype of the female parent?

b) What is the genotype of the unknown male parent?

Solution: a) Since the gene for vermilion is recessive and X-linked and, since vermilion-eyed male progeny were

123

observed, the female parent must have been heterozygous, with a genotype of $\underline{v}^+\underline{v}$.

b) Since the male can only transmit his X-chromosome to his daughter progeny, and since the female parent was heterozygous, the only way vermilion-eyed female progeny could occur would be for the unknown male to have been $\underline{v}_\wedge$ in genotype.

In turkeys, the gene for short wattle (ℓ) is X-linked recessive. Its wild-type allele (L) is responsible for producing a long wattle. In turkeys, like in all birds, the female is the heterogametic sex, possessing an X and a Y chromosome. The male has two X chromosomes.

The sex of a female can be reversed to male if the one functional ovary is destroyed or removed. Assuming that such a reversal can yield a fertile male, what will be the phenotypic ratio of a cross between a short-wattled reversed male and a long-wattled female?

♀ \ ♂	$\underline{\ell}$	$\wedge$
$\underline{L}$	L $\underline{\ell}$ long ♂	L $\wedge$ long ♀
$\wedge$	$\underline{\ell}\ \wedge$ short ♀	probably dies

Solution: For this problem, we will represent long-wattled females as L∧, the ∧ standing for the Y chromosome. Normal long-wattled males will be LL. When the short wattled allele is present, L is replaced by ℓ.

Because the reversed male was once a female, its genotype will be ℓ∧ in this case. The genotype of the female in this problem is L∧. In setting up a Punnett square, we get the following:

The phenotypic ratio is 1 long ♂ : long ♀ : 1 short ♀.

124

In Drosophila melanogaster, the gene for white eyes, w, is recessive and X-linked. Red eyes result from the wild-type allele at this locus.

(a) On chromosomes, symbolize the genotypes of a white-eyed male, a red-eyed female (both possible types), and a white-eyed female.

(b) Diagram a cross between a homozygous red-eyed female and white-eyed male. Carry this to the F_2 generation and give phenotype ratios for each sex.

(c) Show a cross between an F_1 female and white-eyed male. Give phenotype ratios.

(d) Show a cross between an F_1 female and wild-type male. Also give ratios.

(a) $\dfrac{w}{} \rightarrow$, $\dfrac{w^+}{} \rightarrow$, $\dfrac{w^+}{w^+}$, and $\dfrac{w^+}{w}$, $\dfrac{w}{w}$.

(b) $\dfrac{w^+}{w^+} \times \dfrac{w}{} \rightarrow$ P

$\dfrac{w^+}{} \quad \dfrac{w}{} \quad \underline{} \rightarrow$ gametes

$\dfrac{w}{w^+} \quad \dfrac{w^+}{} \rightarrow$ $F_1 \times F_1$ (all red-eyed)

$\dfrac{w}{} \quad \dfrac{w^+}{} \quad \dfrac{w^+}{} \quad \underline{} \rightarrow$ F_1 gametes

$\dfrac{w}{w^+} \quad \dfrac{w^+}{w^+}$ F_2 females, all redeyed

$\dfrac{w}{} \rightarrow \quad \dfrac{w^+}{} \rightarrow$ F_2 males, ½ red, ½ white

(c) $\dfrac{w}{w^+} \rightarrow \times \dfrac{w}{} \rightarrow$ females, ½ red, ½ white; males, ½ red, ½ white

(d) $\dfrac{w}{w^+} \times \dfrac{w^+}{} \rightarrow$.   females, all red males, ½ red, ½ white

Solution: X-chromosomes are usually represented by a "———" and Y chromosomes by a "———→". Since only X chromosomes carry this gene, letters symbolizing the eye color gene are only on the "———→". Crosses are then completed in the usual way.

In man, the gene (i) for ichthyosis is sex-linked and recessive to the gene (I) for normal skin. Ichthyosis is a disease which produces scaley skin. Diagram on chromosomes the genotypes of the following crosses and summarize the expected phenotypic ratios:

(a) a normal man, and a woman with ichthyosis;
(b) a man with ichthyosis and a normal heterozygous woman;
(c) a man with ichthyosis and a normal homozygous woman.

Solution: This problem can be worked out in the same manner as the previous one involving crosses diagramed on chromosomes.

(a)

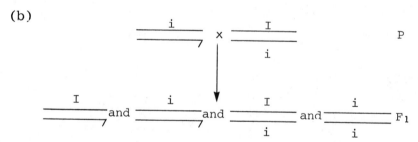

Phenotypically, all normal in F1 generation.

(b)

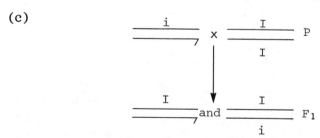

F_1 sons: 1/2 normal, 1/2 with ichthyosis.
F_1 daughters: 1/2 carriers, 1/2 with ichthyosis.

(c)

All phenotypically normal in F_1 generation.

One pair of genes for coat color in cats is sex-linked. The gene B produces yellow coat, b produces black coat, and the heterozygous Bb produces tortoise-shell coat. What kind of offspring will result from the mating of a black male and a tortoise-shell female?

Solution: Sex determination and sex linkage in cats is similar to that found in man, and indeed, in most animals and plants that have been investigated. So for cats, we can assume that if a gene is sex-linked, it is carried on the X chromosome. We can also assume that the Y chromosome carries few genes, and none that will mask the expression of a sex-linked gene or an X chromosome. Female cats, like female humans, are XX, and male cats are XY.

Let X^B represent the chromosome carrying the gene for yellow coat, and let X^b represent the chromosome carrying the gene for black coat. The male parent in this problem is black, so his genotype must be X^bY. The female is tortoise-shell, which means that she is carrying both the gene for yellow color and the gene for black color. Her genotype is X^BX^b. In the cross:

P $\qquad X^bY \quad \times \quad X^BX^b$ ♀

Gametes $\qquad X^b;Y \quad \downarrow \quad X^B; X^b$

F₁

♀	X^b	Y
X^B	X^BX^b	X^BY
X^b	X^bX^b	X^bY

Phenotypically, the offspring consist of:

1/4 tortoise-shell females (X^BX^b),

1/4 black females (X^bX^b),

1/4 yellow males (X^BY), and

1/4 black males (X^bY).

Note that there can never be a tortoise-shell male, because a male can carry only one of the two possible alleles at a time.

The barred pattern of chicken feathers is inherited by a pair of sex-linked genes, B for barred and b for no bars. If a barred female is mated to a non-barred male, what will be the appearance of the progeny?

Solution: This is an example of a sex-linked cross. Using the notations for the sex-linked traits, let X^B be the chromosomes carrying the gene for the barred pattern, and let X^b be the chromosome carrying the gene for the non-barred pattern.

Since B is a dominant gene, a barred female could have one of the 2 genotypes: $X^B X^B$ or $X^B X^b$. The only possible genotype for a non-barred male is $X^b Y$. Therefore, there are two possible crosses between a barred female and a non-barred male:

i)   P   ♀ $X^B X^B$ x $X^b Y$

   Gametes X^B ↓ X^b; Y

   F_1 $X^B X^b$: $X^B Y$

                barred female   barred male.

Phenotypically, all the progeny of this cross have the barred feather pattern.

ii)   P   ♀ $X^B X^b$ x $X^b Y$

     Gametes X^B; X^b ↓ X^b; Y

	X^b	Y
X^B	$X^B X^b$	$X^B Y$
X^b	$X^b X^b$	$X^b Y$

Phenotypically: $X^B X^b$ is a barred female,

$X^b X^b$ is a non-barred female,

$X^B Y$ is a barred male, and

$X^b Y$ is a non-barred male.

● **PROBLEM 4-24**

In pedigree charts a circle represents females and squares represent males. Blackened boxes indicate that the trait is expressed in that individual. If a trait appear in the following patern, what is the mode of inheritance?

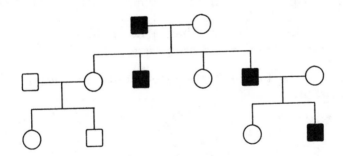

Solution: Because this trait appears in different frequencies in the two sexes, it is probably sex-linked. It cannot be X-linked if it is passed from father to son, since sons only get Y chromosomes from their fathers. Because the trait appears in all males whose fathers had the trait, it is probably Y-linked.

In man, Y-linked inheritance of 17 different genes has been suggested, but only one case has been proven. This is the one causing hairy pinnae in humans (long hair growing on the ears). Y-linked genes are called holandric genes.

VARIATIONS OF SEX LINKAGE

Is there a genetic basis for baldness?

Solution: Baldness has been explained by several different modes of inheritance by different investigators. Pattern baldness appears to be a sex-influenced trait. Genes governing sex-influenced traits may reside on any of the autosomes or on the homologous portions of the sex chromosomes. The dominant or recessive properties of the alleles of sex-influenced traits is dependent upon the sex of the bearer, due largely to sex hormones.

The gene for pattern baldness is dominant in men, but exhibits recessiveness in women. Indications are that a single pair of autosomal genes control pattern baldness, acting in the following fashion:

Genotype	Male	Female
BB	bald	bald
Bb	bald	not bald
bb	not bald	not bald

The allele seems to exert its effect only in the presence of testosterone.

Pattern baldness and short index fingers are both sex-influenced. Both are dominant in men and recessive in women. Determine the phenotypic ratios of the F_1 generation resulting from a cross between a heterozygous short-fingered man without the balding trait and a short-fingered woman heterozygous for the balding trait.

<u>Solution</u>: It often helps to make up a table showing the phenotypic expression of the traits in each sex.

Genotype	Male	Female	Geno-type	Male	Female
BB	bald	bald	ℓℓ	short-fingered	short-fingered
Bb	bald	nonbald	Lℓ	short-fingered	long-fingered
bb	nonbald	nonbald	LL	long-fingered	long-fingered

According to the chart our parental genotypes are:

P: Lℓbb   X   ℓℓBb
         short-fingered   short-fingered,
         non-bald man   non-bald woman

We can then use the forked-line method to determine the progeny.

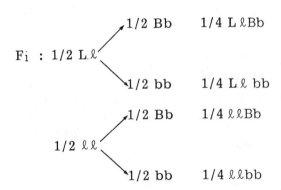

1/2 Bb   1/4 LℓBb

Fᵢ : 1/2 Lℓ

1/2 bb   1/4 Lℓ bb

1/2 Bb   1/4 ℓℓBb

1/2 ℓℓ

1/2 bb   1/4 ℓℓbb

Following the chart, the following phenotypes result:

<u>Men</u>   <u>Women</u>

LℓBb short-fingered, bald   long-fingered, nonbald

Lℓbb short-fingered, nonbald   long-fingered, nonbald

ℓℓBb short-fingered, bald   short-fingered, nonbald

ℓℓbb short-fingered, nonbald   short-fingered, nonbald

ratios: Men: 1/2 short-fingered and bald
1/2 short-fingered and nonbald

Women: 1/2 long-fingered and nonbald
1/2 short-fingered and nonbald

In the domestic fowl. males and females may exhibit pronounced differences in plumage. In the Leghorn breed, all males are "cock-feathered" and all females are " hen-feathered". In the Sebright bantam breed, birds of both sexes are "hen-feathered". In other breeds, like the Hamburg or Wyandotte, all females are "hen-feathered", but males can be either "hen-" or "cock-feathered". What mode of inheritance is operating? How is it different from sex linkage?

Solution: This is an example of a sex-limited inheritance pattern. Sex-limited genes are genes whose phenotypic expression is determined by the presence or absence of a sex hormone, thus limiting their affect to one sex or the other.

Feathering types in fowls are known to be controlled by a single gene pair. The recessive allele h controls the "cock-feathering" type in which the birds have long, pointed, curved, fringed feathers on tail and neck. "Hen-feathering", in which the feathers are shorter, rounder, straighter, and without fringe is controlled by the allele H. Following this, Leghorns must be all hh, Hamburgs and Wyandottes may be HH, Hh or hh, and Sebright bantams must be HH. Remember that "cock-feathering" is limited to the male sex.

Insight into the behavior of allele h was gained from chickens that had had their gonads removed. These birds all became "cock-feathered", regardless of genotype.

In summary, H produces "hen-feathering" in the presence of either sex hormone, and "cock-feathering" in the absence of a sex hormone. This allele is dominant to h, which produces "hen-feathering" in the presence of a female hormone, and "cock-feathering" if it is absent. This explains the differential expressions of the gene between the sexes.

Sex-limited traits are principally responsible for secondary sex characteristics. For example, beard development in humans occurs normally only among men. Sex-limited inheritance is quite different from sex-linked inheritance. Sex-limited genes are usually found on autosomal genes, yet they express development only in one sex. This action is clearly related to the sex hormones, as expression can sometimes be reversed if the hormonal environment is altered.

SHORT ANSWER QUESTIONS FOR REVIEW

Choose the correct answer.

1. Which one of the following statements does
    not apply to human sex chromosomes?
    Human sex chromosomes _____ (a) carry
    allelic pairs. (b) determine individual sex.
    (c) are identical in women. (d) are identical
    in men. (e) both a and d   e

2. The Y chromosome determines that an
    individual will be male by (a) stimulating
    the sex organs to become male gonads. (b)
    stimulating the brain to secrete male hormones.
    (c) inducing the X chromosome to cease
    estrogen production. (d) destroying one X
    chromosome.   a

3. Barr bodies result from (a) inactivation of
    one X chromosome by the Y chromosome. (b)
    a third X chromosome. (c) inactivation of one
    X chromosome for dosage compensation. (d)
    both b and c   c

4. The long arm of the Y chromosome and the
    short arm of the X chromosome seem to be
    homologous. What accounts for this? (a)
    An $X(X^S X^S)$ female and an $X(Y^L Y^L)$ male
    have sexual characteristics. (b) AN $X(X^S X^S)$
    female and an $X(Y^S Y^S)$ male have Turner's
    characteristics. (c) An $X(X^L X^L)$ female
    and an $X(Y^L Y^L)$ male have sexual char-
    acteristics. (d) all of the above   a

5. In the asparagus plant, sex is determined by
    a gene which is dominant for maleness. Only
    homozygous recessive plants are females.
    What would be the percentage of females if
    a female plant was crossed with a homozygous
    male plant? (a) 25% (b) 50% (c) 75% (d)0%   d

6. A man and a woman are both affected by
    vitamin D resistant rickets which is a
    dominant sex-linked allele. All of the female
    offspring of these people are affected with
    rickets, but some of the males are not.

What are the possible genotypes of the
parents? (a) Both are homozygous for the
trait. (b) The woman is heterozygous and
the man is homozygous. (c) The woman
is homozygous, and the man is heterozygous. (d) This is not possible.

b

7. Pseudohypertrophic muscular dystrophy is a
disease determined by a sex-linked recessive
allele. What are the possible genotypes of a
woman and man whose offspring are all
affected with this disease? (a) Woman is
homozygous dominant and man is heterozygous.
(b) Woman is homozygous recessive and man
is homozygous dominant. (c) Woman is homozygous recessive and man is heterozygous
recessive. (d) None of the above

c

8. A cross between a trihybrid plant with the
genotype AaBbCc and a dihybrid plant with
the genotype AaBBCc produces nine different
genotypes. How many of the offspring would
be sexual, yielding polyploids? (a) 36 (b)
18 (c) 12 (d) 6 (e) 4

c

9. The fly Drosophila melanogaster has the gene
that codes for white eyes as recessive and
x-linked. Red eyes result from the wild type
allele at the same locus. A cross between a
heterozygous red eyed female and a white
eyed male would produce (a) all red eyed
progeny. (b) all white eyed males and all
red eyed females. (c) one red eyed male
and one white eyed male. (d) one red eyed
female and one white eyed female. (e) both
c and d

e

10. The gene for pattern baldness is dominant
in men, but exhibits recessiveness in women.
The difference in expression results from (a)
the gene for baldness being x-linked. (b)
the gene for baldness being y-linked. (c)
the expression of the gene depending upon the
hormonal balance of the individual. (d) both
a and c (e) none of the above

c

The pedigree chart below represents a trait which appeared in the following pattern.

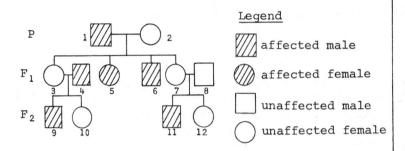

Legend

⊘ affected male

⊘ affected female

☐ unaffected male

○ unaffected female

Based on this pedigree answer questions 11-13

11. What is the possible genotype of the mother (individual 2)? (a) heterozygous dominant (b) homozygous recessive (c) heterozygous recessive (d) there is not enough information   c

12. In the F_1, what is the possible genotype of individual 7? (a) heterozygous dominant (b) homozygous recessive (c) heterozygous recessive (d) there is not enough information   c

13. What is the mode of inheritance of this trait? (a) x-linked (b) dominant in men, recessive in women (c) y-linked (d) none of the above   b

Fill in the blanks.

14. Men have _____ pairs of autosomes and one _____ pair of sex chromosomes.   22, XY

15. Women have _____ pairs of autosomes and one _____ pair of sex chromosomes.   22, XX

16. The fertilization of an egg by a Y sperm results in a _____ offspring.   male

17. A plant which produces only one type of gamete is called _____.   dioecious

18. Some plants of the _____ species produce only staminate flowers and others produce only pistillate flowers.   asparagus

|

19. The parasitic wasp <u>Habrobracon</u>, as all other insects, develops into a male by_____.

   partheno-genesis

20. Sex determination of the parasite in question 19 is also accomplished by fertilization and a diploid male results only when _____ for a given allele.

   hemizygous

21. In the turkey, as in most birds, the female is the _____sex, which possesses an XY chromosomal pair.

   hetero-gametic

22. Genes which are Y-linked are called _____.

   holandric

23. Sex limited genes are those whose phenotypic expression is determined by the presence or absence of sex _____.

   hormones

24. Beard development in humans is generally limited to one sex (male), yet studies indicate that there is no real difference in the number of hairs per unit area of skin between men and women. This indicates that beard development is a _____trait.

   sex-limited

Determine whether the following statements are true or false.

25. Since two X ova are produced for every Y sperm, the number of females born in a population is twice the number of males born.

   False

26. Barr bodies are found in all tissues of a female mammal that has two or more X-chromosomes.

   True

27. A person with Klinefelter's Syndrome has an XXY karotype and is usually a phenotypically sterile male.

   True

28. Male bees develop from unfertilized eggs which undergo DNA replication and give rise to diploid individuals.

   False

29. Sex-linked traits are carried mostly on the X chromosome. Since females have two X chromosomes, they have twice the chance of expressing a recessive sex-linked trait.

   False

To be covered
when testing
yourself

30. Color blindness is an inherited disorder
    produced by a sex-linked recessive allele.   True

31. If a phenotypically normal couple has a son
    with hemophilia, there is a chance that some
    of their daughters will be carriers.   True

In questions 32 through 36 match the terms in
column A with their appropriate descriptions in
column B.

A	B	
32. Dosage compensation	a) sex chromatin	b
	b) inactivation of	
33. Turner's syndrome	one X chromosome	e
	c) inactivation of one	
34. Klinefelter's syndrome	X chromosome so as	f
	to reduce to half the	
35. Barr body	allele	a
	d) inactiviation of	
36. Lyon hypothesis	all but one X	d
	chromosome	
	e) phenotypical	
	female (X,O)	
	f) phenotypical male	
	(XXY)	

In questions 37 through 45 match the following
terms in column A to its appropriate description
in column B.

It is given that honey bees have 32 chromosomes.

A	B	
37. XXY	a) 32 chromosomes	f
	b) 16 chromosomes	
38. XYY	c) 8 chromosomes	e
	d) 4 chromosomes	
39. XO	e) phenotypical male	g
	f) phenotypical male with one	
40. XX	or more barr bodies	h
	g) phenotypical female with-	
41. XXX	out barr bodies	i
	h) phenotypical female	
42. Queen bee	with one barr body	a
	I) female with no barr	
	bodies	

SHORT ANSWER QUESTIONS FOR REVIEW

43. Male drone   b

44. Female worker   a

45. Unfertilized egg   b

CHAPTER 5

MUTATIONS AND ALLELES

MUTATIONS

● **PROBLEM** 5-1

> Mutation rates may be increased by chemical mutagens. How do chemicals induce mutations?

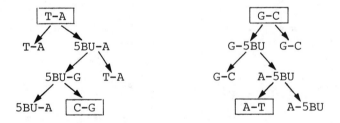

Fig. 1: 5-Bromouracil

Solution: Chemicals can induce mutations in DNA by incorporating themselves into the DNA structure or by chemically altering the existing nucleotides. Base analogues and acridine dyes can mutate a stretch of DNA by the former method and nitrous acid and alkylating agents act in the latter way.

A base analogue has a chemical structure that is similar to the naturally occuring bases. These analogues have critical differences that lead to changes in pairing so that a base substitution can occur at the next replication. An analogue of thymine is 5-bromouracil (5BU). This analog can incorporate opposite adenine or guanine.

The arrows in Figure 1 represent the fates of each strand upon replication. This diagram shows how a T-A base pair can be changed to a C-G base pair and how a G-C base pair can be changed to A-T. Such mutations are called transitions if a purine replaces a purine (adenine and guanine are purines) or if a pyrimidine replaces a pyrimidine (thymine, cytosine, and uracil are pyrimidines). If a purine replaces a pyrimidine or vice versa, then a transversion has occurred.

Nitrous acid acts on the DNA in a very different way. Nitrous acid (HNO_2) removes the amino group ($-NH_2$) of the nucleotide and substitutes a keto group ($=0$) instead. This transformation creates differences in hydrogen bonding properties which can lead to transitions.

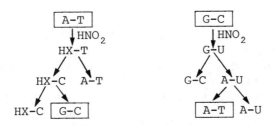

Fig. 2: Nitrous Acid

Thymine and uracil are not affected by nitrous acid since they do not contain amino groups.

Alkylating agents, such as ethyl methane sulfonate (EMS) and ethyl ethanesulfonate (EES) add a methyl or ethyl group to one of the carbons (carbon 7) of guanine. The guanine linkage is weakened and it can be lost from the DNA, leaving a gap. Transitions or transversions can arise in this gap. If the alkylated guanine is not lost from the strand, it pairs like adenine, creating a GC to AT transition.

Acridine dyes can be responsible for frameshift mutations. They intercalate between adjacent bases and can cause additions or deletions.

These are a few of the chemicals that can cause mutations in DNA. Many chemicals are mutagens, but their mechanisms are poorly understood.

a) How are mutations detected?

b) How are potential mutagens tested?

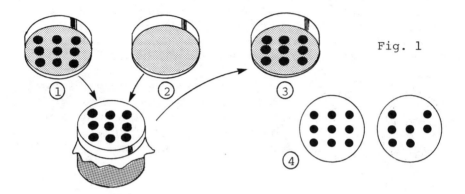

Fig. 1

Solution: Since mutations are changes in the DNA, they can be detected as abnormalities among a population of organisms. The study of mutations is very important to the study of genetics because it is through a comparison of these abnormalities that many conclusions regarding gene structure, function and regulation have been reached. Mutations can be observed through visible phenotypic differences and through altered nutritional requirements. Mutagens are agents that can induce mutations. Using bacteria with a specific mutation, the Ames test can detect chemical mutagens.

(a) Different mutations manifest themselves in different ways. Mutations in structural genes can lead to visible phenotypic differences in an individual. Mutations in genes used in metabolic or catabolic pathways may lead to changes in nutritional requirement. Drosophila has been used extensively to study how mutations that produce visible alterations, such as wing structure or eye color, are inherited. Mutations that affect biochemical pathways have been studied in E.coli and other bacteria. Specific clones of cells can be followed through a technique called replica plating as shown in Figure 1.

In replica plating a plate of cells growing on normal medium(1) is pressed onto a velveteen-covered block. Cells from each colony stick to the velveteen when plate(1) is removed. Plate(2), with a special medium, such as a medium lacking one nutrient, is now pressed onto the velveteen. When this plate is removed it has the colonies in the same places as the original, (3). Step (4) shows a comparison of the original plate to that of the plate with a deficient medium. The colonies that grow on the original, but not on the deficient medium, are those clones that contain a mutation. This technique can be used to test other types of mutations, such as those leading to antibiotic resistance.

(b) A very powerful way to test potential mutagens is by the Ames test. This procedure involves subjecting a strain of <u>Salmonella typhimurium</u>, that has a specific frameshift or base pair mutation that makes it His$^-$, to chemicals. Those chemicals that can mutate the bacteria to His$^+$ are mutagenic. Some chemicals become mutagenic only when a liver extract, S-9, is added to the medium. This extract oxidizes the chemicals to a mutagenic form much as the mammalian system inadvertantly does. The Ames test has proven to be a useful primary test to screen for potential mutagens and carcinogens. The chemicals can be further tested in more expensive animal tests.

● PROBLEM 5-3

How are frameshift mutations produced?

<u>Solution</u>: Frameshift mutations are caused by the addition or subtraction of one or several base pairs in the DNA. This alteration in the nucleotide sequence will change the reading frame of the mRNA transcript. A changed amino acid sequence in the protein could result.

Let us look first at the results that an addition and a subtraction (deletion) have on the genetic sequence. Then we can examine some mechanisms for such mutations. And finally, we can discuss some corrections.

Figure 1 shows how the amino acid sequence can change by the addition or deletion of one base pair. If the addition or deletion consisted of a multiple of three bases, the frame would not be altered since it is read in groups of threes.

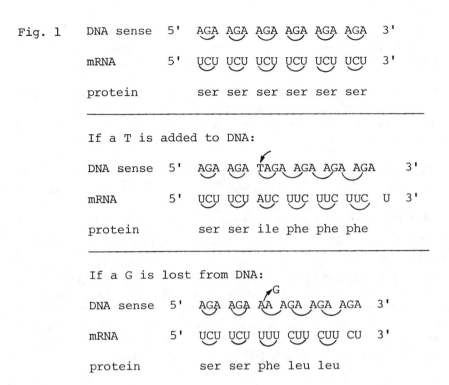

Fig. 1

DNA sense 5' AGA AGA AGA AGA AGA AGA 3'

mRNA 5' UCU UCU UCU UCU UCU UCU 3'

protein ser ser ser ser ser ser

If a T is added to DNA:

DNA sense 5' AGA AGA TAGA AGA AGA AGA 3'

mRNA 5' UCU UCU AUC UUC UUC UUC U 3'

protein ser ser ile phe phe phe

If a G is lost from DNA:

DNA sense 5' AGA AGA AA AGA AGA AGA 3'

mRNA 5' UCU UCU UUU CUU CUU CU 3'

protein ser ser phe leu leu

Fig. 2: Phase-shift mutations produced by errors in the mutation-repair mechanism

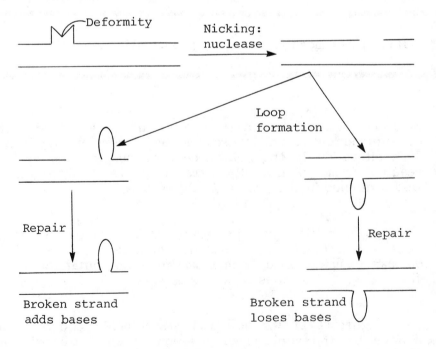

Deformity

Nicking: nuclease

Loop formation

Repair

Repair

Broken strand adds bases

Broken strand loses bases

Such additions and deletions can be produced by errors made during repair or replication or by the action of certain chemicals. Figure 2 shows how a frameshift

144

mutation can be produced by mistakes made during repair. The formation of a loop during the repair process can result in either the addition or the loss of bases. When the loop forms in the strand that is being repaired, extra bases may be added to this strand since the loop is shorter in length than the outstretched piece. Thus, enzymes can add extra bases that they sense are missing, although they have only been misplaced by the loop. A loop in the unbroken strand of the duplex can pull the two broken strands closer together, 'thus losing bases. When each of the strands in both cases are later replicated, normal duplexes will be formed as well as duplexes that have gained or lost nucleotides.

Acridine dyes are chemical mutagens that can insert (intercalate) into DNA. If they insert into a strand that is replicating, a deletion will occur:

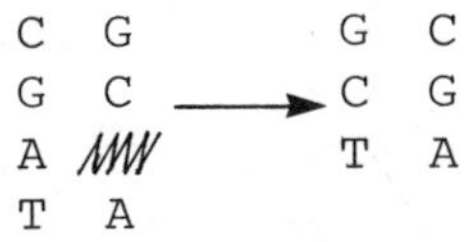

```
C  G        G  C
G  C ──────► C  G
A MWV        T  A
T  A
```

If the intercalation occurs in the template strand (that one that is not replicating) an addition occurs:

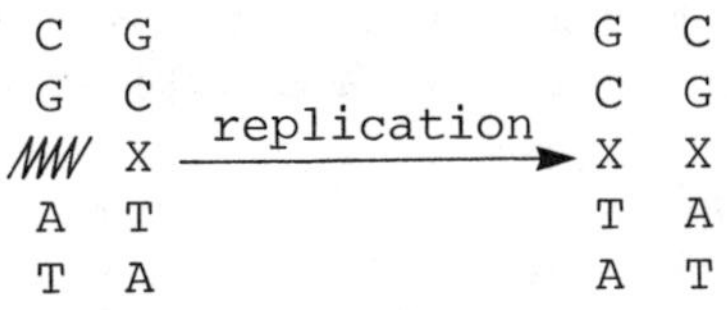

```
C  G                    G  C
G  C    replication     C  G
MWV X  ─────────────►   X  X
A  T                    T  A
T  A                    A  T
```

Thus, frameshift mutations can be produced in a variety of ways. Serious frameshift mutations can be minimized, however. If there is an addition in a strand of DNA, a deletion further down the strand can shift the frame back (provided it involves a proper number of nucleotides). If the frame is shifted back, the mutation still exists, but it is not as debilitating since some of the amino acid sequence has been restored, see Figure 3.

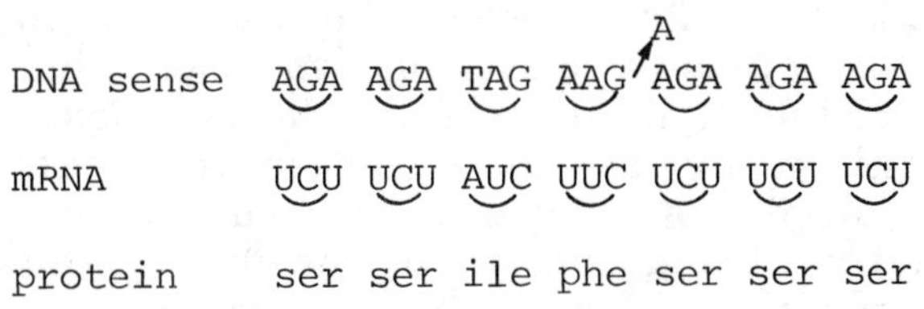

```
                                     A
                                      ⁄
DNA sense   AGA AGA TAG AAG AGA AGA AGA

mRNA        UCU UCU AUC UUC UCU UCU UCU

protein     ser ser ile phe ser ser ser
```

Fig. 3

An addition can mask a deletion in a similar manner.

How does ultraviolet light damage DNA?

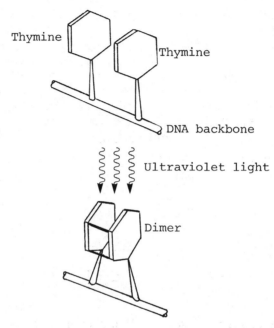

Fig. 1: Thymine dimerization between adjacent
thymine bases in a single strand of DNA.

Solution: Ultraviolet light is a nonionizing form of radiation. It has several effects on DNA, but the major damage of DNA, induced by UV light, is the production of thymine dimers. Thymine dimers are chemical bonds between two adjacent thymine residues as shown in Figure 1. These dimers distort the DNA helix by interrupting the hydrogen bonding between the thymine residues and their complementary adenine residues on the other strand. This interferes with strand replication and leads to mutation or cell death.

Fortunately, thymine dimers are recognized by certain enzymes. The dimers can be made into thymine monomers by photoreactivating enzymes which need a photon of visible light to perform the reaction. Dimers are also recognized by an endonuclease that cuts the helix near the dimer. An exonuclease can then digest the portion of the strand containing the dimer, thus leaving a gap. The gap is filled by a DNA polymerase that uses the complementary strand as a template. Ligase seals the remaining nick. This process is called excision repair.

Most of the dimers induced by UV light are repaired. A faulty excision repair system has been implicated in humans who have xeroderma pigmentosum. Such individuals are homozygous for the mutant allele and are very sensitive to the UV light of sunlight.

A bacterial culture is divided into two halves, A and B, and both halves receive large but equal amounts of ultraviolet light. Culture B is then wrapped in brown paper to isolate it from any light. Culture A is left unprotected from the incident visible light. After 24 hours the cultures are examined. Culture A shows much more growth than culture B. Explain.

Solution: Ultraviolet light creates thymine dimers in DNA molecules. These dimers disrupt the replication of the DNA. Unless these dimers are repaired, they are lethal to the cell. There exist two mechanisms capable of dimer repair: photoreactivation and excision repair. Photoreactivation requires visible light for the activation of the system's enzymes. The excision repair system does not require light energy; hence, it is a dark reaction.

Cultures A and B are identical - they are half of the same original culture. They are exposed to the same amount of UV light, so they probably have comparable amounts of damage in their DNA. Culture A was exposed to visible light and showed much more growth than culture B which was left in the dark. Culture A's photoreactivation system was allowed to work because of its exposure to light. Culture B, because it was left in the dark, had to rely on its excision repair system alone. Since the mortality of culture B was so much greater than that of culture A, culture B's excision repair system may have been damaged by the dose of UV light. If the gene for one of the enzymes of the excision repair system was damaged by the UV light, the system would be inoperative. Culture B, therefore, would be unable to use either of its UV damage repair systems. The excision repair system may have been damaged in culture A also but it could use its photoreactivation system since it was supplied with the necessary light.

This experiment demonstrates the existence of molecular systems that can repair DNA damage. This is of utmost importance since the survival of the cell is dependent on the fidelity of its DNA.

How is the DNA damaged by ultraviolet light repaired?

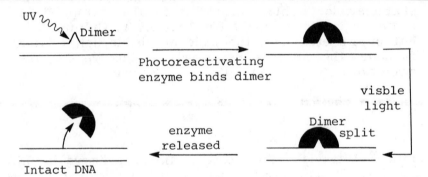

Fig. 1: Photoreactivation

Solution: The solution to the previous question mentioned two repair systems in the bacterial cell which can remove the dimers formed by UV light. These systems are photoreactivation and excision repair.

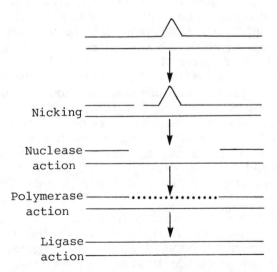

Fig. 2: Excision repair

Photoreactivation can only occur when a photon of visible light is absorbed by the photoreactivation enzyme. This enzyme can bind to a dimer and split it leaving an intact strand of DNA, see Figure 1.

Excision repair is a more complex process because it does not simply break the covalent bond in the dimer. This repair system uses four enzymes to remove the dimer entirely and then to fill in the resulting gap. Figure 2 shows the process. An endonuclease is needed to make a single-stranded nick in the dimer-bearing strand. An exonuclease then digests a length along the strand, including the dimer. A DNA polymerase uses the complementary strand as a template to fill in the missing piece. Ligase then binds the newly copied piece to the original. Base pair substitutions may occur when the DNA polymerase resynthesizes the strand. Such substitutions, however, are not as immediately harmful as the dimers.

● **PROBLEM** 5-7

Photoreactivation and excision repair are two efficient repair mechanisms available to a cell which has undergone UV irradiation. However, extremely high doses of UV elicit a third type of repair system that greatly increases the rate of mutation. What is this system and why does it increase the mutation rate?

Solution: A cell that has been severely damaged by the dimerization of its thymine residues may resort to the SOS repair system. This repair system is highly error-prone so it leads to a high mutation rate.

The SOS system promotes cell survival by allowing DNA synthesis past the pyrimidine dimers during replication. This leaves gaps to be filled in where the dimers originally were. These gaps are filled in by any base regardless of the sequence of the other strand of DNA. These incorrect bases increase the mutations of the cell. However, at least the cell is able to pass some information on to the next generation. A mutated genome is a small step above a genome that is unable to be replicated at all.

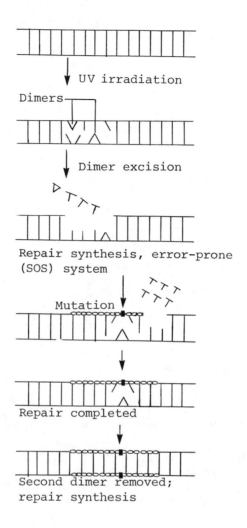

Fig. 1

A DNA molecule contains the following tetranucleotide sequence:

C-G
G-C
A-T
T-A

The molecule is subjected to the following mutagenic agents:

(a) 5-Bromourcil;
(b) nitrous acid;

(c) hydroxylamine;

(d) ethyl ethanesulfonate;

(e) 2-aminpurine.

What mutagenic changes will these agents produce in replicates of the DNA chain?

Thymine

Fig. 1

5-Bromouracil
(Keto)

(enol)

Solution: Each of these chemicals can induce mutations in DNA. 5-Bromouracil and 2-aminopurine are base analogues which can incorporate into the DNA as if they were bases. Nitrous acid, hydroxylamine and ethyl ethanesulfonate chemically alter the existing bases.

(a) 5-Bromouracil is a base analogue that resembles thymine, see Figure 1.

When 5-Bromouracil is in its enol tautomeric form, it can pair with guanine. This results in a change from TA to GC. One altered sequence of this problem would be:

C – G	C – G	C – G	C – G
G – C	G – C	G – C	G – C
A – T $\xrightarrow{5-BU}$	A – 5BU $\longrightarrow$	G – 5BU $\longrightarrow$	G – C
T – A	T – A	T – A	T – A

Another sequence could be:

C – G	C – G	C – G	C – G
G – C	G – C	G – C	G – C
A – T $\xrightarrow{5-BU}$	A – T $\longrightarrow$	A – T $\longrightarrow$	A – T
T – A	5BU – A	5BU – G	C – G

(b) Nitrous acid alters adenine and cytosine by replacing their amino groups with keto groups. When adenine is deaminated and given a keto group it becomes hypoxanthine. Hypoxanthine can pair with cytosine. When

151

cytosine is treated with nitrous acid, it becomes uracil and therefore can pair with adenine.

C – G		U – G	U – A	T – A
G – C		G – U	A – U	A – T
A – T	HNO$_2$	H – T ⟶	H – C ⟶	G – C
T – A		T – H	C – H	C – G

(c) Hydroxylamine causes hydroxylation of the amino group of cytosine. The new molecule can pair with adenine.

C – G		OH‚C – G	OH‚C – A	T – A
G – C		G – C‚OH	A – C‚OH	A – T
A – T	NH$_2$OH	A – T ⟶	A – T ⟶	A – T
T – A		T – A	T – A	T – A

(d) Ethyl ethanesulfonate causes the addition of ethyl groups to guanine. This altered base now acts as a base analogue of adenine so it can bind either to cytosine or to thymine. EES can also cause gaps to be made by the affected purine being excised. This could cause additional mutations, since any base may be placed in the gap. Disregarding the mutations caused by gaps, the changes to DNA would be:

C – G		C – G^{CH_2CH_3}	T – G^{CH_2CH_3}	T – A
G – C	CH$_2$CH$_3$‚	G – C ⟶	G – T	A – T
A – T	EES	A – T	CH$_3$CH$_2$‚ A – T	A – T
T – A		T – A	T – A ⟶	T – A

(e) 2-Aminopurine is a base analogue that incorporates as a substitute of adenine. It can pair with cytosine.

C – G		C – G	C – G	C – G
G – C		G – C	G – C	G – C
A – T	2 – AP	2AP – T ⟶	2AP – C ⟶	G – C
T – A		T – 2AP	C – 2AP	C – G

● PROBLEM 5-9

Is the affect of background radiation in producing spontaneous mutations more significant in humans or in fruit flies? Why?

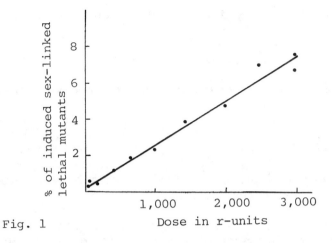

Fig. 1

Solution: Radiation doses are cumulative with respect to induced mutations. This is because radiation produces ions when it is absorbed by a cell. Any one of the millions of ions that are produced can be responsible for a genetic change. So the length of time over which an organism absorbs radiation, even if it is background radiation, will be important in analyzing how effective the radiation is in inducing mutations.

A fruit fly has an average life span of four weeks. A human has an average life span of about 75 years. Even if the human being does not live out his expected life span, he will probably live 20 or more years. Since the question stated that the radiation was background radiation, the day-by-day exposure of the human and the fly can be expected to be the same. Thus the human, with his much longer life span, can be expected to absorb more radiation to induce more mutations than the fruit fly.

● **PROBLEM 5-10**

E.coli sensitive to streptomycin was inoculated into a large flask containing liquid culture medium and allowed to multiply for one week. Ten equal samples of this culture were plated onto agar plates containing streptomycin. A second experiment was performed. The same streptomycin-sensitive E.coli strain was, this time, inoculated into ten separate flasks. After one week equal portions of each flask were poured onto ten agar plates containing streptomycin. What would be the results of this experiment if

(a) streptomycin resistance was postadaptive in origin?

(b) streptomycin resistance was preadaptive in origin?

Solution: This is an actual test used to determine if mutations pre-exist in a population or if a potential mutagen causes the mutations. It is called the fluctuation test and was first derived by S. Luria and M. Delbrück to find whether the presence of a bacteriophage elicited the formation of phage-resistant bacteria.

(a) If the resistance to streptomycin was postadaptive (meaning that the presence of streptomycin in the medium induced resistance) the mutation to streptomycin resistance would occur when the bacteria encountered the antibiotic in its environment. The E.coli strain is not introduced to any streptomycin until it is put on the plates. If this is a postadaptive mutation the mutation will occur on the plates. The bacteria on each plate should have the same chance of becoming resistant to the antibiotic. Therefore, in both parts of the experiment, similar numbers of streptomycin resistant colonies would grow on all of the plates.

(b) If the mutation was preadaptive (occuring randomly before the introduction of the antibiotic) very different results would be expected. The first part of the experiment should show similar colony counts of resistant clones on each plate. This is because any cell that mutates in the large flask will divide. The mutant cells are free to move in the large flask, and when the plates are inoculated an even distribution of mutants will result. However, in the second part of the experiment this is not allowed to happen. The ten flasks at the start of the experiment confine any mutant cell to its own flask. It is possible for a mutation to occur in one cell at an early part of its life cycle and in another cell in a different flask at a much later stage. The first cell can undergo more divisions to produce more resistant clones than the cell of the second flask. When samples are plated some plates may contain more streptomycin resistant colonies than others. This noticeable fluctuation points to the resistance-producing mutation arising randomly at any time of the bacteria's life cycle. This is a preadaptive type of resistance.

Actual experiments of this type have shown that streptomycin resistance and the phage resistance mentioned earlier are both preadaptive mutations. The presence of the antibiotic or the phage does not greatly affect the number of resistant mutants.

Suppose that a wild-type bacterium has a sequence of ten genes that codes for the ten enzymes necessary for the biosynthesis of tyrosine.

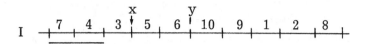

I

The numbers represent the genes, and the long arrow indicates the direction of transcription. A mutant is isolated that has a perfect inversion of the genes 5 and 6. Breakage and rejoining occurred at X and Y in such a way that the rest of the gene sequence was preserved.

II

7   4   3   6   5   10   9   1   2   8

a) Does the mutant have a normal phenotype (Tyr$^+$) or does it require tyrosine for growth (Tyr$^-$)?

b) How, if at all, could the mutation affect:
    1) the transcription of Gene 9?
    2) the translation of the message of Gene 9?

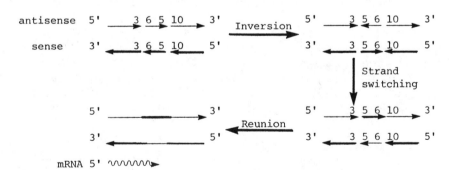

Fig. 1

Solution: A wild-type bacterial strain can grow on a minimal medium that contains such basic materials as glucose and inorganic salts. This strain of bacteria can synthesize all of the essential amino acids and nutrients that it needs to grow. It is called prototrophic. On the other hand, mutant strains exist that require one or more nutritional supplements for growth. Such an organism is called an auxotroph.

a) In this problem we are asked to find out if the mutant bacteria is prototrophic (Tyr$^+$) or auxotrophic (Tyr$^-$). We must find out the effect that the inversion has on the structure of the genes. To do this we must look at both strands of the DNA duplex. Figure 1 shows the breakage and reunion that produced the inversion.

Figure 1 shows that when the inversion occurred, the 5' → 3' polarity of the strands was destroyed. In order to regain the proper chain polarity portions of the sense and antisense strands switched. This has very important consequences. The sense strand of a DNA duplex is the strand from which the mRNA is transcribed. The antisense strand is not used in this process; it is used to generate a complementary sense strand upon replication. Therefore, the important sequence that codes for the amino acid sequence of a polypeptide is the sense strand. The antisense strand will contain complementary nucleotides but it does not have a meaningful sequence. The inversion creates a sense strand that has a piece of antisense strand where the genes 5 and 6 are located. When these genes are transcribed, a garbled sequence will be transcribed to the mRNA. The resulting polypeptides will contain improper amino acids, if any, and therefore be nonfunctional. Since all ten of the enzymes in this pathway are needed for the synthesis of tyrosine, the mutant bacteria will be Tyr$^-$ and auxotrophic. This bacterial strain requires tyrosine in its medium in order to grow.

b) The antisense portion of the mutated sense strand may contain a sequence that could signal chain termination. For instance, an inverted repeat followed by a string of T residues signals the polymerase and transcript to dissociate. In that case none of the genes downstream from the inversion, including gene 9, would be transcribed.

The translation of gene 9 could be affected even if its transcription proceeded normally. The mRNA sequence that was transcribed from the antisense strand containing genes 5 and 6 could contain stop codons. If the codons UAA, UAG or UGA occur anywhere along the stretch of mRNA, the translation will be stopped. None of the genes downstream from the stop codon will be translated.

The effects of an inversion of two genes can drastically change the functioning of the DNA. This problem illustrates how dependent mRNA and proteins are on the fidelity of DNA.

A wild-type male <u>Drosophila</u> is irradiated. How could you tell if this has caused a lethal mutation on the X chromosome?

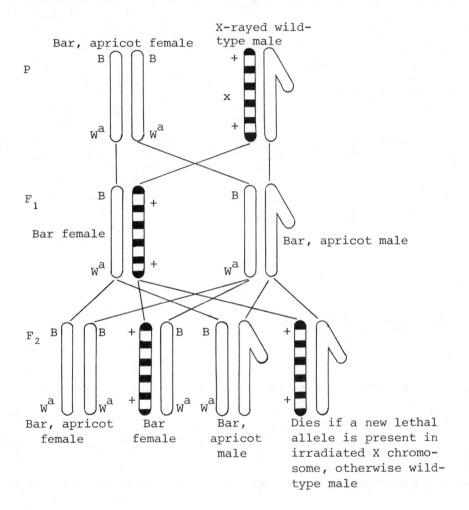

Fig. 1: Diagram of the Muller-5 method. The irradiated X chromosome and its descendants are black- and white- striped.

<u>Solution</u>: The Muller-5 method is used to test the X chromosome. Muller-5 stock female flies have a complex system of inversions on their X chromosome that prevents crossovers along the entire chromosomal length. In addition, this chromosome carries two marker genes, one for apricot eye color (w^a) and one for bar-shaped eyes (B). When this female is mated with the irradiated male,

the progeny of the F_2 generation indicate whether or not a lethal mutation occurred on the male's X chromosome. As shown in Figure 1, the Muller-5 method can detect this type of mutation. Half of the females are Muller-5 flies (with apricot-colored and bar-shaped eyes) and half of the females are wild-type. Half of the males will also be Muller-5 and half will be wild-type. However, if a lethal mutation occurred on the X chromosome, no wild-type males would survive. The wild-type male contains the irradiated X chromosome. If a lethal mutation occurred, it would be expressed. The inversions that prevent the Muller-5 X chromosome from crossing over ensure that the irradiated X chromosome doesn't change its sequence by recombination with the only other homologous chromosome in the experiment. This guarantees that the lethal mutation stays on one chromosome. If it moved to the Muller-5 X chromosome, the results would be inconclusive because the experiment depends on the phenotypic counts of the progeny. Any recombination would introduce uncontrolled change that would alter these counts. In this way, various substances can be tested for their ability to produce lethal mutations on the X chromosome of Drosophila.

MUTATION RATE

● PROBLEM 5-13

What are the causes of conditions such as Huntington's disease and hemophilia A in humans? Are the frequencies of these diseases the same?

Table 1: Frequencies of some human disorders caused by spontaneous mutations

Trait	Mutations per 10^6 cells or gametes
Huntington's disease	1
Aniridia (absence of iris)	5
Retinoblastoma (tumor of retina)	20
Hemophilia A	30
Achondroplasia (dwarfness)	40-140
Neurofibromatosis (tumor of nervous tissue)	130-250

Solution: Both Huntington's disease and hemophilia A arise from spontaneous mutations. Huntington's disease is a fatal disease that leads to the degeneration of the nervous system. It has variable expressivity: one person may develop symptoms in childhood while another may develop symptoms at age 60. This disease manifests when the individual is heterozygous for the dominant allele Ht. Hemophilia A is a sex-linked disorder. People with hemophilia A cannot synthesize antihemophilic globulin (AHG) which is required for the formation of thromboplastin which initiates blood clotting. Hemophilia A has existed in some members of the royal families in Europe over the past century. It is believed that Queen Victoria was the first carrier of the mutant gene which arose either in the sperm or the egg from which she developed. Queen Victoria was probably the source in this family since none of her male ancestors showed the disorder while many of her male descendants did.

The frequencies of these diseases are not the same (see Table 1) since spontaneous mutations are rare and random events. Some genes are more susceptible to mutations than others, hence, mutation rates will differ.

The specific causes of these diseases are not known. Spontaneous mutations may be the result of occasional mistakes made during DNA replication that are missed by the proofreading enzymes. Radiation and chemicals in the environment contribute to DNA damage, but calculations have shown this to be insufficient for the observed mutation rates. Mutagens, can however, increase the mutation rate in laboratory experiments in bacteria and mice. Although radiation release and chemical pollution have not scientifically been proven to undeniably cause mutations in humans, they have shown effects in controlled laboratory studies in other organisms. Since DNA is chemically similar in all of the organisms studied, from bacteria to corn to humans, such laboratory results should not be taken lightly.

● **PROBLEM** 5-14

In a population in Denmark, the relative fitness of the allele for chondrodystrophy is 0.1963. The data of the Lying-in Hospital shows that there were 10 dwarfs out of 94,075 births. What is the mutation rate?

Solution: Chondrodystrophy or achondroplasia is a type of dwarfism where the long bones do not develop properly, resulting in a person with a normal sized trunk and head but short arms and legs. The condition is caused by an autosomal dominant allele that is lethal when homozygous.

For an autosomal dominant trait, the mutation rate can be calculated with the formula:

$$\mu = 1/2(1-f)x$$

where μ is the mutation rate, f is the reproductive fitness of the abnormal gene (the frequency that the abnormal allele is passed to the next generation) and x is the frequency of the abnormality in the individuals in one generation.

We are given f and asked to find μ. First, we must find x. We are given that 10 dwarfs are born in 94,075 births. This is the frequency of the generation.

$$x = \frac{10 \text{ dwarfs}}{94,075 \text{ births}} = 0.00012$$

Now, we can simply plug our given numbers into the formula:

$$\mu = 1/2(1-f)x$$

$$\mu = ? \qquad f = 0.1963 \qquad x = 0.00012$$

$$\mu = 1/2(1-0.1963)(.00012)$$

$$\mu = 0.0000427 = 4.27 \times 10^{-5}$$

This number means that 4.27 mutations occur in 100,000 (10^5) gametes. Or, dividing by 4.27: 1 out of 23,400.

● **PROBLEM** 5-15

A dominant trait has a fitness of 0.6. The frequency in a population of this trait is 1 in 8,000. What is the mutation rate?

Solution: This problem can be solved by using the equation:

$$b = \frac{2\mu}{1-w}$$

where   b = frequency at equilibrium
         μ = mutation rate
         w = fitness of a dominant trait.

We are given that the frequency is 1 in 8,000 and the fitness of the trait is 0.6, so:

$$b = \frac{1}{8000}$$

w = 0.6
μ = ?

Plugging these numbers into the formula, we can find the mutation rate, μ:

$$b = \frac{2\mu}{1-w}$$

$$\frac{1}{8000} = \frac{2\mu}{1-0.6}$$

Cross multiplying gives us:

$$16000\mu = 1 - 0.6$$

$$\mu = 2.5 \times 10^{-5}$$

The frequency of this trait is 2.5 for every 100,000 gametes.

• PROBLEM 5-16

A strain of Salmonella typhimurium has a base pair substitution which makes it His⁻. This strain's rate of spontaneous reversion to His⁺ is 5×10^{-8}. Chemical X is added to the growth medium of a culture of these cells. Solutions are diluted and plated onto minimal medium, (a 10^{-2} dilution) and onto nutrient rich medium (a 10^{-3} dilution). The plates are incubated for 48 hours. The colonies are counted: 50 colonies on the minimal medium and 1,000 colonies on the nutrient rich medium. What can you conclude from this experiment?

Solution: This experiment attempts to discover the effect of chemical X on the spontaneous mutation rate of an organism. The procedure is the basis of the Ames test, which tests potential carcinogens. To discover the effects, if any, of chemical X on the mutation rate of this bacterial strain, we must calculate the mutation rate after the addition of chemical X. Since we know the spontaneous mutation rate when no chemical has been added, we can compare the rates. To find the mutation rate we need to know:

$$\text{mutation rate} = \frac{\text{number of mutants}}{\text{total number of cells}}$$

In our experiment, the mutants are those cells which revert to His$^+$ and thus are able to grow on minimal media. The total cell count is taken from the nutrient rich plate which supports the growth of both His$^-$ and His$^+$ cells. 50 colonies grew on the minimal medium. To find the number of cells, we divide the number of colonies by the dilution:

$$\frac{50}{10^{-2}} = 5 \times 10^3 \text{ revertant cells}$$

The same procedure is used to find the total cell count:

$$\frac{1000}{10^{-3}} = 1 \times 10^6 \text{ cells}$$

We can now find the mutation rate:

$$\frac{\text{\# mutants}}{\text{total cells}} = \frac{5 \times 10^3}{1 \times 10^6} = 5 \times 10^{-3} \quad \text{(or 1 out of 200)}$$

Compare the original rate of 5×10^{-8} (or 1 out of 2 x 10^7) to this chemically induced rate. The frequency of mutations after the addition of chemical X is much higher than the frequency when no chemical is added. We can conclude that chemical X is highly mutagenic and should be studied further.

ALLELES

● PROBLEM 5-17

How can allelism be tested?

Fig. 1

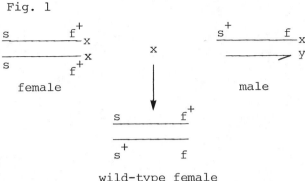

wild-type female

Solution: When several genes are discovered that affect the same trait it is important to decide if the genes are alleles or not. This is important because occasionally genes at different loci may affect the same trait. Allelism can be tested through genetic crosses. Alleles will not be able to cross over since they are at the same genetic locus on the chromosome map. Only genes at different loci will be able to recombine. To demonstrate how the results of genetic crosses can be used to test allelism, we will describe the cross of two marked strains of Drosophila.

There are two genes on the X chromosome that cause similar abnormalities in the wings of Drosophila: forked (f) and singed (s). If a homozygous singed female is crossed with a forked male all of the female progeny will be normal, see Figure 1.

Since the forked chromosome carries the normal gene of singed, s^+, and the singed chromosome carries the normal gene of the forked, f^+, these traits are mutant forms of different genes. They are not alleles.

If they were mutant alleles, however, no crossing over would occur and all of the daughters would be mutant. Neither chromosome would have the normal allele of the other.

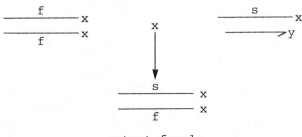

mutant female

Thus, we can formulate a rule:

If the hybrid of two recessive mutants is normal, then the mutations are at different loci and are not alleles; if the hybrid of the two is abnormal, the mutations are alleles.

● **PROBLEM** 5-18

Distinguish between penetrance and expressivity.

Solution: A recessive gene produces a given trait when it is present in the homozygous state. A dominant gene produces its effect in both the homozygous and heterozygous states. Geneticists, however, have found that many genes do not always produce their phenotypes when they should. Genes that always produce the expected phenotype in individuals who carry the gene in an expressible combination are said to have complete penetrance. If only 70 percent of such individuals express the character phenotypically, then the gene is said to have 70 percent penetrance. Penetrance is thus defined as the percentage of individuals in a population who carry a gene in the correct combination for its expression (homozygous for recessive, homozygous or heterozygous for dominant) and who express the gene phenotypically.

Some genes that are expressed may show wide variations in the appearance of the character. Fruit flies homozygous for the recessive gene producing shortening of the wings exhibit variations in the degree of shortening. Expressivity is defined as the degree of effect or the extent to which a gene expresses itself in different individuals. If it exhibits the expected trait fully then the gene is said to be completely expressed. If the expected trait is not expressed fully, the gene shows incomplete expressivity.

The difference between the two terms - penetrance and expressivity - lies in the fact that the former is a function of the gene at the population level, while the latter varies on an individual level. Thus, a given gene having a certain penetrance within a population may have varying expressivity in individuals of that population who express it.

Both penetrance and expressivity are functions of the interaction of a given genotype with the environment. Changes in environmental conditions can change both the penetrance and expressivity of a gene. For example, a given gene may code for an enzyme required for the synthesis of a given metabolite in bacteria. If that metabolite is provided in the organism's nutrient environment, the organism might not produce the enzymes needed for its synthesis and the gene will not be expressed. If, however, the nutrient is depleted from the media, the organism will begin to manufacture the enzyme and thus express the gene. In humans, it is thought that allergy is caused by a single dominant gene; the different types of allergies are due to the varying expressivity of the gene, as a result of the interaction of the gene with both the environment and a given individual's genetic and physical makeup.

● **PROBLEM** 5-19

Osteogenesis imperfecta is associated with bone, eye and ear defects. Some persons show only one defect and others show any combination of the remaining defects. Explain.

Solution: Osteogenesis imperfecta is an autosomal dominant disease that expresses itself in bone abnormality. The bones of affected people are very brittle. The eye and ear defects that are also associated with the allele are expressed in only some of the carriers. The variance in the expressivity is termed just that - expressivity. Expressivity refers to the degree to which the phenotype of an allele is expressed.

The allele for osteogenesis imperfecta also shows pleiotropy. Pleiotropy occurs when a single gene locus has more than one phenotypic effect. Thus, a single dominant allele may express itself in numerous variations.

● **PROBLEM** 5-20

What are multiple alleles and how do they originate?

Solution: Multiple alleles are three or more genes that control a single trait. They presumably have arisen from mutations in the same gene of different individuals. Most series of multiple alleles are associated with gradation in a phenotype. For instance, Drosophila has a series of mutations in eye color that vary from the wild-type red to the mutant white. Mutants can have apricot, buff, eosin, coral, honey, pearl or blood colored eyes. In humans, the blood type locus has multiple alleles.

● **PROBLEM** 5-21

An actress with O type blood accused a producer with B type blood of being the father of her child in a paternity suit. The child was also O type. What does the blood type evidence suggest about his guilt?

Solution:

Blood types	Genotypes
A	AA or Aa
B	$A^B A^B$ or $A^B a$
AB	$A^B A$
O	aa

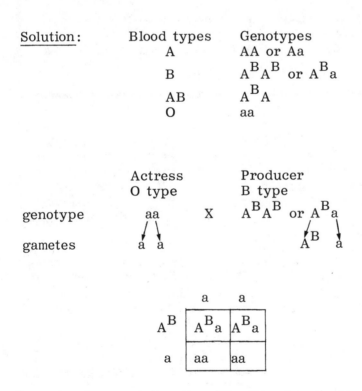

If the producer were heterozygous for A^B he could father an O type child. This evidence indicates that he could have been the father but does not prove it.

If a person with O type blood marries a person with AB type blood what will be the expected results in the progeny?

Solution:

Blood types	Genotypes
A	AA or Aa
B	$A^B A^B$ or $A^B a$
AB	AA^B
O	aa

Phenotypes	O type		AB type
Genotypes	aa	X	AA^B
Types of gametes	a a		A A^B

	a	a
A	Aa	Aa
A^B	$A^B a$	$A^B a$

1/2 Aa   A type

1/2 $A^B a$ B type

Mrs. Doe and Mrs. Roe had babies at the same hospital at the same time. Mrs. Roe brought home a baby girl and named her Nancy. Mrs. Doe received a baby boy and named him Richard. However, she was sure she had had a girl and brought suit against the hospital. Blood tests showed that Mr. Doe was type O, Mrs. Doe was type AB, and Mr. and Mrs. Roe were both type B. Nancy was type A and Richard type O. Had an exchange occurred?

Solution: Inheritance of blood groups is an example of a trait controlled by multiple alleles. The term "multiple alleles" is applied to three or more genes that control a single trait; different combinations of any two genes may be present in a gene pair determining that trait in an individual. Any individual in the population may have any two of the possible alleles, but never more than two, because only two genes for a particular trait can be carried by an individual. Any gamete may have only one of the possible alleles. However, in the population as a whole, three or more different alleles will occur.

The blood types of man - O, A, B and AB - are coded for by multiple alleles. Gene I^A provides the code for the synthesis of a specific protein, agglutinogen A, in the red cells. Gene I^B leads to the production of a different protein, agglutinogen B. Gene i produces no agglutinogen. Gene i is recessive to the other two genes, but neither gene I^A nor I^B is dominant to the other. The symbols I^A, I^B and i are used to emphasize that all three are alleles at the same locus. Individuals with genotypes $I^A I^A$ and $I^A i$ make up blood group A, and produce agglutinogen A. Those with genotypes $I^B I^B$ and $I^B i$ compose blood group B, and produce agglutinogen B. Blood group O individuals have genotype ii, and produce no agglutinogens. When an individual has the genetic makeup of $I^A I^B$, he has both agglutinogens A and B and he belongs to blood group AB. These blood types are genetically determined and do not change during an individual's lifetime.

In reference to the problem given, it is possible to determine if an exchange occurred by comparing the blood types of the babies with the possible bloodtypes that could be found in any offspring of each set of parents. In other words, we can cross the genotypes of each set of parents and determine what genotypes are possible for their offspring. Then we can see if the bloodtypes of the babies that each family brought home is compatable with the possibilities, and if the parents could then have indeed produced a child with that given bloodtype.

We are told that Mrs. Doe is type AB. Therefore, her genotype must be $I^A I^B$. Mr. Doe is type O, so his genotype is ii. The possible bloodtypes of any Doe family offspring are obtained as follows:

P   ♀ $I^A I^B$ x   ii

Gametes I^A; I^B i

F_1 $I^A i$ $I^B i$

blood
group   A   B

Thus, Mr. and Mrs. Doe can only produce offspring having bloodtypes A or B.

In the Roe family, we are told that Mr. and Mrs. Roe are both type B. Therefore, each parent has one of two possible genotypes, $I^B I^B$ or $I^B i$. Taking each possibility:

1)   P   ♀ $I^B I^B$ x $I^B I^B$

     gametes I^B ↓ I^B

     F_1 $I^B I^B$

     blood group = B

2)   P   ♀ $I^B i$ x $I^B I^B$

     gametes $I^B ; i$ ↓ I^B

     F_1 $I^B I^B$: $I^B i$

     blood group = B

3)   P   ♀ $I^B i$ x $I^B i$

     gametes $I^B ; i$ ↓ $I^B ; i$

♀	I^B	i
I^B	$I^B I^B$	$I^B i$
i	$I^B i$	ii

     F_1 $1\ I^B I^B$: $2\ I^B i$: $1\ ii$

     blood groups = B   O

Thus, the Roes can produce only offspring having bloodtype B or O.

Now let us look at the bloodtypes of the babies that each family brought home. The Does brought home Richard, who is type O. But, as we have seen, the Does can produce only offspring of type A or B. The Roes brought home Nancy, who is type A. But it would be impossible for the Roes to have a child with bloodtype A, for the only possible bloodtypes for their offspring are B and O. Therefore Richard, who is type O, must be their child, and Nancy who is type A, must be the Doe's daughter. We see that an exchange did indeed take place.

● **PROBLEM** 5-24

Consider the following three loci in humans, each of which is considered to be a complex locus with multiple alleles: ABO locus (6 alleles), Rh locus (8 alleles) and MN locus (4 alleles). Assuming that each locus is independent of the other two, how many different genotypic combinations can there exist in a given population?

Solution: We first use the formula $\frac{x(x+1)}{2}$, where x = the number of alleles for a given locus to determine the number of possible genotypes for each locus.

For the ABO locus, $\frac{6(6+1)}{2}$ = 21 genotypes,

the Rh locus gives $\frac{8(8+1)}{2}$ = 36 genotypes, and

for the MN locus, there are $\frac{4(4+1)}{2}$ = 10 genotypes.

Since we assume that the three loci are all independent, the total number of different genotypic combinations can be found by multiplying the number of genotypes for each. Thus, 21 x 36 x 10 = 7,560 different genotypic combinations that can exist for these loci.

● **PROBLEM** 5-25

Consider the ABO blood group locus in humans, which has six (6) alleles reported for it, of which three are most prominent, I^A, I^B and i. The I^A and I^B alleles are both dominant to i and codominant to each other.

A woman of blood group O marries a man who has blood group B. There are four children in the family: a son and daughter of blood group O; a daughter who has A blood type; and a son who has B blood type. One of the children is adopted. Which child is the adopted child?

Solution: Since the mother belongs to blood group O, she and her O daughter and son have the genotype ii. Her husband, who is of blood group B, has to have the genotype $I^B i$, as does the B son. Therefore, the daughter who has blood group A must be the adopted child, for neither parent is a source for allele, I^A.

● **PROBLEM 5-26**

A recent court case used the following evidence as Exhibit A:

Woman	A, M, cde/cde
Child	A, MN, cde/cde
Man 1	O, M, CDe/CDe
Man 2	A, N, cdE/cde

Which man can be the father of the child?

Fig. 1

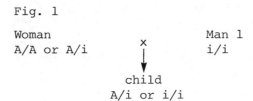

```
Woman                          Man 1
A/A or A/i          x          i/i
                    |
                    ↓
                  child
               A/i or i/i
```

Solution: Exhibit A shows three blood group systems. Comparisons of the mother's and child's phenotype to that of the two men can exclude one of the men from the possibility of being the father of the child. The ABO blood system, the MNS system and the Fisher-Race system for classifying the Rh factor are all shown in Exhibit A. Systematically we can compare the phenotypes and eliminate one of the men.

There are four types of blood in the ABO system: A, B, AB and O. Each of these describes the type of cellular antigens present on the erythrocytes. The antigens, A and B, are passed codominantly as alleles of the same gene. Blood type O has no antigens and is designated by the homozygous genotype i/i. A person with the blood type A can either be homozygous, A/A, or heterozygous, A/i. Thus, from this evidence, either of the men could have fathered the child as shown by the segregation of alleles in Figure 1.

The MNS system is similar to the ABO system. It is a system of alleles that are codominant and that code for another set of cellular antigens. Since the child is MN, and the mother is simply M, the father must have an allele for the N antigen. This excludes Man 1.

We can verify the exclusion of Man 1 by looking at the Rh factor alleles. Numerous alleles contribute to the presence or absence of the Rh factor. The following list shows how these alleles can combine:

$$\left.\begin{array}{l} CDe \\ cDE \\ cDe \\ CDE \end{array}\right\} Rh^+$$

$$\left.\begin{array}{l} cde \\ Cde \\ cdE \\ CdE \end{array}\right\} Rh^-$$

Both the child and the mother are Rh^-; they carry a homozygous set of Rh^- alleles. The father must also be Rh^- since no Rh^+ alleles are present in the child. Man 1 is CDe/CDe; that means that he is homozygous for the Rh^+ condition. He could not be the father of this child. Thus, Man 2 may be the father. However, we can never know definitely who the father is - we can only know who the father is not.

● PROBLEM 5-27

Consider that coat color in rabbits is controlled by a complex locus with a series of four (4) alleles. The alleles arranged in order of their dominance are: c^+ = agouti, c^{ch} = chinchilla, c^h = himalayan and c = albino.

Predict for the following crosses the phenotypes of the progeny and their expected proportions:

a) agouti ♀   X   himalayan ♂

$$\underline{c^+}\underline{c^{ch}} \qquad\qquad \underline{c^h}\underline{c}$$

b) agouti ♀   X   chinchilla ♂

$$\underline{c^+}\underline{c} \qquad\qquad \underline{c^{ch}}\underline{c^h}$$

Solution: a) By constructing the Punnett square, we can determine the types of progeny that this cross will produce.

♀ \ ♂	$\underline{c^h}$	$\underline{c}$
$\underline{c^+}$	$\underline{c^+}\underline{c^h}$ agouti	$\underline{c^+}\underline{c}$ agouti
$\underline{c^{ch}}$	$\underline{c^{ch}}\underline{c^h}$ chinchilla	$\underline{c^{ch}}\underline{c}$ chinchilla

Thus, the predicted phenotypic ratio will be 1 agouti: 1 chinchilla even though all four alleles are segregating in this cross.

b) Construction of the Punnett square for this cross will be as follows:

♀ \ ♂	$\underline{c^{ch}}$	$\underline{c^h}$
$\underline{c^+}$	$\underline{c^+}\underline{c^{ch}}$ agouti	$\underline{c^+}\underline{c^h}$ agouti
$\underline{c}$	$\underline{c^{ch}}\underline{c}$ chinchilla	$\underline{c^h}\underline{c}$ himalayan

For this cross, even though all four alleles are segregating, the predicted phenotypic ratio will be 2 agouti : 1 chinchilla : 1 himalayan.

In a certain animal species, four alleles (a^+, a^1, a^2 and a^3) have a locus on chromosome 1. Another series of alleles (b^+, b^1 and b^2) have their locus on chromosome 2. Theoretically, how many genotypes are possible with respect to these two allelic series?

Solution: This problem involves two sets of multiple alleles. To find out how many genotypes are possible, we must use a binomial expansion. A binomial expansion can be used to calculate the number of different allelic combinations. The form that the expansion takes is:

$$\frac{n!}{(n-k)!\,k!}$$

where n = the number of different alleles and k = number of alleles per genotype (k = 2 in a diploid cell).

In a population there are both heterozygotes and homozygotes, so the formula becomes:

$$\frac{n!}{(n-k)!\,k!} + n \quad \text{where} \quad \frac{n!}{(n-k)!\,k!} = \text{number of hetero-zygotes and n = number of homo-zygotes.}$$

This formula can be simplified by factoring and substituting k = 2:

$$\frac{n!}{(n-2)!\,2!} + n = \frac{n(n-1)!}{2(n-2)!} + n = \frac{n(n-1)(n-2)!}{2(n-2)!} + n =$$

$$\frac{n(n-1)}{2} + n = \text{number of genotypes}$$

Now, we can use this formula to find the answer. Since we have two series of alleles, we must solve each separately and then multiply the results to find the total number of possibilities.

The first locus has four alleles: a^+, a^1, a^2 and a^3. So, n = 4:

$$\frac{n(n-1)}{2} + n = \frac{4(4-1)}{2} + 4 = 10 \text{ genotypes.}$$

The second locus has three alleles: b^+, b^1 and b^2; so here n = 3:

$$\frac{n(n-1)}{2} + n = \frac{3(3-1)}{2} + 3 = 6 \text{ genotypes.}$$

The total number of genotypes possible with respect to both loci is the product of the two:

$$10 \times 6 = 60 \text{ possible genotypes.}$$

Thus, from only two series of alleles, 60 genotypes are possible. The great variability that diploid organisms possess is clearly evident if you bear in mind that thousands of such genes exist.

● **PROBLEM 5-29**

Four alleles in rabbits, listed in order of dominance, are: c^+, colored; c^{ch}, chinchilla; c^h, Himilayan; and c, albino. What phenotypes and ratios would result from the following crosses:

(a) $c^+c^+ \times cc$;

(b) $c^+c \times c^+c$;

(c) $c^+c^{ch} \times c^+c^{ch}$;

(d) $c^{ch}c \times cc$;

(e) $c^+c^h \times c^+c$;

(f) $c^hc \times cc$?

Solution: This problem uses an example of multiple alleles. The order of dominance is given as: c^+, c^{ch}, c^h, c. The possible genotypes and their corresponding phenotypes are:

Phenotypes	Genotypes
color	$c^+c^+, c^+c^{ch}, c^+c^h, c^+c$
chinchilla	$c^{ch}c^{ch}$
light gray	$c^{ch}c^h, c^{ch}c$
Himalayan	c^hc^h, c^hc
albino	cc

175

Therefore, a rabbit with genotype c^+c^h would phenotypically be colored since c^+ is dominant to c^h. However, a c^hc rabbit would be Himalayan since c^h is dominant to c. An albino rabbit will only occur in a homozygous genotype, cc, since this is the recessive allele. Each part of this problem involves simple genetic crosses that can be done using Punnett squares.

(a) The rabbits here are c^+c^+ (colored) and cc(albino). Their cross would yield the following:

	c^+	c^+
c	c^+c	c^+c
c	c^+c	c^+c

All of the progeny of this cross are colored since c^+ is dominant to c.

(b) Both rabbits of this cross are colored, c^+c. Their cross yields:

	c^+	c
c^+	c^+c^+	c^+c
c	c^+c	cc

This time there are 3 colored rabbits and 1 albino. The phenotypic ratio is 3:1.

(c) Both rabbits of this cross are, again, colored although their genotypes differ from the cross in (b). Here the rabbits are c^+c^{ch}. The cross yields:

	c^+	c^{ch}
c^+	c^+c^+	c^+c^{ch}
c^{ch}	c^+c^{ch}	$c^{ch}c^{ch}$

Three of these rabbits are colored and one is chinchilla, $c^{ch}c^{ch}$. The phenotypic ratio is 3:1.

(d) The next cross is with a light gray rabbit, $c^{ch}c$ and an albino, cc. Their progeny are:

	c^{ch}	c
c	$c^{ch}c$	cc
c	$c^{ch}c$	cc

This cross yields two light gray rabbits, $c^{ch}c$ and two albino rabbits, cc. The phenotypic ratio is 2:2 or 1:1.

(e) This cross involves two colored rabbits. But in this cross, both parents have different recessive alleles. One is c^+c^h and the other is c^+c. This cross produces:

	c^+	c^h
c^+	c^+c^+	c^+c^h
c	c^+c	c^hc

The progeny are three colored rabbits with different genotypes and one Himalayan rabbit, c^hc. The phenotypic ratio is 3:1.

(f) This problem crosses a Himalayan rabbit, c^hc with an albino rabbit, cc. Their progeny would be as follows:

	c^h	c
c	c^hc	cc
c	c^hc	cc

These are two Himalayan rabbits, c^hc, and two albino rabbits, cc. The phenotypic ratio is 2:2 or 1:1.

From these crosses, we can make some generalizations. When both parents are homozygous for an allele, all of the progeny are identical for that trait. When one parent is homozygous and the other is heterozygous with the same allele as the homozygous parent, then half of the progeny will be phenotypically and genotypically like one parent and half will be like the other parent. If both parents contain an allele for one of the more dominant traits then the phenotypic ratio will be 3:1 as long as all of the other alleles in the cross are recessive to that common allele.

Both Mr. and Mrs. Brown suffer from an autosomal recessive condition that makes them anemic. Mr. Brown has one amino acid substitution in the β-chain of his hemoglobin molecules and Mrs. Brown has a similar defect in her α-chain. Neither Betsy nor Boopsy, their children, are anemic. Explain.

Solution: The adult human hemoglobin is comprised of four polypeptide chains, 2 α-chains and 2 β-chains. There are six known human globin chains: α, β, δ, γ, ε, and ζ. All six of these chains are structurally similar. A hypothesis exists that says that these chains arose from a single globin gene that duplicated. Each copy of the gene then evolved through mutations so that the gene products are now dissimilar enough to produce slightly different polypeptide chains. The α- and β- chains have genes that are on separate chromosomes; thus, alleles of the same gene do not code for the different hemoglobin chains. Since the globin genes code for very similar polypeptides, they are called a gene family.

Mr. and Mrs. Brown have anemia because one of their hemoglobin genes carries a defect that arises from an autosomal recessive condition. Thus, the genes for the defective α- and β-chains can be represented as aa and bb, respectively. Similarly, the normal homozygous states are AA and BB and the normal heterozygous states are Aa and Bb.

Mrs. Brown, whose α-chain is defective, could have the genotype aaBB. Mr. Brown, whose β-chain is defective, could be AAbb. One of them could also have the heterozygous condition in their normal globin chain; Mr. Brown could be Aabb or Mrs. Brown could be aaBb. Thus, if Betsy or Boopsy were conceived by the cross AAbb x aaBB, their possible genotypes would be:

	Ab	Ab
aB	AaBb	AaBb
aB	AaBb	AaBb

All of these genotypes have normal hemoglobin chains. Thus, any child born of such a cross would not be anemic. If Betsy or Boopsy were the result of the fusion of a different pair of gametes AAbb x aaBb, then one of them may have inherited anemia.

	Ab	Ab
aB	AaBb	AaBb
ab	Aabb	Aabb

This cross shows two progeny with defective β-chains. It also shows two progeny with normal chains; so the Brown children could have been conceived in a cross such as this.

Thus, in a case like this, two parents with a homozygous trait may or may not pass the disorder to their children.

● **PROBLEM** 5-31

A cross of <u>Drosophila</u> yielded two heterozygous females with <u>very different</u> phenotypes: $\dfrac{w\ +}{+\ apr}$ had pale, apricot eyes and $\dfrac{+\ +}{w\ apr}$ had the wild-type red eyes. Explain these phenotypes.

<u>Solution</u>: By examining these two genotypes, we can answer this question. First we notice that the wild-type trait is expressed when the alleles are on the same homologous chromosome. A different, and presumably mutant, phenotype is exhibited when the alleles are on separate homologues. These are the conditions found when pseudoalleles are involved. Pseudoalleles are very closely related genes which can undergo recombination. When pseudoalleles are in trans, on different homologous chromosomes, the mutant phenotype is expressed. When these pseudoalleles are in cis, on the same chromosome, the wild-type phenotype is expressed.

There are two explanations for the variance in phenotype when the cis-trans effect is involved. E.B. Lewis and M.M. Green have proposed that each gene in a pseudoallelic series produces a gene product that interacts with the next gene in the series which in turn produces a gene product that interacts with the next gene and so on. The mutant phenotype is expressed because the gene products cannot operate in trans to interact with the other genes. Either the distance between the chromosomes is too great, the gene product is too unstable or not enough is produced to travel so far. G. Pontecorvo suggested an alternative explanation. His explanation is that the pseudoalleles represent mutations at different sites within a cistron. A gene would then function normally if it was nonmutant. But a mutation would result in a changed or absent gene product. Pontecorvo also said that a single gene (cistron) could break by recombination. Thus, the recombination could account for these pseudoalleles appearing on both the same and different chromosomes. Although both interpretations are valid, the second has been more widely accepted, since proof of interaction of gene products must be identified for the first explanation to hold.

SHORT ANSWER QUESTIONS FOR REVIEW

In questions 1-3 match the chemical to its method of mutation

1. Base analogues
2. Alkylating agents
3. Acridine dyes

   (a) cause deletions and additions of bases in DNA
   (b) structure mimics those of the naturally occuring DNA bases
   (c) alter base pair properties by adding such chemical groups as methyl and ethyl

b

c

a

Choose the correct answer.

4. A frameshift mutation (a) is caused by the addition or subtraction of one or more of the DNA base pairs. (b) will result in a change of the mRNA transcript. (c) a and b (d) none of the above

c

5. The two ways thymine dimers can repair themselves are (a) photoreactivation and endonucleation. (b) endonuleation and ligation. (c) photoreactivation and incision repair. (d) photoreactivation and excision repair.

d

6. The most rarely used system of repair a cell can use when it has been severely radiated by ultraviolet light is the (a) ligation system. (b) SOS system. (c) base lipidization system. (d) spindle system.

b

7. Nitrous acid (HNO_2) alters which of the following bases? (a) thymine and guanine (b) adenine and guanine (c) adenine and cytosine (d) cytosine and thymine

c

8. Which of the following is a base analogue of adenine? (a) 2-Aminopurine (b) 2-Mercaptovaline (c) 56-Dimethylamine (d) 4-Fluorouracil

a

9. Prototrophic bacteria (a) require a large amount of supplemental nutrients. (b) are virtually self sustaining. (c) cannot reproduce (d) none of the above

b

SHORT ANSWER QUESTIONS FOR REVIEW

10. The _____ is calculated by using the
    formula $\mu = \frac{1}{2}(1-f)X$, where f is the
    reproductive fitness of the abnormal gene
    and X is the frequency of the abnormal
    individual in one generation. (a) Romberg
    rate (b) mortality rate (c) morbidity rate
    (d) mutation rate

    d

11. Alleles are (a) any genes controlling the
    same trait. (b) genes on the same locus of
    a chromosome controlling the same trait. (c)
    genes controlling one trait that are able to
    recombine. (d) genes unable to control the
    same trait.

    b

12. A man with type A blood marries a woman
    with type AB blood. What are the different
    blood types their children could have? (a)
    A only (b) AB only (c) A and AB (d)
    A, B, and AB

    d

13. In a certain species these three alleles have
    a locus on chromosome 1. $(g+, g^1, g^2)$.
    Another series of alleles have their locus
    on chromosome $2(K^1, K^2, K^3, K^4, K^5)$.
    Theoretically there should be _____
    genotypes with respect to these two allelic
    series. (a) 45 (b) 90 (c) 135 (d) 180

    b

14. If intercalation of a chemical mutagen occurs
    on the template strand, a(n) _____ occurs.
    (a) transcription (b) translation (c)
    addition (d) depletion

    c

15. Ethyl ethanesulfonate causes (a) addition
    of an ethyl group to cytosine. (b) addition
    of an ethyl group to guanine. (c) additioon
    of an ethyl group to adenine. (d) addition
    of an ethyl group to thymine.

    b

Fill in the blanks.

16. The _____ involves the addition of possible
    chemical mutagens to a specific strain of
    Salmonella typhimurium.

    Ames test

17. When _____ is induced into DNA, thymine
    dimers result.

    ultra-violet
    light

SHORT ANSWER QUESTIONS FOR REVIEW

18. In order for photoreactivation to occur, at least one _____ must be present.

photon

19. 5-Bromouracil is a _____ that closely resembles _____.

base analogue, thymine

20. _____ resistance occurs randomly before the introduction of the chemical.

Preadaptive

21. The _____ method tests for mutations on the X chromosome.

Muller-5

22. Mutations are _____ occurences, some of which do not appear for many generations.

rare

23. Allelism can be tested for through _____.

genetic crosses

24. Penetrance differs from expressivity in that penetrance deals with the function of the gene at the _____ level, while expressivity deals with the function of each gene _____.

population, individually

25. _____ occurs when a single gene locus has more than one phenotypic effect.

Pleiotropy

26. _____ are agents that can induce mutations.

Mutagens

27. Both penetrance and expressivity are functions of the interactions of a given _____ with the environment.

genotype

28. A good example of a trait with _____ in humans is blood type.

multiple alleles

Determine whether the following statements are true or false.

29. The only way to detect a mutation is through visible differences.

False

30. Radiation doses are not cumulative with respect to induced mutations.

False

31. Postadaptive resistance occurs when the presence of a chemical in a medium induces resistance.

True

183

| Answer

To be covered
when testing
yourself

32. Hemophilia A differs from Huntington's disease in that Hemophilia A occurs as a spontaneous mutation while Huntington's disease has a gradual onset. | False

33. Multiple alleles are three or more genes that control a certain trait. | True

34. It is possible for a man with type B blood and a woman with type O blood to have a child with type A blood. | False

35. Mendelian inheritance cannot be applied to organisms containing multiple alleles. | False

36. If there are more than 2 alleles controlling a trait, there will be an order of dominance. | True

37. There are some cases where both parents have a recessive trait yet their children do not. | True

38. Acridine bases intercalate two adjacent bases causing additions and depletions. | True

39. Some mutations occur without any alterations of the amino acid sequence. | False

40. A prototroph is also called the wild type. | True

41. If a cross between two recessive mutants is normal, the mutations are on the same loci and are alleles. | False

42. Adenine and guanine are pyrimidines. | False

43. During replica plating, the colonies that grow on the original medium only contain a mutation. | True

CHAPTER 6

GENETIC INTERACTIONS

CODOMINANCE

● **PROBLEM** 6-1

In snapdragons, plants homozygous for red have red flowers; those homozygous for white have white flowers, and those which are heterozygous have pink. If a pink flowered snapdragon is crossed with a white flowered plant, what will be the expected phenotypic results in the progeny?

Solution: This is a case of incomplete dominance. Red (R), White (R') Heterozygous pink individuals are RR'.

	Pink flowered		White flowered
Genotypes	RR'	X	R'R'
Types of gametes:	R R'		R' R'

Types of gametes

	R	R'
R'	RR'	R'R'
R'	RR'	R'R'

Phenotypic results:

1/2 R'R   pink

1/2 R'R'   white

The color and shape of radishes is controlled by 2 pairs of alleles that sort independently and show no dominance. Round shape is controlled by the L' allele; length is controlled by the L allele. Heterozygous radishes (LL') are oval. The R alleles produces red radishes and the R' allele produces white. Purple flowers are produced by RR' heterozygous plants. Using the checkerboard method, diagram a cross between red long (RRLL) and white round (R'R'L'L') radishes to get the F1 phenotypic and genotypic results. Then using a Punnett square, show a cross between F1 progeny to obtain F2. Summarize the F2 phenotypic and genotypic results.

<u>Solution</u>: P: RRLL X R'R'L'L

Gametes: RL X R'L'

F1: RR'LL'

All of the F1 progeny are purple and oval.

F1 cross: R'RLL' X RR'LL'

Gametes	RL	RL'	R'L	R'L'
RL	RRLL	RRLL'	RR'LL	RR'LL'
RL'	RRLL'	RRL'L'	RR'LL'	RR'L'L'
R'L	RR'LL	RR'LL'	R'R'LL	R'R'LL'
R'L'	RR'LL'	RR'L'L'	R'R'LL'	R'R'L'L'

F2 results:

Phenotypes	Genotypes	Genotypic ratio	Phenotypic ratio
red, long	RRLL	1	1
red, oval	RRLL'	2	2
red, round	RRL'L'	1	1
purple, long	RR'LL	2	2
purple, oval	RR'LL'	4	4
purple, round	RR'L'L'	2	2
white, long	R'R'LL	1	1
white, oval	R'R'LL'	2	2
white, round	R'R'L'L'	1	1

Because dominance is not expressed, the genotypic and phenotypic ratios are identical.

EPISTASIS

● **PROBLEM** 6-3

What is epistasis? Distinguish between the terms epistasis and dominance.

Genotypes	A_B_	A_bb	aaB_	aabb
Classical ratio	9	3	3	1
Dominant epistasis	12		3	1
Recessive epistasis	9	3	4	
Duplicate genes with cumulative effect	9	6		1
Duplicate dominant genes	15			1
Duplicate recessive genes	9	7		
Dominant and recessive interaction	13		3	

Solution: Several genes are usually required to specify the enzymes involved in metabolic pathways leading to phenotypic expression. Each step in the pathway is catalyzed by different enzymes specified by different wild-type genes. Genetic interaction occurs whenever two or more genes specify enzymes involved in a common pathway. If any one of the genes is mutant, the pathway is blocked and genes after it in the pathway cannot have any phenotypic effect. We normally say that the mutant gene is epistatic to the suppressed gene.

When epistasis is involved in a dihybrid cross, the classical 9:3:3:1 ratio is modified into ratios which are various combinations of the classical groupings, resulting in less than four phenotypes. Six types of epistatic ratios are commonly recognized. A summary of them appears in the table.

Epistasis can involve any of these ratios. Examples of them will be shown in following problems.

Dominance involves <u>intra-allelic</u> gene suppression, where masking effects are seen between alleles at the same locus. Epistasis involves <u>inter-allelic</u> gene suppression between genes of different loci.

● **PROBLEM 6-4**

Two independently assorting loci, (c) and (a), control coat color in mice. Mice which are homozygous for recessive (c) cannot synthesize pigment, and thus have white hair (albino). Mice which are homozygous for (a) have completely black hair. It is thought that the (a) locus is involved in pigment placement, because in the case of (aa), melanin is distributed throughout the hair; but, when the dominant allele A is present, the melanin only goes to parts of the hair, resulting in a grayish coat called "agouti". Of course, this color cannot occur when the mice have the albino alleles, (cc), no matter what (a) alleles are present. Consider a cross between black with (CCaa) genotypes and white mice carrying (ccAA) genes. What are the phenotypic ratios for the F1 and F2 generations?

	black CCaa	x	albino ccAA
P			

(Ca) (cA)

	agouti CcAa	x	agouti CcAa
F₁			

F₂

	(CA)	(Ca)	(cA)	(ca)
(CA)	CCAA agouti	CCAa agouti	CcAA agouti	CcAa agouti
(Ca)	CCAa agouti	CCaa black	CcAa agouti	Ccaa black
(cA)	CcAA agouti	CcAa agouti	ccAA albino	ccAa albino
(ca)	CcAa agouti	Ccaa black	ccAa albino	ccaa albino

Summary: 9/16 agouti, 3/16 black,
4/16 albino

188

Solution: When genes exhibit epistasis, the genotypes are exactly the same as in other multihybrid crosses. Only the phenotypic ratios are different. The Punnett square for the cross is shown in the diagram.

The F1 progeny are all (CcAa). They express the agouti pattern because (Aa) is producing the pigment and (Cc) is distributing it to parts of the hairs.

F2 progeny were classified as 9 agouti, 3 colored, and 4 albino. This is a recessive epistasis ratio. cc is epistatic to A_ in this case. The pigment-distributing gene (A) cannot be expressed because there is no pigment to distribute. (A_) is masked when (cc) is present and results in the same phenotype as (ccaa) does. This produces the 9:3:4 ratio.

● PROBLEM 6-5

A walnut-combed rooster is mated to three hens. Hen A, which is walnut-combed, has offspring in ratio of 3 walnut : 1 rose. Hen B, which is pea-combed, has offspring in the ratio of 3 walnut : 3 pea : 1 rose : 1 single. Hen C, which is walnut-combed, has only walnut-combed offspring. What are the genotypes of the rooster and the three hens?

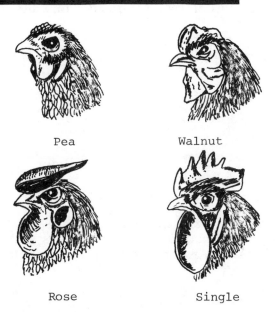

Pea   Walnut

Rose   Single

Types of combs in chickens.

Solution: This problem is an illustration of crosses in which there is gene product interaction. Interaction is usually indicated when the ratios observed in the offspring cannot be explained by simple dominant-recessive or codominant relationships or linkage. The usual method of interaction is one in which one gene or gene pair masks the expression of another non-allelic gene or gene pair. This is called epistasis. Epistasis can occur in conjunction with dominant-recessive and/or codominant relationships, as it does in this problem. This can best be illustrated by looking at the different genotypes that are possible.

Let R be the dominant allele for rose comb, and r its recessive allele, and let P be the dominant allele for pea comb and p its recessive allele. These four alleles interact in the following manner: the alleles R and P act codominantly to produce walnut comb (they are called coepistatic alleles). Each is dominant over both recessive alleles. When neither dominant allele is present, the single comb trait is expressed by the recessive alleles. In summary:

$$
\begin{array}{lll}
\text{R-pp (RRpp;Rrpp)} & = & \text{rose comb} \\
\text{rrP- (rrPP;rrPp)} & = & \text{pea comb} \\
\text{R-P-(RRPP; RRPp; RrPP; RrPp)} & = & \text{walnut comb} \\
\text{rrpp} & = & \text{single comb}
\end{array}
$$

Let us look at each cross and see what they tell us about the possible genotypes of the rooster and hens involved. Then we can coordinate what we have learned from each cross to determine the exact phenotypes.

In the cross between the rooster and Hen A (each walnut andR-P-):

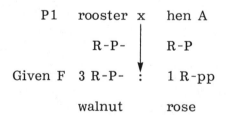

Since rose-combed offspring (R-pp) were produced, each parent must have had one recessive P gene to donate. This tells us that the rooster is R-Pp and the Hen R-Pp.

In the cross between the rooster (now known to be R-Pp) and Hen B (pea-combed and therefore rrP-):

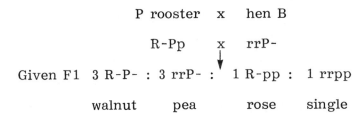

P rooster   x   hen B

R-Pp   x   rrP-

Given F1   3 R-P- : 3 rrP- : 1 R-pp : 1 rrpp

walnut   pea   rose   single

The fact that single-combed progeny resulted means that each parent must have both an r and a p to donate. Therefore, the R-Pp rooster has to be RrPp and the rrP- hen has to be rrPp.

In the cross between the rooster (RrPp) and hen C (walnut-combed and R-P-):

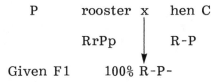

P   rooster x   hen C

RrPp   R-P

Given F1   100% R-P-

Here, since only walnut-combed progeny resulted, hen c can carry no recessive alleles; otherwise, pea (R-pp) or rose (rrP-) would have been produced. Therefore, c is RRPP.

We can now go back and solve the first cross. If the rooster is RrPp:

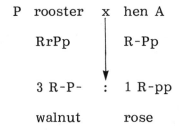

P rooster   x   hen A

RrPp   R-Pp

3 R-P-   :   1 R-pp

walnut   rose

If Hen A had an r gene at (-), then the progeny of the rrP- or pea-combed type would have been produced; but none were. So Hen A must be RRPp. Note that we also know that no single-combed progeny were produced. Therefore, all 4 recessive alleles cannot be present in the total genotypes of both parents. Since we already have 3 recessive known alleles (-) must be R, and again, Hen A is RRPp.

Summarizing:

       rooster   is   RrPp,
       hen A   is   RRPp,
       hen B   is   rrPp, and
       hen C   is   RRPP.

Doing the crosses verifies the results with the ratios obtained.

1)   P   rooster x   hen A

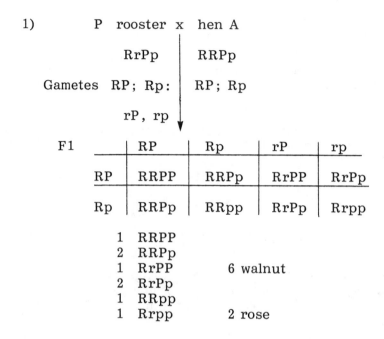

                RrPp | RRPp

      Gametes RP; Rp: | RP; Rp

                rP, rp ↓

F1		RP	Rp	rP	rp
RP		RRPP	RRPp	RrPP	RrPp
Rp		RRPp	RRpp	RrPp	Rrpp

```
1  RRPP
2  RRPp
1  RrPP        6 walnut
2  RrPp
1  RRpp
1  Rrpp        2 rose
```

Since 6/2 = 3/1, the ratio is 3 walnut : 1 rose.

2)   P   rooster   hen B

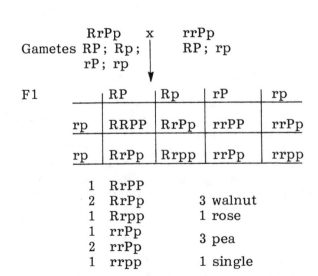

            RrPp   x   rrPp
      Gametes RP; Rp; | RP; rp
            rP; rp ↓

F1		RP	Rp	rP	rp
rp		RRPP	RrPp	rrPP	rrPp
rp		RrPp	Rrpp	rrPP	rrpp

```
1  RrPP
2  RrPp        3 walnut
1  Rrpp        1 rose
1  rrPp
2  rrPp        3 pea
1  rrpp        1 single
```

The ratio is 3 walnut : 3 pea : 1 rose : 1 single.

3)   P   rooster   x   hen C

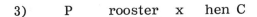

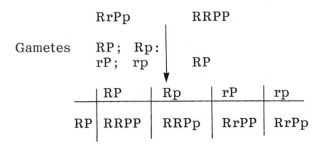

	RP	Rp	rP	rp
RP	RRPP	RRPp	RrPP	RrPp

All the offspring are walnut.

In snapdragons, the genes R and T are necessary for tall plants. In the absence of either or both genes, a plant will be dwarf. For the following crosses, determine the phenotypic ratio for the progeny:

a) Rr   tt   x   Rr   Tt ♂

b) Rr   Tt   x   rr   tt ♂

Solution: a) We use the Punnett square to get:

♀ \ ♂	RT	Rt	rT	rt
Rt	RR Tt tall	RR tt dwarf	Rr Tt tall	Rr tt dwarf
rt	Rr Tt tall	Rr tt dwarf	rr Tt dwarf	rr tt dwarf

Thus, the phenotypic ratio will be 5 swarf : 3 tall.

b) The Punnett square constructed for this cross will yield:

♀ \ ♂	rt	
RT	Rr Tt	tall
Rt	Rr tt	dwarf
rT	rr Tt	dwarf
rt	rr tt	dwarf

Thus, the phenotypic ratio will be 3 dwarf : 1 tall.

In cultivated flowers, called "stocks", pigment is controlled by two independently assorting alleles. When the dominant allele A is present at one locus, C at the other locus leads to red; cc leads to cream. The double recessive aa at the first locus produces a white flower regardless of alleles at the second locus.

(a) If a homozygous red stock is crossed with a white variety, what phenotypic and genotypic ratios are expected in the F1 and F2 generations?

(b) If a cross between a red stock and a white stock produces progeny of all three phenotypes, what are the genotypes of the parents?

(c) Come up with a possible mechanism to explain this phenotypic action.

Solution: (a) A cross between an AACC stock and an aacc stock will result in the following:

P: AACC   x   aacc

       red   white

Gametes: AC   x   ac

     F1: AaCc, all cream

     F1 gametes: AC, Ac, aC, ac

     F2 genotypes:

194

	AC	Ac	aC	ac
AC	AACC	AACc	AaCC	AaCc
Ac	AACc	AAcc	AaCc	Aacc
aC	AaCC	AaCc	aaCC	aaCc
ac	AaCc	Aacc	aaCc	aacc

F2 phenotypes: 9 red : 3 cream : 4 white

This is an example of recessive epistasis, known because of the phenotypic ratio. The recessive aa is epistatic to the C-locus.

(b) For a flower to be red it must be AACC, AACc, AaCC, or AaCc. The white parent has to be aaCC, aaCc, or aacc. Looking at the possible red parents, we can eliminate AACC and AaCC because cream (A_cc) progeny cannot come from these parents. They both have CC genotypes and cannot give their progeny to the c allele needed for cream color. The white aaCC can also be eliminated as a possible parent for the same reason.

The red parent of the AACc genotype can also be eliminated, since its progeny can never be white. White flowers are homozygous for aa, but flowers will not be white if a parent is homozygous for AA since a parent cannot give any a alleles.

When the remaining possibilities are crossed, all three phenotypes result. These two crosses are AaCc x aaCc and AaCc x aacc. Punnett squares can be worked out for these and all possible crosses to prove that these two crosses are the only ones that produce red, cream, and white progeny.

(c) One mechanism that explains recessive epistasis is shown in the diagram.

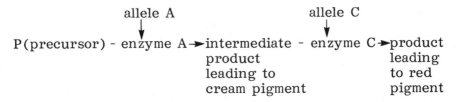

The A and C alleles are needed in the pathway leading to red flowers. If enzyme A is not produced because of a homozygous aa condition, the pathway is blocked and all flowers are white. Enzyme A produces pigment for cream flowers. If enzyme C is present, the pathway is completed and all flowers are red. If enzyme C is not present in this case, the pathway is stopped at this point and flowers are cream colored.

● **PROBLEM** 6-8

How may a classic Mendelian 9:3:3:1 ratio be converted into a (a) 9:7 or a (b) 15:1 ratio?

Solution: When epistasis is operating between two gene loci the number of phenotypes in F2 generations is less than four. When two phenotypes are seen in a 9:7 ratio, duplicate recessive genes are acting to produce identical phenotypes; two dominant genes are necessary to complement each other and express the trait. For example, if both A and B were needed for pigment formation, the following results would be expected:

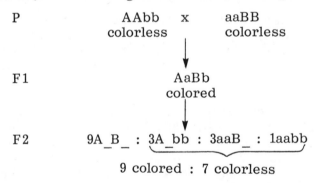

P   AAbb   x   aaBB
                  colorless   colorless

F1   AaBb
                          colored

F2   9A_B_ : 3A_bb : 3aaB_ : 1aabb

               9 colored : 7 colorless

When a 15:1 ratio is seen, duplicate dominant genes are producing the same phenotype without a cumulative effect. When either dominant allele is present the trait is expressed. If the genes suppressed pigment formation, the following would result:

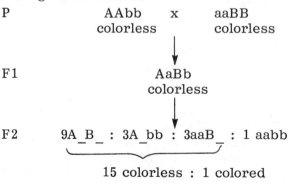

P   AAbb   x   aaBB
                  colorless   colorless

F1   AaBb
                          colorless

F2   9A_B_ : 3A_bb : 3aaB_ : 1 aabb

               15 colorless : 1 colored

196

In chickens, comb shape is controlled by two pairs of independent genes, R vs. r and P vs. p. The following genotypic combinations represent the interactions and the phenotypes that result:

R_ P_ = walnut   rr P_ = pea

R_ pp = rose   rr pp = single

Determine the expected phenotypic ratios of the progeny for each of the matings below:

a) rr Pp ♀ x Rr Pp ♂

b) Rr pp ♀ x rr Pp ♂

Solution: a) We construct the Punnett square for this cross to get:

♀ \ ♂	RP	Rp	rP	rp
rP	Rr PP walnut	Rr Pp walnut	rr PP pea	rr Pp pea
rp	RrPp walnut	Rr pp rose	rr Pp pea	rr pp single

Thus, the phenotypic ratio is 3 walnut : 3 pea : 1 rose : 1 single.

b) The Punnett square for this cross yields:

♀ \ ♂	rP	rp
Rp	Rr Pp walnut	Rr pp rose
r p	rr Pp pea	rr pp single

The phenotypic ratio observed is 1 walnut : 1 rose : 1 pea : 1 single.

POLYGENIC INHERITANCE

Kernel color in wheat is determined by the action of two pairs of polygenes that produce colors varying from dark red to white. If AABB (dark red) and aabb (white) are crossed,

(a) What fraction of the F2 generation can be expected to be like either parent?

(b) How many F2 phenotypic classes result?

Solution: This problem is based on the principle of polygenic inheritance. Polygenic inheritance differs from the classical Mendelian pattern in that the whole range of variation is covered in a graded series. In polygenic inheritance certain assumptions are made:

1. Each contributing gene in the series produces an equal effect.

2. Effects of each contributing allele are cumulative.

3. There is no dominance.

4. There is no epistasis among genes of different loci.

5. No linkage is involved.

6. Environmental effects are either absent or may be ignored.

(a) If we symbolize the genes for red with the capital letters A and B, and the alleles resulting in lack of pigment production by a and b, the cross can be diagrammed like this:

P: AABB   x   aabb
       dark red   white

Gametes: AB   x   ab

F1:   AaBb
              intermediate red

F2	AB	Ab	aB	ab
AB	AABB	AABb	AaBB	AaBb
Ab	AABb	AAbb	AaBb	Aabb
aB	AaBB	AaBb	aaBB	aaBb
ab	AaBb	Aabb	aaBb	aabb

Assuming each capital allele increases the depth of color equally, we can classify the F2 generation in this way:

Number of Genes for Red	Genotype	Phenotype	Fraction of F2
4	AABB	dark red	1/16
3	AABb, AaBB	medium red	4/16
2	AAbb, aaBB, AaBb	intermediate red	6/16
1	aaBb, Aabb	light red	4/16
0	aabb	white	1/16

We can see that 2/16 of the F2 generation resembles either parent from the P generation, 1/16 of white and 1/16 of dark red.

(b) As shown in the above table, there are a total of 5 phenotypic F2 classes.

● **PROBLEM 6-11**

Skin color in humans is an example of a polygenic trait. What is a polygenic trait, and why were the early results of the Davenports' experiments with skin color found to be oversimplified?

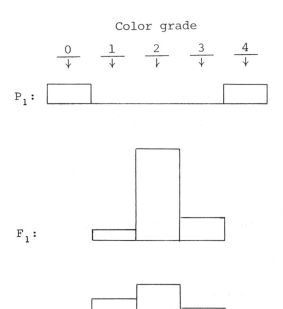

Color grade

0   1   2   3   4

P_1:

F_1:

F_2:

Solution: Polygenic traits are traits that show a continuous variation in phenotypes instead of distinct classifications such as red and white. When polygenes are in operation, pinks are also present.

A quantitative basis for skin color measurement was postulated by G.C. and C.B. Davenport in 1913. The Davenports measured the grades of color by matching them to a rotating color wheel in which various proportions of different colors could be obtained. The colors were graded on a scale from 0 (very light) to 4 (very dark) depending on the size of the black area on the color wheel. They then measured skin color in 29 F1 offspring which had one black and one white parent and in 32F2 progeny from two mulatto parents. The results are shown diagramatically in the figure.

The F2 generation consisted of approximately a 1:4:6:4:1 ratio, the one expected if they were dealing with two independently assorting gene pairs showing incomplete dominance and additivity. If we consider Mendel's law of segregation and assortment and each F2 grade is considered a genotype, then 0 grade can be taken as aabb, grade 1 can be taken as Aabb or aaBb, grade 2 can be taken as AaBb, AABb, AaBB, or AABB, and so on.

Recent studies using a fixed wavelength of light and measuring skin reflections show a continuous distribution of skin color instead of a series of discrete classes. Determination of skin color is more complicated than the

Davenports' model. More genes are probably involved, and it is not likely to be a simple case of incomplete dominance.

Height in a certain plant species is controlled by two pairs of independently assorting alleles, with each participating allele A or B adding 5 cm to a base height of 5 cm. A cross is made between parents with genotype AABB and aabb. Disregarding environmental influences,

(a) What are the heights of each parent?
(b) What is the expected height of the members of the F1 generation?
(c) What are the expected phenotypic ratios in the F2 generation?

Solution: Base height = 5 cm

Since each allele contributes an additional 5 cm, we use the following formula:

Total height = (each effective allele x 5cm) + base height

(a) Height of AABB = (4 x 5cm) + 5 cm

Height of AABB = 25 cm

Height of aabb = 0 + 5 cm

Height of aabb = 5 cm

(b)   P: AABB   x   aabb

Gametes: AB   x   ab

F1:   AaBb

Height of AaBb = (2 x 5) + 5

= 15

201

(c) The possible F2 progeny are:

	AB	Ab	aB	ab
AB	AABB	AABb	AaBB	AaBb
Ab	AABb	AAbb	AaBb	Aabb
aB	AaBB	AaBb	aaBB	aaBb
ab	AaBb	Aabb	aaBb	aabb

The genotypes and phenotypes of the F2 can be arranged in tabular form.

Genotype	Number of Genes for Height	Fraction of F_2	Height
AABB	4	1/16	25
AABb, AaBB	3	4/16	20
AAbb, aaBB, AaBb	2	6/16	15
aaBb, Aabb	1	4/16	10
aabb	0	1/16	5

● **PROBLEM 6-13**

The weight of the fruit in one variety of squash is determined by three pairs of genes. The homozygous dominant condition, AABBCC, results in 6-pound squashes, and the homozygous recessive condition, aabbcc, results in 3-pound squashes. Each dominant gene adds 1/2 pound to the minimum 3-pound weight. When a plant having 6-pound squashes is crossed with one having 3-pound squashes, all the offspring have 4 1/2-pound fruit.

What would be the weights of the F2 fruit, if two of these F1 plants were crossed?

Solution: This problem deals with polygenic inheritance; that is, the situation in which two or more independent pairs of genes have similar and additive effects on the same characteristic. Examples of such inheritance are height and skin color in man, and commercially important characteristics in animals and plants, such as the amount of eggs and milk produced, the size of fruit, and so on.

In the cross between a 6-pound squash plant and a 3-pound squash plant:

P1	AABBCC	x	aabbcc
Gametes	ABC		abc

F1   100% AaBbCc

We are told that each dominant gene adds 1/2 pound to the weight. The presence of 3 dominant genes in F1 (A, B, and C) would increase the weight by 1/2 + 1/2 + 1/2 or 1 1/2 lbs. Therefore, each squash from F1 weighs

3 + 1 1/2   or   4 1/2 pounds.

In the cross between two F1 plants, we must first determine the possible gametes from each plant. The number of possible gametes is obtained using the 2^n rule, where n is the number of heterozygous traits and 2^n is the total number of different gametes formed. For each parent, n is equal to 3. Therefore, the number of gametes is 2^3 or 8.

The genotypes of these gametes can be obtained by dichotomous branching, which ensures that all possible combinations are considered. Each possible gene from each allelic pair is matched to every possible gene combination of the other two pairs as follows:

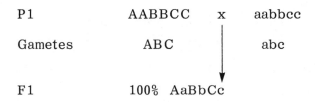

Gametes

			Gametes
	B	C	ABC
		c	ABc
A			
	b	C	AbC
		c	Abc
	B	C	aBC
		c	aBc
a			
	b	C	abC
		c	abc

Looking at the cross:

	1 2 3		1 2 3
P1	Aa Bb Cc	x	Aa Bb Cc

Gametes	ABC;ABc;AbC;Abc;	ABC;ABC;AbC;Abc,
	aBC;aBc'abc;abc;	aBC;aBc;abC;abc

Separating the trihybrid cross into three monohybrid crosses, and then using dichotomous branching to determine all possible combinations of the results of these crosses, one obtains:

1 x 1 results	2 x 2 results	3 x 3 results	Genotypes	Phenotypes (weight in pounds)
		1CC	1 AABBCC	6
	1BB——2Cc		2 AABBCc	5 1/2
		1cc	1 AABBcc	5
		1CC	2 AABbCC	5 1/2
AA——2Bb——2cc	4(2x2)	AABbCc	5
		1cc 1CC	2 AABbcc	4 1/2
	1bb——2Cc		1 AAbbCC	5
		1cc	2 AAbbCc	4 1/2
		1cc	1 AAbbcc	4
	1BB——2Cc		2 AaBBCC	5 1/2
		1cc 1CC	r(2x2)	AaBBCc	5
2Aa——2Bb——1Cc			2 AaBBcc	4 1/2
		1cc 1CC	4(2x2)	AaBbCC	5
	1bb——2Cc	8(2x2x2)	AaBbCc	4 1/2
		1cc	4(2x2)	AaBbcc	4
			2 AabbCC	4 1/2
		4(2x2)	AabbCc	4
		1CC		
	1BB——2Cc		2 Aabbcc	3 1/2
		1cc	1 aaBBCC	5
		1cc	2 aaBBCc	4 1/2

204

```
1aa ——— 2Bb ——— 2Cc
                  1cc                    1 aaBBcc        4
                  1cc                    2 aaBbCC        4 1/2
        1bb ——— 2Cc                        aaBbCc        4
                       4(2x2)            2 aaBbcc        3 1/2
                  1cc
                                         1 aabbCC        4
                                         2 aabbCc        3 1/2
                                         1 aabbcc        3
```

Summarizing: 1/64   weighs 6 pounds
                6/64   weighs 5 1/2 pounds
                15/64   weighs 5 pounds
                20/64   weighs 4 1/2 pounds
                15/64   weighs 4 pounds
                6/64   weighs 3 1/2 pounds
                1/64   weighs 3 pounds

It is important to be able to associate quantitative characteristics with polygenic inheritance. The cross itself is not difficult but may at times be tedious. (Note: this problem could also have been done using the Punnett square, but dichotomous branching is more frequently used in crosses involving three or more traits.)

● PROBLEM 6-14

Two 30" plants are crossed, resulting in progeny of the following ratio: one 22", eight 24", twenty-eight 26", fifty-six 28", seventy 30", fifty-six 32", twenty-eight 34", eight 36", and one 38". Starting with "A" and going through the alphabet to represent different alleles, what are the most probable genotypes of the parents?

Solution: The total number of phenotypic classes in the F2 generation is given by the formula:

$$\text{\# of phenotypes} = 2n + 1,$$

where n = the number of pairs of polygenes.

There are 9 phenotypic classes, so:

205

$$2n + 1 = 9$$

$$n = \frac{8}{2} = 4 = \text{total number of pairs of polygenes}$$

We can symbolize the genes for height with the capital letters "A" through "D" and their corresponding alleles with the lower case letters "a" through "d". Because the height of both parent plants is 30" their genotypes must be identical. The only genotypes that could have produced the phenotypes in the same ratio as resulted are AaBbCcDd x AaBbCcDd. If you are not convinced of this, work this cross out with a Punnett square or the forked-line method to prove it.

● **PROBLEM** 6-15

Two races of corn averaging 48 and 72 inches in height are crossed. The height of the F1 generation does not vary very much, averaging 60 inches. When 500 of these plants were classified, two were 48 inches, and two were 72 inches, the rest falling between these in height. What is the number of polygenes involved, and how many inches does each contribute?

Solution : The fraction of the F2 generation, like a single parent, is given by the formula $(\frac{1}{4})^n$ where n=the number of pairs of polygenes.

In the F2 generation, two out of 500 are 48" in height and two are 72". Therefore, the fraction of F2 like a single parent

$$= \frac{2}{500} = \frac{1}{250}$$

Considering the formula $(\frac{1}{4})^n$ we see that the series goes $\frac{1}{4}$ when n = 1, 1/16 when n = 2, 1/64 when n = 3, etc. 1/250 is closest to 1/256, when n = 4. Therefore, we must be dealing with four pairs of alleles, or eight polygenes.

The total height difference between the shortest and tallest plants in the F2 is 72-48-24. Dividing 24 into the total number of polygenes, 8, we can find how much height each polygene contributes to the plant:

$$\frac{24''}{8} = 3''$$

Flower length varies between two strains of a certain plant. This is due to a specific number of polygenes. Using the data given below, find approximately how many genes are in the series.

Group	Mean $(\bar{X})$	Variance (s^2)	Cause of variation
Strain A	21 mm	1.43 mm^2	Environment
Strain B	39	1.16	Environment
F1(AxB)	30	1.80	Environment
F2(F1xF1)	30	5.10	Genes, environment

Solution: The number of genes can be calculated by the formula:

$$n = \left(\frac{1}{8}\right) \left(\frac{R}{V_F - V_F}\right)$$

R is the difference between the mean values of the two inbred strains.

V_{F1} and V_{F2} are the variances of the F1 and F2 generations produced as a result of a hybrid cross of the two strains.

Substituting the values from the table into the problem,

$$n = \left(\frac{1}{8}\right) \left(\frac{(39 - 21)^2}{5.10 - 1.80}\right)$$

$$= \left(\frac{1}{8}\right) \left(\frac{324}{3.30}\right)$$

$$= \left(\frac{324}{(8)(3.30)}\right)$$

$$= 12.27 \text{ or } \sim 12 \text{ gene pairs}$$

207

One must be careful in using such a formula. The formula assumes that each gene in a series either affects the trait completely or not at all. It also assumes that the affect of any allele is equal to that of any other allele. These assumptions are not necessarily true. Therefore, the answer can only be an estimate of the actual number.

● **PROBLEM 6-17**

Although it is possible to categorize eye color in humans into blue or brown phenotypic classes, there are clearly many variations in hue within the 2 classes. What type of inheritance mechanism may be working to produce eye color?

Solution: Human eye color can be regarded as controlled by one principal gene that is influence by other genes called modifiers. The main gene has two alleles - dominant B for brown eyes and recessive b for blue eyes. Blue eyes (b/b) owe their color to the scattering of white light by the almost colorless cells of the outer iris. This affect is greatest in the shorter wavelengths, the blues, thus giving the iris its blue appearance. Brown-eyed people (B/B or B/b) have melanin on the front layer of the iris and, thus, do not scatter as much light through their irises. One gene controls whether the eye will be blue or brown, but many modifier genes produce variations on the shade. Some affect the amount of pigment in the iris, some the tone of the pigment, and some the distribution of the pigment. These modifiers can lead to variations on the blue tone, as in the case of gray or green eyes; or, they can change brown pigment, leading to brown variations such as black. Two blue-eyed people can occassionally have a brown-eyed child because one of them has a lack of pigmentation due to modifier genes and actually has the B/b genotype.

● **PROBLEM 6-18**

What is meant by the term transgressive segregation? How can it be explained?

Solution: Transgressive segregation is seen when the variability of an F2 generation is so great that some individuals show more extreme development than either parental type. Assuming all of the contributing alleles act with equal and cumulative effects, transgressive segregation can be demonstrated with this example:

Let capital letters stand for active growth alleles and small letters stand for noncontributing alleles. Considering three loci, transgressive segregation is possible if the parental genotypes are as follows:

P: aaBBCC   x   AAbbcc

F1:   AaBbCc

F2:
      AABBCC _____aabbcc

(positive transgression)   (negative transgression)

In this case one parent has four active alleles and the other has two. All F1 are intermediate with three active alleles. Genotypes of F2 have segregated out so that some individuals have six active alleles and some have none. Both of these types are more extreme than the parental generation F2. The progeny's five or six active alleles represent positive transgression because they contain more active alleles than the parents. F2, with zero or one active allele, represents negative transgression.

PLEIOTROPISM

● PROBLEM 6-19

How can a single gene pair have more than one phenotype effect? Use sickle cell anemia as an example.

Fig. 1

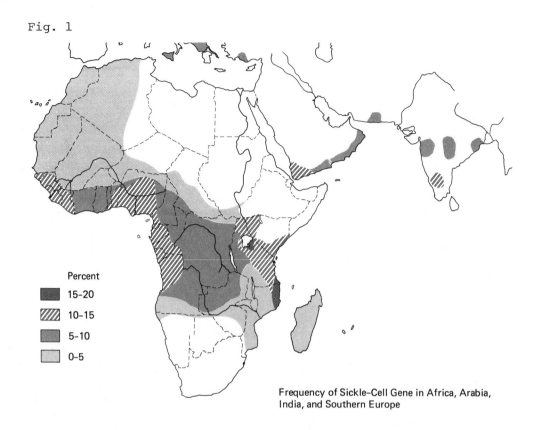

Percent
- 15–20
- 10–15
- 5–10
- 0–5

Frequency of Sickle–Cell Gene in Africa, Arabia, India, and Southern Europe

Solution: This problem is based on the phenomenon known as pleiotropism. A pleiotropic condition is one in which a single gene pair influences more than one trait.

Sickle cell anemia is a mutation that exhibits pleiotropy. It is present in the heterozygous state in about one out of every ten U.S. blacks. In sickle cell anemia, an amino acid in the sixth position of the beta chain is changed from glutamic acid to valine. People with the homozygous condition suffer from sickle cell anemia; those with the heterozygous condition have the sickle cell trait, a much less serious problem than the disease.

The change in the beta chain is produced as a result of a codon transversion from AT to TA. As a result the mutant mRNA replaces the base U for A as the middle base in the triplet code. The altered triplet code then codes for the amino acid valine.

The phenotypic effects resulting from this amino acid change are varied. Sickling crises occur in homozygous people when red blood cells, with their irregular spindle shape, clog small blood vessels and cut off oxygen supply to certain tissues as a result of decreased oxygen-carrying capacity. The chain of reactions occurring as a result of the transversion mutation are shown in Figure 2.

Fig. 2

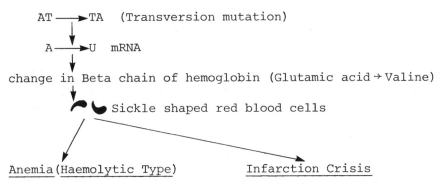

AT ——▶TA   (Transversion mutation)

A——▶U mRNA

change in Beta chain of hemoglobin (Glutamic acid → Valine)

Sickle shaped red blood cells

Anemia (Haemolytic Type)

Secondary folate deficiency

Growth retardation

Delayed puberty

Aplastic crisis

Fatigue

Infection

Leg ulcers

Cardiomegaly

Cholelithiasis

Marrow hyperplasia

Infarction Crisis

Spleen and bone infarction

Abdominal pain due to
        mesenteric infarction

Papillary necrosis of the
        kidney

Aseptic necrosis of head
        of femur

Another of the pleiotropic effects of the trait is an increased resistance to malaria. This explains why the mutation, which can result in death, has remained in gene pools, and why it is especially prevalent in malaria-ridden areas of Africa.

● **PROBLEM** 6-20

A cross between 2 yellow-haired mice results in an F1 ratio of: 2 Yellow: 1 non-yellow: 1 yellow (dies). Diagram a cross to explain these results.

$$P_1 \qquad \begin{array}{c} \text{yellow} \\ Y^l y^L \end{array} \qquad \times \qquad \begin{array}{c} \text{yellow} \\ Y^l y^L \end{array}$$

$$G_1 \qquad \tfrac{1}{2}Y^l, \ \tfrac{1}{2}y^L \qquad\qquad\qquad \tfrac{1}{2}Y^l, \ \tfrac{1}{2}y^L$$

$$F_1 \qquad \left(\begin{array}{c} \tfrac{1}{4}Y^l Y^l \\ \text{dies} \end{array}\right) \qquad \begin{array}{c} \tfrac{1}{2}Y^l y^L \\ \text{yellow} \end{array} \qquad \begin{array}{c} \tfrac{1}{4}y^L y^L \\ \text{nonyellow} \end{array}$$

Solution: This F1 ratio of 1:2:1 is characteristic of a cross between 2 monohybrids, not of a dihybrid cross. Therefore, pleiotropism must be considered. Hair color and viability both seem to be affected by the same allele pair. From the F1 ratio it can be assumed that the allele dominant for one effect is recessive for the other.

Both traits can be represented as base letters with superscripts indicating the secondary trait. Let Y symbolize the allele for the dominant gene leading to yellow and let y represent its recessive counterpart. Let the superscript l stand for the recessive lethal affect of the dominant allele Y, and let the superscript L represent the normal dominant viable affect of the recessive allele y. The surviving yellow mice can be represented genotypically as $Y^l y^L$ and the non-yellow mice can be represented as $y^L y^L$. The cross involving 2 yellow mice can be summarized as follows:

$$P \quad \begin{array}{c} Y^l y^L \\ \text{yellow} \end{array} \qquad \times \qquad \begin{array}{c} Y^l y^L \\ \text{yellow} \end{array}$$

$$F1 \quad \left[\begin{array}{c} 1 \ Y^L Y^L \\ \text{dies} \end{array}\right] + 2Y^L y^l + 1 \ y^L y^L$$

1(dies):2 yellow:1 non-yellow

● **PROBLEM 6-21**

Plants with red flowers are often observed to also have red stems while the white flowered varieties of the same species have green stems. What is this phenomenon, in which a single pair of alleles has more than one phenotypic affect? What are some other examples?

Solution: This phenomenon is called pleiotropism. The condition in which a single gene has more than one effect on an individual is called pleiotropy. Although in the given example the gene pair only affects 2 different characteristics, it can affect many more as in sickle cell anemia, which was explained in problem 6-19.

In Aquilegia vulgaris there is a gene that elicits red flowers, increases the length of the stems, confers darkness to the endosperm, and increases seed weight. A gene for white eyes in fruit flies also affects the structure and color of internal organs, causes reduced fertility, and reduces longevity.

An example of a pleiotropic affect in man is Marfan's syndrome. One gene causes both an abnormality of the eye lens and extremely long fingers.

ENVIRONMENTAL INTERACTION

● **PROBLEM 6-22**

What is a phenocopy? How can one differentiate between a phenocopy and a mutation?

Solution: A phenotype produced by the environment that simulates the effects of a known mutation is called a phenocopy. It is thought that environmental agents influence the same chemical reactions as mutations do and produce effects similar to the ones produced by mutations. Unlike mutations, phenocopies can not be inherited.

One would test to differentiate between a mutation and a phenocopy by making specific crosses in order to see whether the phenotypic change is transmitted to progeny.

By injecting boric acid into chick eggs at a particular stage of development, chickens with short legs are produced resembling the genetic "creeper" trait. A chick with shortened legs resembling the "creeper" effect can be tested to see if it was caused by a mutation or the teratogenic agent boric acid by crossing it with a normal chicken. If the abnormality was produced by the boric acid, there should not be any "creepers" in the progeny. Presumably, the teratogenic agent interferes with gene function during development but it does not permanently change genes.

● PROBLEM 6-23

Himalayan rabbits are normally white with black ears, nose, feet and tail, but if they are raised in low temperatures they will have completely black fur. Explain how this can be possible.

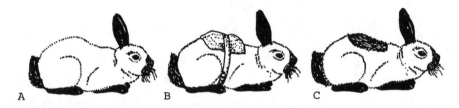

Effect of temperature on expression of a gene for coat color in the Himalayan rabbit. (A) Normally, only the feet, tail, ears, and nose are black. (B) Fur is plucked from a patch on the back, and an ice pack is applied to the area. (C) The new fur grown under the artificially low temperatures is black. Himalayan rabbits are normally homozygous for the gene that controls synthesis of the black pigment, but the gene is active only at low temperatures (below about 92^0F).

Solution: The expression of the gene for coat color in the Himalayan rabbit is temperature dependent. The Himalayan allele codes for a specific enzyme which controls pigment formation. This enzyme is temperature responsive and active only at low temperatures. In the normal environment the temperature of the extremities is below the critical temperature, but the body temperature is higher and the fur on the body remains white.

When the rabbits are reared in colder climates the enzyme is active throughout the body, producing a uniform black color. This temperature-dependent expression is also seen in Siamese cats and sun-red maize.

Himalayan rabbits reared at low temperatures are phenotypically similar to the genetically black rabbit. The two are phenocopies as a result of nongenetic factors that have changed the phenotype.

● **PROBLEM** 6-24

The mean number of abdominal bristles in a population of Drosophila melanogaster is 38. Flies with an average of 42.8 bristles were used to breed the next generation. The mean number of bristles in the F1 generation was 40.6. What is the heritability of this trait?

Solution: Heritability is a population-specific measurement. It measures the relative contributions of genetic and environmental effects on phenotypic variation. If either the genetic or environmental factors change, heritability will also change. Thus, measuring heritability for a group of organisms in two different environments, or for two different populations in the same environment, is likely to yield different results. Heritability values can range from 0 to 1. Something that is highly influenced by environment, like intelligence, will have a low heritability. Bloodtype, however, is never changed by the environment, and will have a heritability of 1. The fraction of phenotypic variation a trait exhibits due to genetic differences can be measured by the heritability of the trait. Heritability can be calculated by the formula:

$$H = \frac{G}{D}$$

G represents the selection gain - the difference between the mean of the F1 generation and the mean of the population. D stands for selection differential - the difference between the mean of the parents and the mean of the population.

Using this formula, the heritability of the bristles can be calculated for the population.

Population mean = 38

Mean of parents = 42.8

Mean of F1   = 40.6

$$D = 42.8 - 38 = 4.8$$

$$G = 40.6 - 38 = 2.6$$

Therefore, heritability can be estimated as

$$H = \frac{G}{D}$$

$$= \frac{2.6}{4.8} = 0.54$$

EXTRANUCLEAR INHERITANCE

● PROBLEM 6-25

The leaf colors resulting from crosses between different branches on variegated <u>Mirabilis</u> <u>jalapa</u> ("four o'clock") plants are shown below:

Branch of Origin of the Male parent	Branch of Origin of the Female parent	Progeny
Green	Green	Green
	Pale	Pale
	Variegated	Green,pale,variegated
Pale	Green	Green
	Pale	Pale
	Variegated	Green,pale,variegated
Variegated	Green	Green
	Pale	Pale
	Variegated	Green,pale,variegated

What is the most likely mode of inheritance?

Solution: The distribution of green pigment in leaves of the "four o'clock" plant varies from branch to branch.

216

Three basic patterns of pigment distribution have been observed: leaves on certain branches may be solid green, other branches may be variegated (green interspersed with pale spots), and still others may be completely pale. Pigment in most plants is carried by cytoplasmic organelles known as plastids. The most significant plastid is the chloroplast. Chloroplasts contain a green pigment, known as chlorophyll. Besides being responsible for the characteristic green color of many plants, it is of paramount importance in photosynthesis. Pale leaves and the pale patches of variegated leaves cannot carry out photosynthesis but they receive sustenance from chloroplast-abundant green areas.

In the early part of the 1900's a scientist named C. Correns was following the inheritance of pigment distribution traits in the "four o'clock" plant. In 1909 Correns discovered that the progeny inherit the phenotype of the female parent. In other words, ovules from fully green branches of the female plant will only grow into fully green plants, regardless of the pollen source. Ovules from a fully pale female branch will only become white plants, even if the male is green or variegated. If the mother is fully green or pale, variegated plants will never result, even in subsequent generations.

If the female is variegated, however, 3 seed types will be produced, regardless of the male phenotype: green, white and variegated. The most widely held theory assumes that a variegated ovule contains normal and abnormal plastids. An ovule with only normal plastids would yield a green plant; an ovule with abnormal plastids would yield a white plant, and a mixture of both would yield variegated plants (in majority).

This case is a classic study of cytoplasmic (maternal) inheritance. This phenomenon, when found in plants, is caused by the inheritance of chloroplastic DNA (cp DNA) from the mother.

The reason why cp DNA is maternally inherited probably lies in the mechanism of fertilization. Both animal eggs and plant embryo sacs are very large cells with much organell rich cytoplasm whereas the sperm (pollen) contains and contributes only nucleic material during fertilization.

Paramecium cells can maintain a type of bacterial species called kappa particles within their cytoplasm. Maintenance of the kappa particles is dependent upon the presence of a dominant nuclear gene K. Bacteria that have kk alleles lose the kappa particles after mitosis. A KK strain of Paramecium harboring kappa particles is crossed with a kk strain. (a) Assuming normal conjugation without cytoplasmic transfer and autogamy in the exconjugants, what are the genotypic and phenotypic results of this cross?

Fig. 1

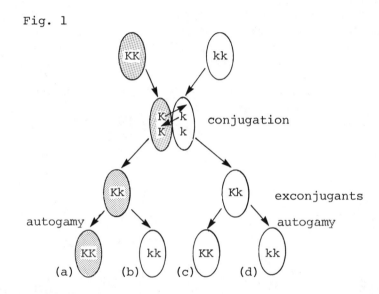

Solution: Using shading to represent the presence of kappa particles, the cross is diagrammed in Figure 1.

In this case, the conjugation exchanges genes only. The exconjugants have identical genes, but only one has kappa particles. This is because only one cell had them before, and there was no exchange of cytoplasm. Following autogamy only one cell still contains kappa particles, cell (a). Cell (b) had them immediately following autogamy, but could not maintain them without the K allele. Although cell (d) could maintain kappa particles, none were present for it to maintain. Cytoplasmic exchange would have to take place for it to obtain any. Cell (d) does not have kappa particles and could not maintain them if it did.

218

The hermaphroditic snail <u>Limnaea</u> <u>peregra</u> can reproduce either by self-fertilization, or by crossing. When snails are crossed, all the progeny are the same with respect to shell coiling. A cross between a dextral female and sinistral male yields an all dextral F1, which when self-fertilized produces all dextral progeny. When these F2 offspring are selfed, 3/4 of them give rise to dextral F3 while 1/4 produce sinistral F3. The reciprocal cross (dextral male and sinistral female) produce all sinistral F1 and all dextral F2. The F3 generation results in the same ratios as the reciprocal cross. How can these results be explained?

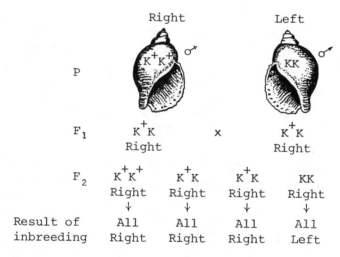

Fig. 1: Cross between K^+K^+ female and KK male

<u>Solution</u>: The direction of the coiling can either be dextral, to the right, or sinistral, going to the left. The genotype of the mother directs the coiling regardless of the genotype of the zygote. If the mother has the dominant K^+ gene for dextral, all her progeny will coil dextrally. If she is of the KK genotype, all her progeny will coil sinistrally. This is an example of maternal effect. The genotype of the father has no influence on the phenotype of the progeny.

The results of the cross described in the problem are diagrammed in Figure 1.

The F_1 are coiled dextrally (to the right) because the mother possesed the dominant K+ gene, not because the offspring's own genotype is K+K. In the F2 generation, all are dextral regardless of their own genotype because the previous generation was K+K. The generations produced after this are in a 3:1 dextral:sinistral ratio determined by the genotypic ratio of the F2 generation.

The reciprocal cross is shown in Figure 2.

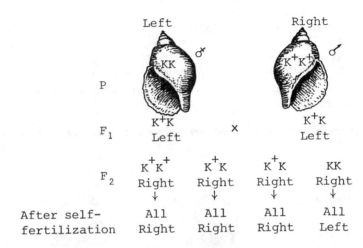

Fig. 2: Cross between KK female and K^+K^+ male

The F1 generation is sinistral (left coiled) because the maternal parent is KK. All F2 are dextral because F1 mothers all have the dominant K^+ allele. After selfing, the 3:1 dextral:sinistral ratio is produced as in the reciprocal cross because the maternal genotypes are K^+K^+ K^+K and KK in a 1:2:1 ratio and dextral is dominant.

As we have seen, a single genetic locus controls the trait for direction of coiling. What is unusual is the effect the maternal genotype has on the phenotype of the progeny regardless of the paternal genotype. Studies have shown that the expression of this locus occurs during oogenesis and that at some time before the second meiotic division the K^+ and K alleles in the maternal genome specify some property of the cytoplasm that will determine the orientation of the first cleavage furrow of the zygote. It has been shown that eggs from sinistral mothers have zygotes which cleave at a 90-degree angle to the plane of cleavage found in eggs from dextral mothers.

SHORT ANSWER QUESTIONS FOR REVIEW

Choose the correct answer.

1. If a hybrid purple radish plant of genotype
   RR' is crossed with another hybrid plant of
   identical genotype , the observed phenotypic
   ratio is one red : two pink : one white.
   What can be concluded from this ratio? (a)
   There was no crossing over. (b) Once a
   hybrid, always a hybrid. (c) Genes assort
   independently. (d) A mutation in the gene
   locus for color produced red and white
   flowers. (e) none of the above   e

2. Mice with the genotypes BB and Bb are
   black, and those with the genotype bb are
   brown. At another locus the genotypes CC
   and cc code for color while the homozygous
   recessive genotype cc codes for albinism.
   What phenotypic ratio would be expected from
   a cross between two mice with the genotype
   BbCc? (a) 9 black : 3 brown : 4 albino (b)
   12 black : 3 brown : 1 albino (c) 9 black :
   6 brown : 1 albino (d) 9 black : 0 brown :
   7 albino   a

3. What mode of inheritance is present in question
   2? (a) codominance (b) epistasis (c)
   multiple allele (d) none of the above   b

4. A 15:1 phenotypic ratio is observed in an
   F_2 generation. This ratio is characteristic
   of (a) duplicate recessive epistasis. (b)
   recessive epistasis . (c) duplicate dominant
   epistasis. (d) both a and b (e) none of the
   above   c

5. In a polygenic interaction (a) each contributing gene in the series produces an equal
   effect. (b) there is no dominance. (c) there
   is no epistasis among genes of different loci.
   (d) there is no linkage. (e) all of the above   e

6. The cross between two plants of equal heights
   results in a progeny with five different
   phenotypes. How many pairs of polygenes
   were involved? (a) 2 (b) 3 (c) 4 (d) 5   a

7. In humans brown eyes are dominant over blue
   eyes. How can two people with blue eyes

produce green eyed offspring? (a) Eye color is a result of incomplete dominance. (b) Modifier genes affect the shade, amount, and tone of pigment. (c) The brown allele is epistatic to blue. (d) none of the above

b

8. In sickle-cell anemia, an amino acid in the sixth position of the β chain is changed from (a) phenylpyruvic acid to glutamic acid. (b) valine to glutamic acid. (c) glutamic acid to phenylpyruvic acid. (d) glutamic acid to valine.

d

9. The sickle-cell trait is very prevalent in malaria-ridden areas of Africa even though this homozygous condition almost always results in death. Why is the frequency of sickle-cell so high in this area? (a) The sickle cell condition and malaria are caused by the same organism. (b) The genes coding for the sickle cell trait also code for an increased resistance to malaria. (c) The gene coding for malaria is epistatic to sickle-cell heterozygosity. (d) none of the above

b

10. How can a phenocopy and a mutation be differentiated? (a) by crossing an unaffected individual with an affected individual. (b) by crossing an affected individual with a carrier. (c) by crossing two affected individuals. (d) none of the above

a

11. What type of progeny should be expected from the cross in question 10, assuming that the condition is a phenocopy? (a) all affected (b) none affected (c) 50% affected (d) 75% affected

b

12. Fur and skin color are usually genetically controlled traits. The Himalayan rabbit changes fur color when the temperature changes. This is because (a) the expression of the gene for color is temperature-dependent. (b) fur color is not genetically controlled in the Himalayan rabbit. (c) fur color is a pleiotropic trait. (d) none of the above

b

13. Two identical (monozygotic) twins are reared apart from the time of birth. At age twenty they are tested for intelligence showing a very large difference in scores. This indicates that intelligence is (a) highly dependent on genes. (b) highly dependent on the environment. (c) inherited differently among twins. (d) none of the above

b

14. It is believed that intelligence is controlled by (a) one dominant gene. (b) two codominant genes. (c) polygenic interactions. (d) all of the above

c

Fill in the blanks.

15. When a homozygous white snapdragon is crossed with a homozygous red snapdragon of the same species, all the progeny are pink. The mode of inheritance exhibited here is hybrid _____.

codominance

16. The ratio of 12:3:1 obtained from a dihybrid cross is indicative of the presence of _____ epistatic genes.

dominant

17. In an epistatic gene interaction, the _____ gene is suppressed, or masked.

hypostatic

18. The ratio of 9:3:4 expresses a _____ epistatic interaction.

recessive

19. A 7:9 ratio exhibited in a dihybrid cross indicates a _____ recessive gene interaction.

duplicate

20. In an epistatic interaction between two gene loci, the number of phenotypes that would be expressed is less than _____.

four

21. Individuals with the sickle-cell trait are _____ for the condition.

hetero-
zygous

22. In Aquilegia vulgaris red flowers always have longer stems, darker endosperm and increased weight. This indicates that a single _____ is providing all these characteristics through a _____ effect.

gene pair
pleiotropic

23. A _____ is a phenotype produced by the
environment which stimulates the effects of
a known mutation.

phenocopy

24. The Himalayan rabbit, the Siamese cat, and
the sun-red maize all exhibit phenotypical
expressions which respond to _____
changes.

temperature

25. In the plant M. jalapa, the transmission of
the chlorophyll pigments occurs through
_____ DNA from the mother to the
daughter cell.

chloroplastic

26. Intelligence is highly influenced by the
environment, therefore its heritability is
very _____ .

low

Decide whether the following statements are true
or false.

27. Epistatic genotypes are exactly the same as
the genotypes produced in multiple hybrid
crosses.

True

28. Polygenic interaction means that several
genes additively affect a given trait
producing multiple graded phenotypes.

True

29. Skin color in humans is a polygenic trait
which produces four different genotypes.

False

30. Human eye color is controlled by two alleles
with brown eye color being dominant over
blue eye color.

True

31. Transgressive segregation is the appearance
in an F_2 generation or later, of more extreme
phenotypes than those of the parents.

True

32. A pleiotropic effect of the sickle-cell trait
is a decreased resistance to malaria.

False

33. Transgressive segregation resembles polygenic
interaction where no single allele is dominant
over another.

False

34. Phenocopies which are produced at a critical
stage of development can be inherited.

False

35. Phenocopies are errors of development produced by slight changes in the RNA structure.

False

36. The heritability of a given trait can be calculated with the formula H = G/D.

False

37. In the palnt M. jalapa, the male parent does not contribute to the transmission of the chlorophyll pigment because it only contributes nucleic material.

True

38. Extranuclear inheritance occurs through cytoplasmic division, rather than through nuclear division.

True

39. In the hermaphroditic snail, Limnaea peregra, the phenotypes of the offspring are influenced solely by the genotype of the mother; the   genotype of the father is unnecessary.

True

In questions 40 through 44 match the terms in column A to their appropriate descriptions in column B.

A	B	
40. Dominance	(a) intra-allelic gene suppression	a
41. Phenocopy	(b) inter-allelic gene suppression	d
42. Epistasis	(c) expression of two or more genes at different loci	b
43. Pleiotropism		e
	(d) environmentally produced phenotypes	
44. Independent Assortment		c
	(e) multiple unrelated effects produced by a single gene	

225

CHAPTER 7

LINKAGE, RECOMBINATION AND MAPPING

LINKAGE AND RECOMBINATION

● PROBLEM 7-1

What is linkage? Illustrate your answer with an example.

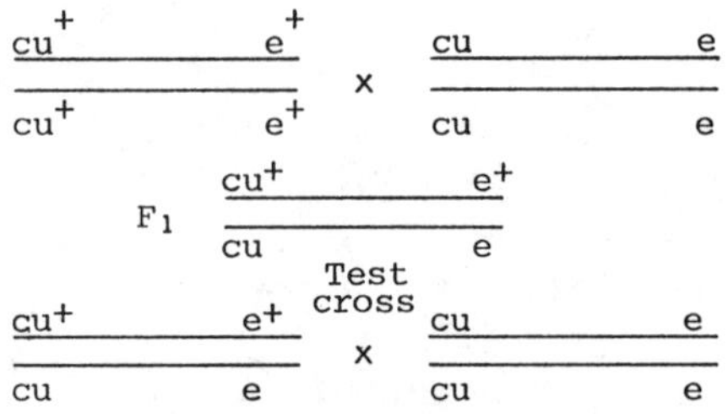

$$\frac{cu^+ \qquad e^+}{cu^+ \qquad e^+} \times \frac{cu \qquad e}{cu \qquad e}$$

$$F_1 \quad \frac{cu^+ \qquad e^+}{cu \qquad e}$$

Test cross

$$\frac{cu^+ \qquad e^+}{cu \qquad e} \times \frac{cu \qquad e}{cu \qquad e}$$

Chromosomes from egg	$\dfrac{cu^+ \quad e^+}{}$	$\dfrac{cu^+ \quad e}{}$	$\dfrac{cu \quad e^+}{}$	$\dfrac{cu \quad e}{}$
Chromosomes from sperm	$\dfrac{}{cu \quad e}$	$\dfrac{}{cu \quad e}$	$\dfrac{}{cu \quad e}$	$\dfrac{}{cu \quad e}$
Proportion	4	1	1	4
Parental or recombination	Parental	Recombination	Recombination	Parental

Fig. 1.
Diagram on the chromosomes of a test cross involving 2 genes in the same chromosome pair. The results show the parental (linkage) and recombination (crossover) groups.

Solution: Genes on the same chromosome tend to stay together during the formation of gametes. This is known as linkage. Neighboring genes are closely linked, and widely separated genes are loosely linked. Loosely linked genes may become separated by recombination. Groups of linked genes are called linkage groups. Markers that assort independently are placed in different linkage groups and those that demonstrate linkage are put into the same linkage group. Genes in different linkage groups follow Mendel's law of independent assortment and show a 9:3:3:1 ratio. Linked genes do not assort independently and they show varied ratios.

Our illustration involves a cross between a homozygous Drosophila female with straight wings and a gray body $(cu^+cu^+;e^+e^+)$ and a male homozygous for the recessive traits, curled wings and ebony body (cu cu; ee). A test cross is performed using a member of the F_1 generation and a fly with both recessive traits homozygous (see diagram). The results show that recombination has produced new combinations of genes along the chromosomes that were not present in the parents. Also, the genes remained linked in some of the progeny; these progeny are of the parental type and are more numerous than the recombinants.

● **PROBLEM** 7-2

In a given organism, two pairs of contrasting genes are under investigation: A vs. a and B vs. b. An F_1 individual resulting from a cross between two homozygous strains was testcrossed, and the following testcross progeny were recovered:

Phenotype	Number
A B	621
A b	87
a B	92
a b	610

a) Are these two genes linked or independent?

b) If linked, what is the amount of recombination that has occurred between them?

c) What are the genotypes of the original homozygous strains?

Solution: a) The determination of linkage or independence can be made very readily. The expected distribution of testcross progeny for independent gene pairs is a 1:1:1:1 ratio for each of the phenotypic classes. A glance at the data reveals that they are not in a 1:1:1:1 ratio; therefore, the two genes must be linked together in the same chromosomal unit.

b) Having determined that the genes are linked, we can find the amount of recombination that has occurred by using the formula:

$$\% \text{ recombination} = \frac{\text{total number of recombinant progeny}}{\text{total number of testcross progeny}} \times 100$$

The recombinant progeny are represented by the phenotypic classes that have the lesser numbers. Looking at our data, we see that the classes Ab and aB have the lowest number of individuals, and are therefore the recombinant classes.

$$\text{Thus, } \% \text{ recombination} = \frac{178}{1,410} \times 100 = 12.6\%$$

c) The genotypes of the original homozygous strains can be determined by finding the parental progeny which are represented by the phenotypic classes that have the larger numbers. These are the classes AB and ab, and since these represent the original combinations of the two genes, the genotypes of the parent stocks were:

$$\frac{A \quad B}{A \quad B} \qquad \frac{a \quad b}{a \quad b} \; .$$

● **PROBLEM** 7-3

A cross is made between an albino strain (al) of Neurospora and a wild-type strain (al$^+$). The albino strain produces light spores and the wild-type strain produces dark spores. The cross results in 129 asci of the parental type - 4 light spores; 4 dark spores - and 141 asci of recombinant types, a 2:2:2:2 sequence or a 2:4:2 sequence. What is the recombination frequency between the al locus and the centromere?

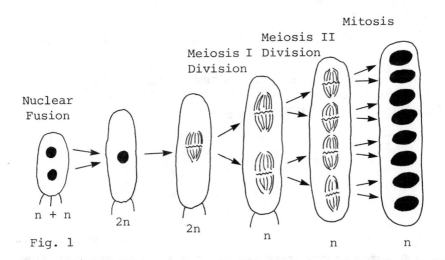

Fig. 1

Solution: <u>Neurospora</u> is an ascomycete (or sac fungus). Eight spores are formed following the fusion of two nuclei, two rounds of meiosis and one of mitosis (see Figure 1). Each pair of chromosomes produces four haploid spores. Since the wild-type strain produces dark spores and the albino strain produces light spores, the segregation of chromosomes can be followed by analyzing the order of light and dark spores. This order will be influenced by segregation and recombination. Figure 2 shows how the parental and recombinant classes of asci were produced in this cross.

Fig. 2

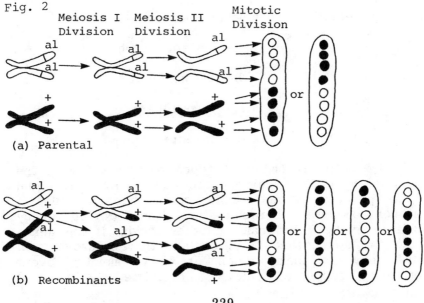

229

To find the frequency with which recombination occurs, we use the following relationship:

$$\text{Frequency of recombination} = \frac{\text{\# recombinants}}{\text{total asci}}$$

$$= \frac{141}{141 + 129} = 0.52 \text{ or } 52\%$$

We have to divide this percentage in half since only two of the four strands underwent recombination. The actual frequency of recombination is then

$$\frac{52}{2} = 26\%.$$

● **PROBLEM 7-4**

Can you distinguish between two gene loci located on the same chromosome that have 50 percent crossing over, and two gene loci each located on different chromosomes?

Solution: When two linked genes have 50 percent crossing over between them, it means that 50 percent of the progeny will be recombinants. For example, a heterozygous parent genotypically $\frac{A\ B}{a\ b}$ will form four types of gametes if a cross occurs between A and B:

A	B	A B - parental type
A	B	A b - recombinant
a	b	a B - recombinant
a	b	a b - parental type

Now, if the recombinant types occurred 50% of the time, this means that they are produced in numbers equal to the parental types. This could happen only if crossover occurred between the genes during every meiosis in every individual. In other words, if the genes are so far apart that it is certain that crossover will occur between them, then in any meiotic event recombinant types will always be formed - in equal numbers in relation to parental types. Therefore, the four types of gametes occur in a 1:1:1:1 ratio. When testcrossed, the progeny will also occur in a 1:1:1:1 phenotypic ratio.

This means that the ratio of the progeny from parents having linked genes showing 50% crossing over is indistinguishable from that of parents with genes that are not linked. Thus, when genes are separated by 50 map units, it is impossible to differentiate between linkage and non-linkage.

Note that no more than 50% recombination is ever expected between any two loci because only two of the four chromatids are involved in crossing over. In fact, the ratio is usually less than 50% because crossover may not always occur and because double or multiple crossovers can reduce the apparent number of crossover events, as shown below.

$$\begin{array}{ccc}
A①\ B & A②b & A\ B \\
\times & \times & \\
a\ \ b & a\ \ B & a\ b
\end{array}$$

● **PROBLEM** 7-5

A cross is made between two strains of <u>Neurospora</u>: one strain requires thiamine in its medium (thi), and the other strain grows in buttonlike colonies (but). The following data is collected:

$$thi\ but^+ \quad x \quad thi^+ but$$

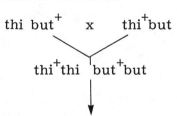

$$thi^+ thi\ \ but^+ but$$

Class	Number of Asci	Spores			
		1+2	3+4	5+6	7+8
A	280	$thibut^+$	$thibut^+$	thi^+but	thi^+but
B	51	$thibut^+$	thi^+but^+	$thibut$	thi^+but
C	19	$thibut^+$	$thibut$	thi^+but^+	thi^+but
D	3	$thibut^+$	thi^+but	$thibut^+$	thi^+but

231

(a) Are these genes linked?

(b) Determine the sequence of the points: centromere, thi locus, but locus.

(c) Calculate the map distances.

Solution: This problem involves the mapping of two genetic loci with respect to the centromere. This can be done through a two-point cross. The recombination frequencies that come from such a cross enable us to determine distances between markers.

(a) Yes, the genes are linked. They are linked because they do not assort independently. If the genes assorted independently, equal numbers of each class would have been observed.

(b) To determine the sequence of the two loci and the centromere we must assume a sequence, examine each class of asci and see if the results match our predictions. Suppose we assume the order to be:

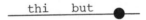

We can look at all chromatids of each class to see how the spore order was formed. For instance, class A has thibut$^+$ thibut$^+$ thi$^+$but thi$^+$but spores. The original cross yielded:

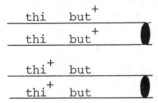

The spores and the chromatids are in the same order, so class A contains nonrecombinant asci.

Class B has spores in this order: thibut$^+$ thi$^+$ but$^+$ thibut thi$^+$but. To go from the original order, as in class A, to this, we must include a crossover event:

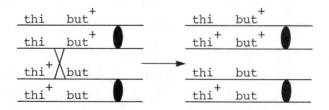

Class C and class D can be examined in the same way.

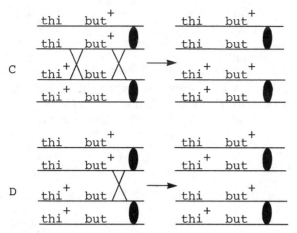

Here we encounter a problem. Double crossover events are rarer than single crossover events. But our data shows that the event of class C occurs 19 times while the event of class D occurs 3 times. The double crossover event of class C cannot occur more often than the single crossover event of class D. Our positional assumption must be wrong.

Another possibility is that the centromere lies between the two markers:

Again, we test this assumption.

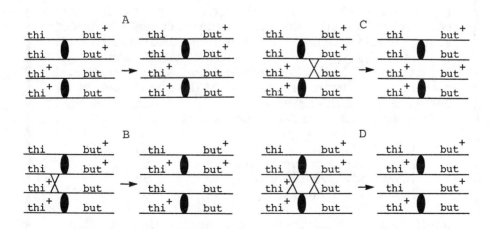

These results are more consistent with our numerical data; the double crossover event, D, occurs the least. Thus we have the sequence:

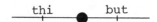

(c) The map distances can be calculated by using the data that we are given. The distance from the thi locus to the centromere can be determined by finding the recombination frequency of the thi locus. Class B and class D involved a crossover event including the thi locus. The total of these events is divided by the total asci of all events and then multiplied by 1/2 because only two of the four chromatids underwent recombination.

$$\frac{51 + 3}{353} \times 1/2 = 0.0764 = 7.64 \text{ map units}$$

The same can be done for the but locus by using classes C and D.

$$\frac{19 + 3}{353} \times 1/2 = 0.0297 = 2.97 \text{ map units}$$

Our final map is:

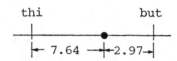

TWO-POINT CROSS

● **PROBLEM 7-6**

In Drosophilia, the dominant gene G codes for gray body color, and the dominant gene N codes for normal wings. The recessive alleles of these two genes result in black body color (g) and vestigial wings (n) respectively. Flies homozygous for gray body and normal wings were crossed with flies that had black bodies and vestigial wings. The F_1 progeny were then testcrossed, with the following results:

Gray body, normal wings	236
Black body, vestigial wings	253
Gray body, vestigial wings	50
Black body, normal wings	61

Would you say that these two genes are linked? If so, how many map units apart are they on the chromosomes?

Solution: To determine if the two genes are linked, we look at the F_2 progeny. We notice that there are two large groups (236, 253) which are approximately equal, and two small groups (50, 61) which are also nearly equal. We can reduce these numbers to small whole number ratios:

gray body, normal wings	236/50	roughly equals 5
black body, vestigial wings	253/50	roughly equals 5
gray body, vestigial wings	61/50	roughly equals 1
black body, normal wings	50/50	roughly equals 1

Since the heterozygous F_2 parent (the result of a cross from two homozygous parents) is crossed with a double recessive, we would expect a 1:1:1:1 phenotypic ratio among the offspring. However, the ratio here is 5:5:1:1. This significant departure from the 1:1:1:1 ratio indicates that linkage is indeed likely. The fact that the ratio divides the progeny into four groups - two large and of equal size, and two small and of equal size - is also a typical result of a cross involving linked genes.

To calculate the distance between the genes, we will have to rely on the fact that the frequency of crossing over depends on this distance. It is logical to assume that the farther apart two genes are on a chromosome, the more likely it is that a crossover will occur because there is a larger possible region in which it can occur. The process of locating genes on chromosomes is called mapping.

The percentage of crossing over or recombination gives us no information about the absolute distances between the genes but it does give us relative distances between them. Suppose, for example, that genes A and B have a recombination frequency of 20% and genes A and C have a frequency of 40%. From this data, we cannot tell the exact distance of B from A or C from A, but, we can say that C must be twice as far from A as B is from A, since twice as much crossing over occurred in the distance between C and A. Instead of having to compare two distances every time we want to refer to the separation of two genes, we have, by convention, established a standard measurement known as a map unit. A map unit is defined as the distance on the chromosome within which a crossover occurs one percent of the time. When genes on a chromosome are allocated their respective positions on that chromosome, we can obtain what we call a genetic map.

To obtain the map distance between two genes, we have to know the frequency of crossing over between them. Recombination frequency is defined as the ratio of the number of recombinants to the whole progeny, that is,

$$\text{recombination frequency (RF)} = \frac{\text{number of recombinants}}{\substack{\text{total number of offspring in} \\ \text{that generation containing} \\ \text{the recombinants}}}$$

Because recombinants can only result from a crossover event, their numbers in the population will be small for closely linked genes. The recombinants in this problem are found in the two smaller groups, and their total is 50 + 61 or 111. The total number of progeny is 236 + 253 + 50 + 61 or 600. Therefore:

$$\text{RF} = \frac{\text{number of recombinants}}{\text{total number of progeny}} = \frac{111}{600} = 0.185.$$

Since the map units are expressed as a percentage of recombination, a RF of 0.185 is the same as 0.185 x 100 or 18.5 map units.

Hence a map distance of 18.5 map units separates the gene for body color from the gene for wing size.

```
G                                    N
|←——————— 18.5 map units ——————→|
```

● PROBLEM 7-7

In fruit flies, black body color (b) is recessive to the normal wild-type body color (b^+). Cinnabar eye (cn) is recessive to the normal wild-type eye color (cn^+). A homozygous wild-type fly was mated to a fly with black body and cinnabar eyes. The resulting heterozygous F_1 fly was mated to a fly with black body and cinnabar eyes. These were the results in the offspring:

  90 wild-type
  92 black body and cinnabar eyes
   9 black body and wild-type eyes
   9 wild-type body and cinnabar eyes.

What is the map distance between the gene for black body and the gene for cinnabar eyes?

Solution: If genes are on the same chromosome they are said to be linked because they will tend to be inherited together. If linkage is involved genes will tend to remain in the original parental combinations. Combinations unlike either of the original parents will tend to be much less frequent than would be expected from independent assortment. In this example the categories containing only 9 individuals represent individuals unlike either of the original parents. These types resulted from crossing over or exchange of chromatid segments between the two gene loci. The amount of crossing over is proportional to the distance between genes. The map distance is determined by dividing the number of crossover types by the total number of offspring.

$$\frac{18}{200} = 0.09$$

This is converted to percent by multiplying by 100; moving the decimal point two places to the right. One percent of crossing over equals 1 map unit. These two gene loci are therefore 9 map units apart.

● **PROBLEM 7-8**

In Drosophila, the genes black (b), and vestigial (vg) are 20 chromosome map units apart. In an original cross between black, normal-winged females and normal-bodied, vestigial males, F_1 flies were recovered. If the F_1 flies are intercrossed, predict the phenotypic classes and the number of flies in each, if 1,500 F_2 progeny were classified.

Solution: Since we know the distance between two loci, we can predict the frequency of both the recombinant and the parental gametes produced. From this we can predict the progeny genotypes and phenotypes, including their respective frequencies in the following manner:

The F_1 females will produce the parental gametes b+ and +vg at a frequency of 0.4 each, and will produce the recombinant gametes b vg and + + at a frequency of 0.1 each. Since there is little or no recombination in the male of Drosophila, the F_1 males will only produce the parental gametes at a frequency of 0.5 each.

We now use the Punnett square to complete our prediction.

♀ \ ♂	b +	+ vg
.4 b +	$\dfrac{b\ +}{b\ +}$ .20	$\dfrac{b\ +}{+\ vg}$ .20
.4 + vg	$\dfrac{b\ +}{+\ vg}$ .20	$\dfrac{+\ vg}{+\ vg}$ .20
.1 + +	$\dfrac{b\ +}{+\ +}$ .05	$\dfrac{+\ vg}{+\ +}$ .05
.1 b vg	$\dfrac{b\ +}{b\ vg}$	$\dfrac{b\ vg}{+\ vg}$ .05

Summarizing the phenotypes that will result from this cross, we have:

+ + .50

b + .25

+ vg .25

b vg 0

Thus, we see that phenotypic distribution will be 2:1:1:0 because of the failure to observe recombination in the male. We can now convert these frequencies into numbers simply by multiplying them by the total number of flies recovered.

$$+\ +\ (.50) \cdot 1500 = 750$$

$$b\ +\ (.25) \cdot 1500 = 375$$

$$+\ vg\ (.25) \cdot 1500 = 375$$

$$b\ vg \qquad\qquad = \ \ 0$$

Total 1,500

● PROBLEM 7-9

The gene r, for rosy eyes, is 12 map units away from the gene k, for kidney-shaped eyes. Both of these genes are recessive to their wild-type alleles. If a heterozygous wild-type fly, resulting from a cross between a homozygous wild-type fly and a fly with rosy, kidney-shaped eyes, is crossed to a fly with rosy, kidney-shaped eyes, what will be the types of gametes and the frequencies of each?

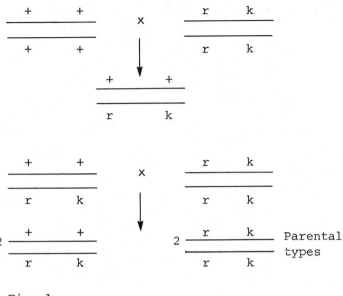

Fig. 1.

<u>Solution</u>: The cross is shown in Figure 1.

Since the distance between the two loci is 12 map units, 12% of the progeny will undergo recombination to produce additional types of gametes:

$$\begin{array}{cc} + & + \\ \hline r & k \end{array} \quad \longrightarrow \quad \begin{array}{cc} + & k \\ \hline r & + \end{array}$$

Since crossing over is a reciprocal exchange there should be two crossover types of equal frequency for both parental and recombinant classes.

$$\text{Recombinants}: 12\% = \frac{12}{100} = 0.12$$

$$\frac{0.12}{2} = 0.06 \text{ for each type of recombinant}$$

The remaining 88% are parental types:

$$88\% = 0.88$$

$$\frac{0.88}{2} = 0.44 \text{ for each type of parental}$$

Thus, our gametes will be as follows:

$$\left.\begin{array}{l} 0.44 + + \\ 0.44\ r\ k \end{array}\right\} \text{Parental types}$$

$$\left.\begin{array}{l} 0.06\ r\ + \\ 0.06\ +\ k \end{array}\right\} \text{Recombinant types}$$

THREE-POINT CROSS

● **PROBLEM** 7-10

Three linked loci in corn are involved in the following cross:

$$\frac{+\quad sh\quad +}{+\quad sh\quad +} \times \frac{c\quad +\quad wx}{c\quad +\quad wx}$$

$$\downarrow$$

$$\frac{+\quad +\quad +}{c\quad sh\quad wx}$$

Then a testcross is performed:

$$\frac{+\quad +\quad +}{c\quad sh\quad wx} \times \frac{c\quad sh\quad wx}{c\quad sh\quad wx}$$

This cross gave the following results:

	Phenotype	Number of progeny
1.	White, shrunken, starchy	116
2.	Colored, full, starchy	4
3.	Colored, shrunken, starchy	2538
4.	Colored, shrunken, waxy	601
5.	White, full, starchy	626
6.	White, full, waxy	2708
7.	White, shrunken, waxy	2

6708

Colored is dominant to white (c); full is dominant to shrunken (sh); and starchy is dominant to waxy (wx). What is the sequence of the genes? What are the map distances?

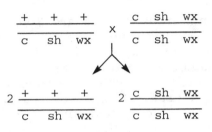

Fig. 1.

Solution: This is a three-point cross. To find the gene sequence, we need to determine which progeny are parental types (noncrossover events) and which are double and single crossover events (recombinants). The frequencies of such occurrences give us map distances.

There are several steps that can be followed to make three-point crosses less monstrous.

1. Carry out the cross (in this case, the testcross) to find the nonrecombinant parental types, see Figure 1.

We can ignore the second two progeny because any crossover event would result in the same homozygous chromosomes.

2. If it is not given, go through the phenotypic results and write each class using symbols. This will make it easier to classify the offspring.

1. White, shrunken, starchy   c sh +

2. Colored, full, starchy   + + +

3. Colored, shrunken, starchy   + sh +

4. Colored, shrunken, waxy   + sh wx

5. White, full, starchy   c + +

6. White, full, waxy   c + wx

7. White, shrunken, waxy   c sh wx

8. Colored, full, waxy   + + wx

3. Classify the progeny as parental (the most numerous class), double crossover (the rarest event), single crossover I, and single crossover II. To determine the crossover events the progeny must be compared to the parental types.

The most numerous classes are 3 and 6. Therefore + sh + and c + wx are the parental class. The double crossover events are 2 and 7 - the least numerous classes. The double crossovers are + + + and c sh wx. From this information we can determine something about the sequence. An examination of the parental classes and the double classes shows that the sh gene is the only gene which moved. To go from the parental type to the double type, a double crossover event moved the sh gene. This, then, must occupy the center position, see Figure 2.

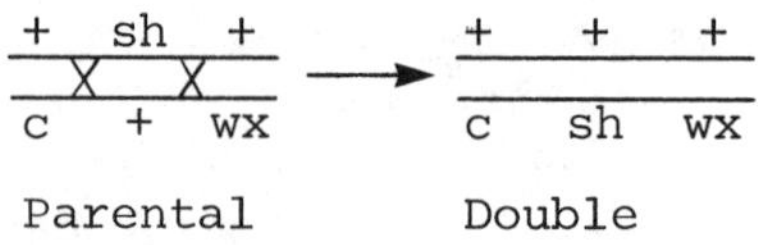

Fig. 2.

The single crossover events are those that show the repositioning of one gene. There are two groups of single crossovers, Single I and Single II, see Figure 3.

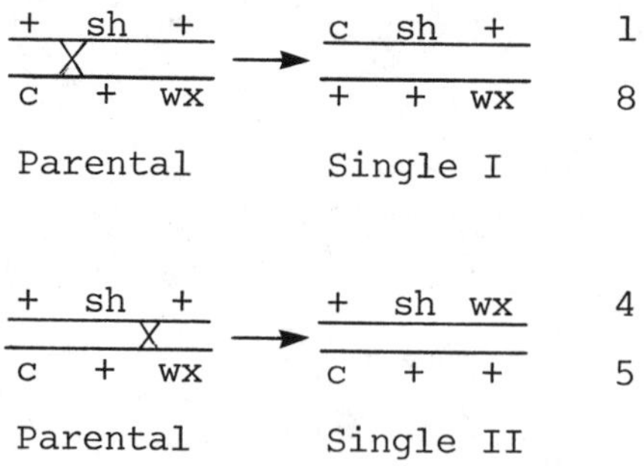

Fig. 3.

4. Count up the progeny in each class.

Parental   3 + 6   2538 + 2708 = 5246

Single I	1 + 8	116 + 113 = 229
Single II	4 + 5	601 + 626 = 1227
Double	2 + 7	4 + 2 = 6

5. Calculate the frequency of each class by dividing by the total progeny in the study.

$$\text{Parental} = \frac{5246}{6708} = 0.782$$

$$\text{Single I (SI)} = \frac{229}{6708} = 0.0341$$

$$\text{Single II(SII)} = \frac{1227}{6708} = 0.183$$

$$\text{Double (D)} = \frac{6}{6708} = 0.0009$$

6. Call the loci a, b and c. Determine the map distances by finding the frequency with which each loci is able to recombine.

R_{ab} is the recombination frequency of the genes a and b (in our case c and sh). These genes undergo recombination in Single I and in Double. The recombination frequency is then:

$$R_{ab} = SI + D$$

$$R_{c\text{-}sh} = 0.0341 + 0.0009$$

$$R_{c\text{-}sh} = 0.035 \text{ or } 3.5 \text{ map units (mu)}$$

Similar steps are used to find the map units between sh and wx and between c and wx.

$$R_{bc} = SII + D$$

$$R_{sh\text{-}wx} = 0.183 + 0.0009$$

$$R_{sh\text{-}wx} = 0.184 = 18.4 \text{ mu}$$

$$R_{ac} = SI + SII$$

$$R_{c\text{-}wx} = 0.0341 + 0.183$$

$$R_{c\text{-}wx} = 0.217 = 21.7 \text{ mu}$$

The final map then is:

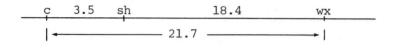

If the two distances are added up, their total, 21.9, is greater than the distance that we calculated for the two outside markers. This is because of double crossovers. If two crossovers occur between the outside markers, their effects cancel each other out; no recombination appears to have occurred. But these double crossovers are seen when the closer markers are used to calculate recombination frequencies. This creates the discrepancy.

● **PROBLEM 7-11**

A cross is made between a heterozygote, +++/rmc, and a recessive homozygote, rmc/rmc. 1280 progeny were analyzed, giving the results below. Determine the order of the three genes r, m and c. Calculate the coincidence and the interference.

+++	413	+mc	170
rmc	426	r++	161
++c	6	+m+	47
rm+	3	r+c	54

Total = 1280

Solution: This problem is a three-point cross. We follow the steps outlined in the previous problem. The coincidence and interference are calculations that compare expected and observed double crossovers.

First we must determine the gene sequence.

1. Perform the cross to find parental type

$$\frac{+++}{rmc} \quad x \quad \frac{rmc}{rmc}$$

$$2\frac{+++}{rmc} \qquad 2\frac{rmc}{rmc}$$

2. Determine parental class and double crossover class by finding the most common and the least common events.

$$\left.\begin{array}{ll} +++ & 413 \\ \\ rmc & 426 \end{array}\right\} \quad 839 \text{ parental}$$

$$\left.\begin{array}{ll} ++c & 6 \\ \\ rm+ & 3 \end{array}\right\} \quad 9 \text{ double crossovers}$$

If we move c in the double crossover class, we get the parental type. Thus, c must be the central gene.

3. Now we can put the progeny into Parental, Single I, Single II and Double classes.

Parental	$\frac{+++}{rmc}$	413 + 426 = 839
Single I(SI)	$\frac{+cm}{r++}$	170 + 161 = 331
Single II(SII)	$\frac{rc+}{++m}$	47 + 54 = 101
Double (D)	$\frac{++c}{rm+}$ or $\frac{+c+}{r+m}$	6 + 3 = 9

4. Find the frequencies

$$\text{Parental} \qquad \frac{839}{1280} = 0.655$$

$$\text{Single I} \qquad \frac{331}{1280} = 0.256$$

Single II $\dfrac{101}{1280} = 0.079$

Double $\dfrac{9}{1280} = 0.007$

5. Calculate the map distances

① $R_{ab} = D + SI$

$R_{rc} = 0.007 + 0.256$

$R_{rc} = 0.263$ or 26.3 mu

② $R_{bc} = D + SII$

$R_{cm} = 0.007 + 0.079$

$R_{cm} = 0.086$ or 8.6 mu

③ $R_{ac} = SI + SII$

$R_{rm} = 0.256 + 0.079$

$R_{rm} = 0.335$ or 33.5 mu

Our map is:

The difference between the observed frequency of double crossovers (0.007) and the expected frequency (SI x SII) occurs because one crossover event interferes somehow with other crossovers. This is known as interference. The coincidence is simply the observed number divided by the expected. Then interference is just:

$$\text{interference} = 1 - \text{coincidence}.$$

$$\text{coincidence} = \dfrac{\text{observed}}{\text{expected}}$$

$$= \dfrac{D}{SI \times SII} = \dfrac{0.007}{0.263 \times 0.086}$$

$$= 0.31 \quad \text{Only 31\% of the expected double}$$
$$\text{crossovers occur.}$$

The interference is then

$$1 - 0.31 = 0.69.$$

Consider the cross:

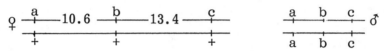

Given the graph below, can you predict the number and types of offspring?

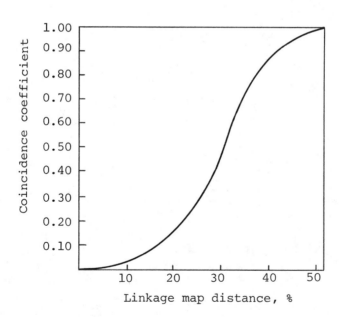

Solution: If we were clairvoyant we could use our powers of perception to solve this problem; however, we are mere scientists and our knowledge of genetics must suffice. We must work backwards to find the types of offspring.

First, find the linkage map distance by adding the distance between markers a and b to the distance between b and c:

$$\text{Linkage map distance} = 10.6 + 13.4$$

$$= 24$$

Find this on the graph's x-axis and go up until you reach the curve. The value of this point on the y-axis is the coincidence coefficient. In this case, the value is 0.25.

Now, go back to the original cross to determine the parental type, single crossover and double crossover progeny.

Only the heterozygote will undergo recombinations that can be observed through these markers.

The single crossover events that can occur in these parental types are:

and

The double crossover event is:

The map distances tell us that the frequency of recombination between a and b is 10.6% or 0.106. That of b and c is 13.4 or 0.134. If these values are multiplied together and then multiplied by the coefficient of coincidence (s) we will get the frequency of double cross over progeny. CO means crossover.

Double CO $=$ Single CO(a-b) x Single CO(b-c) x s

$$= 0.106 \times 0.134 \times 0.25$$

$$= 0.0036 \text{ or } 4 \text{ in } 1000.$$

The single crossover (a-b) can be found by subtracting the double crossover from our recombination frequency. The recombination frequency contains both single and double crossovers that involve a and b. By subtracting the double crossover events, we are left with only the single crossovers. We must first convert 10.6% to a factor over 1000 so that we can subtract 4/1000 from it.

$$\frac{10.6}{100} = \frac{106}{1000}$$

$$\frac{106}{1000} - \frac{4}{1000} = \frac{102}{1000}$$

Thus 102 out of 1000 progeny are single crossover events involving a and b.

A similar procedure is used to find the single crossovers between b and c.

$$\frac{13.4}{100} = \frac{134}{1000}$$

$$\frac{134}{1000} - \frac{4}{1000} = \frac{130}{1000}$$

Thus 130 out of 1000 progeny have undergone single crossover events between b and c.

The number of parental types are those remaining, so by subtracting the sum of the single and double crossover events from 1000 hypothetical progeny, the number of parental types can be obtained.

$$1000 - (4 + 102 + 130) = 1000 - 236$$

$$= 764 \text{ out of } 1000$$

Our final summary of results looks like this:

		+++	
Parental	abc		764

		a++	
Single CO	+bc		102

		++c	
Single CO	ab+		130

		a+c	
Double CO	+b+		4

			1000

This is what we would have seen initially, had we been clairvoyant.

● PROBLEM 7-13

The results from a cross in <u>Drosophila</u> are:

$$♀ \frac{+\quad+\quad+}{sc\quad ec\quad cv} \times \frac{sc\quad ec\quad cv}{\longrightarrow} ♂$$

Phenotype	Number of progeny
1. scute, echinus, crossveinless	1158
2. wild-type	1455
3. scute	163
4. echinus, crossveinless	130
5. scute, echinus	192
6. crossveinless	148
7. scute, crossveinless	1
8. echinus	1
	3248

Construct a map of these three sex-linked genes.

Solution: This three-point cross involves three genes on the X chromosome of Drosophila. Echinus mutants have rough eyes with large facets. Scute is a mutation that manifests itself by the reduction or absence of bristles on some parts of the body. Crossveinless mutants do not develop supporting structures in their wings. We construct this map as we have constructed the others.

1. Perform the cross:

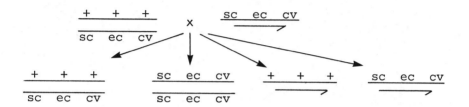

Ignore the homozygous females and the male when considering the recombinant classes since no recombination can occur that involves these three loci.

2. Write out the genotypes

1. scute, echinus, crossveinless   sc ec cv

2. wild-type   + + +

3. scute   sc + +

4. echinus, crossveinless   + ec cv

5. scute, echinus   sc ec +

6. crossveinless   + + cv

7. scute, crossveinless   sc + cv

8. echinus   + ec +

3. Find parentals and double crossovers to determine the middle gene.

$$\frac{sc \quad ec \quad cv}{+ \quad + \quad +} \xrightarrow{} \frac{sc \quad + \quad cv}{+ \quad ec \quad +}$$

Parental   Double
                       crossover

The middle gene is ec.

4. Place into groups: Parental, Single I, Single II, Double and find frequencies.

	sc ec cv		
Parental	+ + +	$\dfrac{1158 + 1455}{3248}$	= 0.804

	sc + +		
Single I(SI)	+ ec cv	$\dfrac{163 + 130}{3248}$	= 0.090

	sc ec +		
Single II(SII)	+ + cv	$\dfrac{192 + 148}{3248}$	= 0.105

	sc + cv		
Double (D)	+ ec +	$\dfrac{1 + 1}{3248}$	= 0.001

5. Find the map distances by finding the recombination frequencies between each loci.

a. R_{ab} = SI + D

R_{sc-ec} = 0.090 + 0.001

R_{sc-ec} = 0.091 or 9.1 mu

b. R_{bc} = SII + D

R_{ec-cv} = 0.105 + 0.001

R_{ec-cv} = 0.106 or 10.6 mu

c. R_{ac} = SI + SII

R_{sc-cv} = 0.090 + 0.105

R_{sc-cv} = 0.195 or 19.5 mu

The completed map for these three loci is:

In <u>Drosophila</u> the genes m, fu and sn reside on the X chromosome. A cross between $\dfrac{\text{m fu sn}}{\text{+ + +}}$ and $\dfrac{\text{m fu sn}}{\longrightarrow}$ produces the following progeny:

m fu sn	3661
m fu +	676
+ fu sn	165
+ fu +	1003
+ + +	3672
+ + sn	665
m + +	173
m + sn	1041

Total = 11,056

Determine the sequence of the genes and calculate the map distances between them.

<u>Solution</u>: This is another three-point cross so we use our step-by-step procedure. Hopefully, the steps are becoming more familiar.

1. Perform the cross:

$$\dfrac{\text{m} \quad \text{fu} \quad \text{sn}}{\text{+} \quad \text{+} \quad \text{+}} \quad \times \quad \dfrac{\text{m} \quad \text{fu} \quad \text{sn}}{\longrightarrow}$$

$$\dfrac{\text{m} \quad \text{fu} \quad \text{sn}}{\text{m} \quad \text{fu} \quad \text{sn}} \qquad \dfrac{\text{m} \quad \text{fu} \quad \text{sn}}{\longrightarrow} \qquad \dfrac{\text{+} \quad \text{+} \quad \text{+}}{\text{m} \quad \text{fu} \quad \text{sn}} \qquad \dfrac{\text{+} \quad \text{+} \quad \text{+}}{\longrightarrow}$$

We can ignore the homozygous female and the males since their recombination events have no bearing on our results.

2. The genotypes are given so we move on.

3. Find the most common (parental) and the rarest

(double crossover) classes. Determine which gene is in the middle

m	fu	sn

```
 m   fu   sn              m   +   sn     But, it        fu   +   sn
 ─X────X──────  ──────►  ─────────────   should be     ─────────────
 +    +    +              +   fu   +                    +    m    +

    Parental                 + fu +                       Double
                                                         crossover
```

But the least common class does not have the above genotype. The gene order must be different. Since m is the only misplaced gene, it must be the middle gene.

```
 fu   m   sn              fu   +   sn
 ─X────X──────  ──────►  ─────────────
 +    +    +              +    m    +

    Parental                 Double
                             crossover
```

4. Place the progeny into the four groups: Parental, Single I, Single II, and Double. Find the frequencies.

	fu m sn	
Parental	+ + +	$\dfrac{3661 + 3672}{11,056} = 0.663$

	+ m sn	
Single I(SI)	fu + +	$\dfrac{1041 + 1003}{11,056} = 0.185$

	fu m +	
Single II(SII)	+ + sn	$\dfrac{676 + 665}{11,056} = 0.121$

	fu + sn	
Double (D)	+ m +	$\dfrac{165 + 173}{11,056} = 0.031$

5. Find the map distances between each gene.

a. $R_{ab} = SI + D$

$R_{fu-m} = 0.185 + 0.031$

$R_{fu-m} = 0.216$ or 21.6 mu

b. $R_{bc} = SII + D$

$R_{m-sn} = 0.121 + 0.031$

$R_{m-sn} = 0.152$ or 15.2 mu

c. $R_{ac} = SI + SII$

$R_{fu-sn} = 0.185 + 0.121$

$R_{fu-sn} = 0.306$ or 30.6 mu

The completed map is:

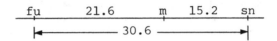

● PROBLEM 7-15

A fully heterozygous fly resulting from a cross between a wild-type fly and a fly showing three recessive traits - rosy eyes (r), ebony body (e), and spineless bristles (s) - was crossed with another fly showing the recessive traits. These were the results in the offspring:

Phenotype	Number of offspring	
1. wild-type	410	
2. ebony, rosy, spineless	411	
3. rosy, spineless	58	
4. ebony	56	
5. ebony, spineless	28	
6. rosy	29	total =
7. spineless	5	1000
8. ebony, rosy	3	

Map these three gene loci.

Solution: This problem can be done like the other three-point crosses.

1. Perform the cross.

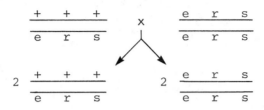

We are only concerned with the heterozygote.

2. Write out the genotypes.

1.	+ + +	410
2.	e r s	411
3.	+ r s	58
4.	e + +	56
5.	e + s	28
6.	+ r +	29
7.	+ + s	5
8.	e r +	3

3. Find the middle gene by comparing parental types to double crossover types.

$$\frac{+\quad+\quad+}{e\quad r\quad s} \longrightarrow \frac{+\quad+\quad s}{e\quad r\quad +}$$

S is the middle gene:

$$\frac{+\quad+\quad+}{e\quad s\quad r} \longrightarrow \frac{+\quad s\quad +}{e\quad t\quad r}$$

4. Put the progeny in recombinant groups and find the frequencies.

256

| | | + + + | | |
| Parental | | e s r | $\dfrac{410 + 411}{1000}$ | $= 0.821$ |

| | | e + + | | |
| Single I(SI) | | + s r | $\dfrac{56 + 58}{1000}$ | $= 0.114$ |

| | | + + r | | |
| Single II(SII) | | e s + | $\dfrac{29 + 28}{1000}$ | $= 0.057$ |

| | | + s + | | |
| Double (D) | | e + r | $\dfrac{5 + 3}{1000}$ | $= 0.008$ |

5. Find the map distances through the recombination frequencies.

    a. R_{ab} = SI + D

        R_{e-s} = 0.114 + 0.008

        R_{e-s} = 0.122 or 12.2 mu

    b. R_{bc} = SII + D

        R_{s-r} = 0.057 + 0.008

        R_{s-r} = 0.065 or 6.5 mu

    c. R_{ac} = SI + SII

        R_{e-r} = 0.114 + 0.057

        R_{e-r} = 0.171 or 17.1 mu

The final map is:

```
  e       12.2        s    6.5    r
--+-------------------+----------+------
  |                                     
  |←————————— 17.1————————→|
```

Given the following testcross data for corn in which the genes for fine stripe ($\underline{f}$), bronze aleurone ($\underline{bz}$) and knotted leaf ($\underline{Kn}$) are involved:

Phenotype	Number
Kn + +	451
Kn f +	134
+ + +	97
+ f bz	436
Kn + bz	18
+ + bz	119
+ f +	24
Kn f bz	86
	1,365

a) Determine the sequence of the three genes.

b) Calculate the amount of recombination that occurred between each pair of loci.

c) Calculate the coefficient of coincidence.

Solution: a) The correct gene sequence can be determined by identifying first the parental gene combinations and then the double crossover gene combinations. The parentals will be the most frequent of the eight phenotypic classes and the double crossovers will be the least frequent. Having determined these classes, the gene in the middle will be in opposite relationship to the two outside genes in the double crossover classes as it was in the parental classes. The parental classes are Kn + + and + f bz, and the double crossover classes are Kn + bz and + f +. The gene $\underline{bz}$ is the middle gene because in the parentals it is in repulsion to $\underline{Kn}$ and in coupling with $\underline{f}$, while in the double crossovers, it is in coupling with $\underline{Kn}$ and in repulsion to $\underline{f}$. Neither of the other two genes, $\underline{Kn}$ and $\underline{f}$, show such a reversal of relationship. Thus, the correct sequence of the three genes is $\underline{Kn}$ $\underline{bz}$ $\underline{f}$ or $\underline{f}$ $\underline{bz}$

$\underline{Kn}$ depending upon their relationship to the centromere and mapping positions.

b) If we arbitrarily establish that the sequence is $\underline{f}$ $\underline{bz}$ $\underline{Kn}$, then we can assign "Region I" to the distance between $\underline{f}$ and $\underline{bz}$, and "Region II" to the distance between $\underline{bz}$ and $\underline{Kn}$.

The amount of recombination for Region I then can be calculated by:

$$\% \text{ recombination} = \frac{\text{total number of recombinants for Region I}}{\text{total number of testcross progeny}}$$

$$= \frac{134 + 18 + 119 + 24}{1,365} \text{ x } 100 = 21.6\%.$$

Similarly, the amount of recombination for Region II is calculated as:

$$\% \text{ recombination} = \frac{\text{total number of recombinants for Region II}}{\text{total number of testcross progeny}}$$

$$= \frac{97 + 18 + 24 + 86}{1,365} \text{ x } 100 = 16.5\%$$

Now the total recombination between $\underline{f}$ and $\underline{Kn}$ can be calculated either by adding the two, $21.6\% + 16.5\% = 38.1\%$, or by calculating directly:

$$\% \text{ recombination} = \frac{\text{total number of recombinant events}}{\text{total number of testcross progeny}}$$

$$= \frac{134 + 119 + 97 + 86 + 2(18) + 2(24)}{1,365} \text{ x } 100$$

$$= 38.1\%$$

The reason for doubling the numbers 18 and 24 is that these represent not one, but two recombination events.

c) The coefficient of coincidence (c.c.) is calculated by the formula:

$$c.c = \frac{\text{observed frequency of double crossovers}}{\text{expected frequency of double crossovers}}$$

$$= \frac{.03077}{.03564} = .86$$

where the expected frequency is determined by multiplying the frequency of Region I recombination times that of Region II.

259

Two true-breeding varieties of unicorns differ with respect to three traits. The first has a straight horn, a green coat, and a straight mane. The other variety has a twisted horn, a blue coat, and a curly mane. When a male of either variety is crossed with a female of the other, all the progeny have straight horns, green coats, and straight manes. These hybrid offspring are then crossed to unicorns with twisted horns, blue coats, and curly manes. This cross produces offspring in the following numbers:

straight horn, green coat, straight mane	855
twisted horn, blue coat, curly mane	855
twisted horn, green coat, straight mane	95
straight horn, blue coat, curly mane	95
straight horn, blue coat, straight mane	50
twisted horn, green coat, curly mane	50
	2000

Construct a linkage map for the three genes involved in this cross.

Solution: This is a complicated problem on linkage. Go over the previous problems on recombination. Some new concepts will be introduced here.

This cross involves three traits (that is, a three-point cross) each governed by a gene. To begin, we have to determine the dominance or recessiveness of the phenotypes. This can be obtained from the F_1 since all the F_1 descendants have a straight horn, green coat, and straight mane; the gene for straight horn is dominant over twisted horn (h); green coat is dominant over blue coat (c); straight mane is dominant over curly mane (m). Since the parents are true-breeding, one of them is

$$\frac{+\ +\ +}{+\ +\ +} \text{ and the other } \frac{h\ \ c\ \ m}{h\ \ c\ \ m}.$$

The actual sequence of the genes has yet to be determined. In the cross between two homozygous parents,

$$P_1 \qquad \frac{+\ +\ +}{+\ +\ +} \qquad x \qquad \frac{h\ c\ m}{h\ c\ m}$$

$$F_1 \qquad all\ \frac{+\ \ +\ \ +}{h\ \ c\ \ m}$$

Note that all the dominant genes are on one chromosome while all the recessive ones are on the other. These are the parental types +++ and hcm. All other combinations of genes are recombinants.

To calculate the recombination frequency we have to know the number of recombinants. There are several ways to do this; one of them begins by translating the F_2 phenotypes to genotypes keeping the F_2 progeny in the same order we get:

1	+ + +	855
2	h c m	855
3	h + +	95
4	+ c m	95
5	+ c +	50
6	h + m	50

Consider a crossover between h and c. The number of recombinants is 95③ + 95④ + 50⑤ + 50⑥ = 290.

The RF between h and c = $\frac{290}{2000}$ = 0.145.

An RF of 0.145 gives 0.145 x 100 = 14.5 map units, meaning h and c are 14.5 map units apart.

Consider a recombination between c and m. By similar reasoning, the number of recombinants

$$= 50⑤ + 50⑥ = 100$$

$$RF = \frac{100}{2000} = 0.05$$

That is, a map distance of 5 units separates c and m.

Finally, consider a crossover between h and m.

The number of recombinants

$$= 95③ + 95④ = 190$$

$$RF = \frac{190}{2000} = 0.095$$

That is, h and m are 9.5 map units apart.

Now that we have calculated a map distance for any two of the three genes, we are ready to plot the linkage map. As our reference points we use h and m, which are 9.5 units apart.

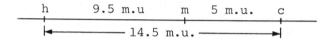

We know that h and m are 14.5 units apart. But c can be to the right or left of h. To determine which side of h c is on, we look at the distance between c and m, which is 5 units. This means c must be on the right side of h.

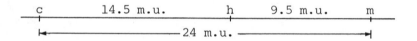

If c were 14.5 units to the left of h, then c and m would be separated by 24 units. This is not the case.

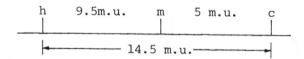

Therefore, the correct linkage map for the three genes is

```
h    9.5m.u.    m    5 m.u.    c
|_____|_____|_____
|                                        |
|———————— 14.5 m.u.————————|
```

MAPPING

● **PROBLEM** 7-18

The actual physical distances between linked genes bear no direct relationship to the map distances calculated on the basis of crossover percentages. Explain.

Solution: In certain organisms, such as Drosophila, the actual physical locations of genes can be observed. The chromosomes of the salivary gland cells in these insects have been found to duplicate themselves repeatedly without separating, giving rise to giant bundled chromosomes, called polytene chromosomes. Such chromosomes show extreme magnification of any differences in density along their length, producing light and dark regions known as banding patterns. Each band on the chromosome has been shown by experiment to correspond to a single gene on the same chromosome. The physical location of genes determined by banding patterns gives rise to a physical map, giving absolute distances between genes on a chromosome.

Since crossover percentage is theoretically directly proportional to the physical distance separating linked genes, we would expect a direct correspondence between physical distance and map distance. This, however, is not necessarily so. An important reason for this is the fact that the frequency of crossing over is not the same for all regions of the chromosome. Chromosome sections near the centromere regions and elsewhere have been found to cross over with less frequency than other parts near the free end of the chromosome.

In addition, mapping units determined from crossover percentages can be deceiving. Due to double crossing over (which results in a parental type), the actual amount of crossover may be greater than that indicated by recombinant type percentages. However, crossover percentages are nevertheless invaluable because the linear order of the genes obtained is identical to that determined by physical mapping.

● **PROBLEM** 7-19

How can human genes be mapped?

Solution: Humans cannot be experimentally bred for moral, physiological (e.g. long gestation period) and practical (e.g. small "litter" size) reasons. We cannot, therefore, map the human genome by doing testcrosses as we do in Drosophila. Mapping of human genes can be done instead through somatic cell genetics, recombinant DNA hybridization probes and studies of pedigrees.

Mouse   Human

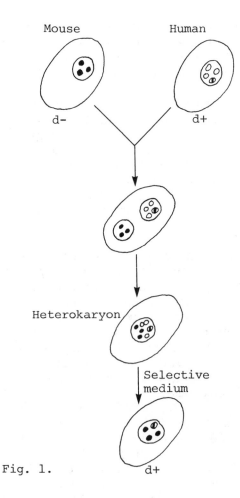

d-   d+

Heterokaryon

Selective
medium

Fig. 1.   d+

Somatic cell genetics involves the fusion of two somatic cells. When the two cell nuclei fuse, one set of chromosomes is preferentially lost. When human and mouse cells are fused, most of the human chromosomes are lost. In this way, specific traits can be selected. For instance, if a mouse cell, mutant for a particular enzyme (d-), is fused to a human cell that is d+, the human d gene can be mapped to a particular chromosome. Most of the human chromosomes are lost from the heterokaryon, but those cells that are d+ have retained the chromosome that we are interested in. All of the d+ cells can be karyotyped and the human chromosome that is common to all of them is the one that carries the d gene.

Recombinant DNA hybridization probes can be used to map a gene to a specific site of a chromosome. Chinese hamster ovary (CHO) cells are a haploid cell line that can be hybridized to human cells. Again, the human chromosomes will be lost preferentially. If we know that a gene is on a chromosome we can select for CHO cells that contain that particular human chromosome. Treatment with clastogens stimulates chromosomal breakage. Subclones with selectable markers on the chromosome and with deficiencies, due to the breakage, are isolated. Lost traits can be matched to lost bands in the karyotype. DNA can then be isolated from each of the subclones. This DNA is cut with restriction enzymes, run on an electrophoretic gel and hybridized with the radioactive cloned gene that was mapped. The gene can be pinpointed to a specific area of the chromosome by the results of the hybridization experiment.

Human-mouse hybrids can also be used in hybridization studies. Hybrids with known human chromosome compostion can be subjected to hybridization with the labelled DNA of a cloned human gene. The labelled chromosome is then identified by autoradiography.

Human mapping can also be done through studies of inherited traits in families. When genes are sex-linked, they are effectively testcrossed each time male offspring are produced (see Figure 2).

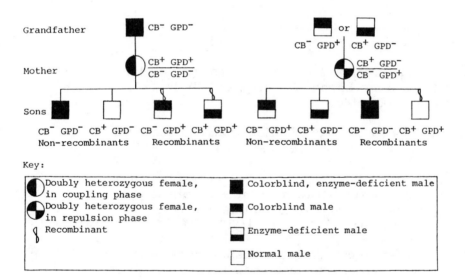

These methods have produced a very complex map of the 24 human chromosomes. The research continues and new information is contributed daily.

SHORT ANSWER QUESTIONS FOR REVIEW

Choose the correct answer.

1. Linked genes (a) sort independently and
    show consistent ratios . (b) sort independently
    and show varied ratios . (c) do not sort
    independently and show consistent ratios. (d)
    do not sort independently and show varied
    ratios.   d

In questions 2 and 3 refer to the data in the chart
below.

Phenotype	Number of Progeny
QR	327
Qr	61
qR	56
qr	342

2. We can determine that the genes (a) are linked.
    (b) are not linked. (c) are partially linked. (d)
    aren't possible.   a

3. The percent recombination that has occurred is
    (a) 10% (b) 15% (c) 30% (d) 50%   b

4. In a cross between two linked genes having 50%
    crossing over between them, what phenotypic
    ratio of the progeny should be expected? (a)
    9:3:3:1 (b) 1:1:1:1 (c) 1:2:1 (d) 2:2   b

5. In order to calculate map distances of genes on
    a chromosome you must know the (a) number
    of mutant genes. (b) crossover percentage.
    (c) recombination frequency of each locus. (d)
    a and c   c

6. A recombinant cross is performed between two
    organisms producing a total of 400 offspring.
    There were two distinct types of recombinants,
    with 36 of the first type and 58 of the second
    type present. The recombination frequency
    of the gene is (a) 0.145 (b) 0.245 (c) 0.345
    (d) 0.445   b

7. Crossing over of the chromosome $\begin{smallmatrix} L & S \\ K & S \end{smallmatrix}$ will

266

yield (a) $\dfrac{L\ \ K}{S\ \ S}$ (b) $\dfrac{S\ \ S}{L\ \ K}$ (c) $\dfrac{L\ \ S}{K\ \ S}$ (d) $\dfrac{K\ \ S}{L\ \ S}$

c

8. Linked genes do not show a 1:1:1:1 phenotypic ratio after being crossed. This is an
example of Mendel's Law of (a) Independent
Assortment. (b) Segregation. (c) both a and b
(d) none of the above

a

9. _____ chromosomes are the giant bundled
chromosomes found in the salivary glands of
the Drosophila . (a) $\propto$ - Helical (b) Polytene
(c) β - Helical (d) Supratene

b

10. One way in which human genes are mapped is
through somatic cell genetics. This refers to
(a) comparing somatic and visceral DNA. (b)
the fission of a somatic cell nucleus. (c) the
addition of cytotoxic agents to somatic cell
nuclei. (d) the fusion of two somatic cells,
allowing specific traits to be studied.

d

11 Two other ways used to map human genes are
(a) DNA hybridization probes and studies of
pedigrees. (b) DNA fission and studies of
pedigrees. (c) DNA hybridization and visceral
cell fission. (d) DNA fission and visceral cell
fission.

a

12. The cross $\dfrac{AOB}{AMB}$ x $\dfrac{AMB}{AMB}$ would yield

(a) 1 $\dfrac{AOB}{AOB}$, 2 $\dfrac{AOB}{AMB}$, 1 $\dfrac{AMB}{AMB}$

(b) 4 $\dfrac{AOB}{AMB}$ (c) 2 $\dfrac{AOB}{AMB}$, 2 $\dfrac{AMB}{AMB}$

(d) 4 $\dfrac{AMB}{AMB}$

c

13. The above cross is known as a (a) two point
cross. (b) three point cross. (c) four point
cross. (d) six point cross.

b

14. The highest percent recombination ever
expected is (a) 50%. (b) 75%. (c) 99%. (d) 100%.

a

SHORT ANSWER QUESTIONS FOR REVIEW

15. In order to determine the gene sequence in a three point cross you must know which of the progeny are (a) parental (non crossover) types. (b) single crossover types. (c) double crossover types. (d) a, b and c

d

16. Which of the following classes of progeny would be most numerous? (a) parental type (b) single crossover type (c) double crossover type (d) triple crossover type

a

Fill in the blanks.

17. Genes in _____ linkage groups follow Mendel's Law of Independent Assortment.

different

18. A gene with a recombination frequency of 0.165 with another gene is _____ map units from the other gene.

16.5

19. The mathematical formula
$$X = \frac{\text{observed frequency of double crossovers}}{\text{expected frequency of double crossovers}}$$
has X representing the _____.

coefficient
of
coincidence

20. Crossover percentage is theoretically _____ proportional to the physical distances observed on linked genes.

directly

21. The linear order of the genes on a chromosome predicted by using the percentage crossover is _____ that of the chromosome as observed by physical methods.

identical
to

22. Along the chromosome there are light and dark banding regions caused by differences in _____ between those regions.

density

23. Most methods of human gene mapping are used because they allow for _____ loss of chromosomes.

preferential

24. The term for exact duplication of human chromosomes is chromosome _____.

cloning

25. Recombination produces new combinations of genes not present in the _____.

parents

26. In a test cross there were 167 recombinants, (81 in one group and 86 in the other) in a total of 1008 progeny. They are _____ map units apart. | 16

27. Linked genes are inherited _____. | together

28. Forty-five percent of crossing over is equal to _____ map units. | 45

29. In a three point crossover, the gene in the center position can be found by comparing the parental type genes and the _____ type genes. | double crossover

Decide whether the following statements are true or false.

30. Neighboring genes are less loosely linked than more distant ones. | False

31. When two linked genes have 50% crossing over between them, 100% of the progeny will be recombinants. | False

32. In a cross between two strains of Neurospora the following data is collected:

Class	# of Asci
F	127
G	135
H	119
I	125
J	130

These data prove that the genes are linked on the original chromosome. | False

33. Ten percent crossing over is equal to one map unit. | False

34. A genetic map is a good representation of the actual structure of a chromosome. | True

35. When performing a double crossover test cross, it is much more likely that the genes are linked. | True

36. Crossover frequency is the same throughout the chromosome. | False

37. In order to do human gene mapping, many test crosses must be performed.

False

38. Genes on the same chromosome tend to stay together during the formation of gametes.

True

39. During a cross in which recombination occurs, more recombinants are found than parental types.

False

40. The ratio of progeny to parents with genes that are not linked is exactly the same as that of parents showing 50% crossing over.

True

41. Double crossover events occur more frequently than single crossovers.

False

42. Either all chromatids of a chromosome undergo recombination, or none of them do.

False

43. By looking at the phenotypes of all progeny of a test cross, as well as the given numerical data, the genotypes of the parents can be determined.

True

CHAPTER 8

POPULATION GENETICS

HARDY-WEINBERG PRINCIPLE AND GENE FREQUENCY

● PROBLEM 8-1

What are the implications of the Hardy-Weinberg Law?

Solution: The Hardy-Weinberg Law states that in a population at equilibrium, both gene and genotype frequencies remain constant from generation to generation. An equilibrium population refers to a large interbreeding population in which mating is random and no selection or other factor which tends to change gene frequencies occurs.

The Hardy-Weinberg Law is a mathematical formulation which resolves the puzzle of why recessive genes do not disappear in a population over time. To illustrate the principle let us look at the distribution in a population of a single gene pair, A and a. Any member of the population will have the genotype AA, Aa, or aa. If these genotypes are present in the population in the ratio of 1/4 AA : 1/2 Aa : 1/4 aa, we can show that given random mating and comparable viability of progeny in each cross, the genotypes and gene frequencies should remain the same in the next generation. Table 1 below shows how the genotypic frequencies of AA, Aa, and aa compare in the population and among the offspring.

Table 1

The Offspring of the Random Mating of a Population Composed of 1/4 AA, 1/2 Aa and 1/4 aa Individuals

Mating Male	Female	Frequency	Offspring
AA x AA		1/4 x 1/4	1/16 AA
AA x Aa		1/4 x 1/2	1/16 AA + 1/16 Aa
AA x aa		1/4 x 1/4	1/16 Aa
Aa x AA		1/2 x 1/4	1/16 AA + 1/16 Aa
Aa x Aa		1/2 x 1/2	1/16 AA + 1/8 Aa + 1/16aa
Aa x aa		1/2 x 1/4	1/16 Aa + 1/16aa
aa x AA		1/4 x 1/4	1/16 Aa
aa x Aa		1/4 x 1/2	1/16 Aa + 1/16aa
aa x aa		1/4 x 1/4	1/16aa
			Sum: 4/16 AA + 8/16 Aa + 4/16aa

Since the genotype frequencies are identical, it follows that the gene frequencies are also the same.

It is very important to realize that the Hardy-Weinberg law is theoretical in nature and holds true only when factors which tend to change gene frequencies are absent. Examples of such factors are natural selection, mutation, migration, and genetic drift.

● **PROBLEM** 8-2

Can complete equilibrium in a gene pool exist in real situations?

Solution: Of the four conditions necessary for the genetic equilibrium described by the Hardy-Weinberg Law, the first, large population size, is met reasonably often; the second, absence of mutations, is never met; the third, no migration, is met sometimes; the fourth, random reproduction, is rarely met in real situations. Therefore, it follows that complete equilbrium in a gene pool is not expected.

With regard to the first condition, many natural populations are so large that chance alone is not likely to cause any appreciable alteration in gene frequencies in their gene pools. Any breeding population with more than 10,000 members of breeding age is probably not significantly affected by random changes.

The second condition for genetic equilibrium - the absence of mutations - is never met in any population because spontaneous mutations are always occurring. Most genes probably undergo mutation once in every 50,000 to 1,000,000 duplications, with the rate of mutation for different genes varying greatly. However, since the rate of spontaneous mutation is usually low, it is usually insignificant in altering the gene frequencies in a large population.

The third condition for genetic equilibrium implies that a gene pool cannot exchange its genes with the outside. Immigration or emigration of individuals would change the gene frequencies in the gene pool. A high percentage of natural populations, however, experience some amount of migration. This factor, which enhances variation, tends to upset the Hardy-Weinberg equilibrium.

The fourth condition - random reproduction - refers not only to the indiscriminate selection of a mate but also to a host of other requirements that contribute to success in propagating the viable offspring. Such factors include the fertility of the mating pair, and the survival of the young to reproductive age. An organism's genotype actually influences its selection of a mate, the physical efficiency and frequency of its mating, its fertility, and so on. Thus, entirely random reproduction in reality is not possible.

We can conclude, therefore, that if any of the conditions of the Hardy-Weinberg Law are not met, then the gene pool of a population will not be in equilibrium and there will be an accompanying change in gene frequency for that population. Since it is virtually impossible to have a population existing in genetic equilibrium, even with animals under laboratory conditions, there must then be a continuous process of changing genetic constitutions in all populations. This is ultimately related to evolution in that evolutionary change is not usually automatic but occurs only when something disturbs the genetic equilibrium.

How can you determine whether or not a given population is in genetic equilibrium?

Solution: In an equilibrium population, both gene frequencies and genotype frequencies remain constant from generation to generation. The best way to determine if a given population is in equilibrium is to compare these frequencies over two generations to see if they are indeed constant. One way to do this is to determine the gene frequencies for a given adult population representative (or a group of that population) and for their offspring. Two generations are thus represented in the sample. For more reliable results, however, more generations should be compared with respect to their gene frequencies.

Suppose one wanted to know if the population of Australian aborigines was in genetic equilibrium. Data from that population concerning the distribution of MN blood groups are gathered and are shown below:

	Phenotype			
Generation (G)	M	MN	N	Total
1	241	604	195	1040
2	183	460	154	797

MN blood groups are determined by two alleles, L^M and L^N, having intermediate or codominant inheritance. Thus M type is coded for by $L^M L^M$, MN type by $L^M L^N$, and N type by $L^N L^N$. We can calculate the genotype frequencies using the data given:

Genotype	Frequency			
	G_1		G_2	
$L^M L^M$	241/1040 =	.231	183/797 =	.230
$L^M L^N$	604/1040 =	.581	460/797 =	.577
$L^N L^N$	195/1040 =	.188	154/797 =	.193
		1.0		1.0

The genotype frequencies are thus found to be essentially the same for both generations.

We could also have determined the allelic frequencies from the data; the number of L^M alleles in the population is twice the number of M individuals ($L^M L^M$) plus the number of MN individuals ($L^M L^N$). The number of L^N alleles is twice the number of N individuals plus the number of MN individuals. Since each individual carries two alleles, the total number of alleles in the population is twice the number of individuals, or the sum of the L^M and L^N alleles. For our population, then, we have the following:

$$\underline{L^M = 2(M) + MN} \qquad \underline{L^N = 2(N) + MN}$$

G_1 $2(241)+604 = 1086$ $2(195)+604 = 994$

G_2 $2(183)+460 = 826$ $2(154)+460 = 768$

Total Alleles($L^M + L^N$)	Frequency L^M	Frequency L^N
G_1 $1086+994=2(1040)=2080$	$1086/2080=.522$	$994/2080=0.478$
G_2 $826+768=2(797)=1594$	$826/1594=.518$	$768/1594=0.482$

As with the genotype frequencies, the allelic frequencies remain nearly the same in both generation. Thus, we can say that, with respect to the MN blood group alleles, the population is in equilibrium. Note that we can only determine equilibrium in a population in reference to a given gene or a small number of genes. Though our population may be in equilibrium for the MN alleles, other allelic systems may not be. For example, migration may be occurring from nearby populations having similar MN allelic frequencies but very different allelic frequencies for color blindness, thus affecting the equilibrium of these genes in the population.

● **PROBLEM** 8-4

In an isolated mountain village, the gene frequencies of A, B and O blood alleles are 0.95, 0.04, and 0.01, respectively. If the total population is 424, calculate the number of individuals with O, A, B and AB type blood.

Solution: Multiple allelic systems establish equilibrium in the same way as single-pair alleles, and the same equilibrium principles can be applied, though naturally the system is more complex. In the inheritance of blood groups, three genes-A, A^B, and a-are involved. Letting p, q, and r, respectively, represent their frequencies, we can say that the total of these frequencies equals 1, (p + q + r = 1). We can represent the total possible gene combinations (genotypes) in the population by means of the same type of expansion used with single-pair allelic systems; in this case, however, three alleles are involved. Thus:

$$(p+q+r)^2 = p^2 + 2pq + q^2 + 2pr + r^2 + 2qr$$

where:

$$p = \text{frequency A}$$

$$q = \text{frequency } A^B$$

$$r = \text{frequency a}$$

The following table summarizes what we know of the genotypes of each blood group and the corresponding allelic and genotypic frequencies.

blood type	genotypes	genotypic frequency
O	aa	r^2
A	AA, Aa	p^2, 2pr
B	$A^B A^B$, $A^B a$	q^2, 2qr
AB	AA^B	2pq

In the given population, p = 0.95, q = 0.04, and r = 0.01. Knowing this we can calculate the blood type frequencies using the results of the expansion. The frequency of type O blood in the population is:

$$r^2 = (0.01)^2 = 0.0001$$

The frequency of type A blood is the sum of the frequencies of the two genotypes comprising this phenotypic blood group:

$$p^2 + 2pr = (0.95)^2 + 2(0.95)(0.01)$$

$$= .9025 + .019$$

$$= 0.9215$$

276

The frequency of type B blood is the sum of the frequencies of the genotypes comprising the group:

$$q^2 + 2qr = (0.04)^2 + 2(0.04)(0.01)$$

$$= .0016 + .0008$$

$$= .0024$$

The frequency of type AB blood is simply:

$$2pq = 2(0.95)(0.04) = .076$$

We can see that the sum of the frequencies is 1:

$$\text{frequency O} = r^2 = .0001$$
$$A = p^2 + 2pr = .9215$$
$$B = q^2 + 2qr = .0024$$
$$AB = 2pq = \underline{.076}$$
$$1.000$$

Converting the frequencies to actual numbers of individuals in the population:

$$O = (r^2)(424) = (.0001)(424) \cong 0 \ (.0424)$$
$$A = (p^2+2pr)(424) = (.9215)(424) = 391$$
$$B = (q^2+2qr)(424) = (.0024)(424) = 1$$
$$AB = (2pq)(424) = (.076)(424) = \underline{32}$$
$$424$$

● PROBLEM 8-5

The dominant gene T controls the ability to taste the chemical phenylthiocarbamide (PTC). Individuals with the T allele find PTC bitter while tt individuals find it tasteless. In a sample of 320 students at Swarthmore College, 218 were tasters and 102 were non-tasters. Assuming this is a random sample from the student body population, estimate (a) gene frequencies and (b) genotype frequencies of the original sample.

$$\underset{\text{N-Phenyl-thiocarbamyl peptide}}{\boxed{}\!\!-\text{NH}-\overset{\overset{\text{S}}{\|}}{\text{C}}-\text{NH}-\overset{\overset{\text{R}_1}{|}}{\text{CH}}-\text{CONH-peptide}}$$

Solution: According to the Hardy-Weinberg equilibrium formula:

$$p^2 + 2\,pq + q^2 = 1,$$

where p^2 represents TT
2pq represents Tt
q^2 represents tt

When p and q represent the frequencies of all alleles in the population, p + q = 1. We use this formula to find the frequencies of both alleles.

Total Sample = 320
Number of non-tasters (tt) = 102

$$\text{Frequency of tt} = \frac{\text{number of non-tasters}}{\text{total sample size}} = \frac{102}{320} = 0.32$$

We can now use this information to find first q and then p. We know that q^2 represents tt, so

$$q^2 = tt = 0.32$$

$$q = \sqrt{0.32} = 0.56$$

Frequency of t = 0.56

We can use our value of q to find p from the formula

$$p = 1 - q$$

$$= 1 - 0.56 = 0.44$$

Frequency of T = 0.44

So the gene frequencies are 0.56 for t and 0.44 for T.

(b) Genotypic frequencies of TT and Tt can be calculated from the gene frequencies.

From the formula $p^2 + 2pq + q^2 = 1$,

$$\text{TT students} = p^2$$

We know that p = 0.44

$$\text{so } p^2 = (0.44)^2 = 0.19$$

Number of TT students = number of TT students x total sample size = 0.19 x 320 = 61.

Again from the formula,

Tt students = 2pq

$$= 2(0.44)(0.56) = 0.49$$

Number of Tt students = 0.49 x 320

$$= 157$$

To check this, we can add all of the different genotypic numbers:

TT	61
Tt	157
tt	102
total students;	320

● PROBLEM 8-6

In a group of students, about 36% could roll their tongues, a trait determined by a dominant gene. The other 64% of the students were nonrollers. Calculate the frequencies of the gene R for tongue rolling and its recessive allele r for nonrolling.

Solution: This problem can be solved by using the Hardy-Weinberg formula.

$$p^2 + 2pq + q^2 = 1 \quad \text{Let p = freq. of R}$$
Let q = freq. of r

p^2 = freq. of homozygous tongue rollers RR

$2pq$ = freq. of heterozygous tongue rollers Rr

q^2 = freq. of non-tongue rollers rr

The percent of nonrollers was given as 64%. Change this to a frequency by moving the decimal two places to the left. .64

$$q^2 = .64$$

$$q = \sqrt{.64} = 0.8 \text{ the frequency of r.}$$

$$p + q = 1 \text{ so } p = 1 - q = 1 - .8 = 0.2 \text{ the frequency of R.}$$

If the frequency of the gene for widow's peak, a dominant trait, is 0.07, what will be the frequency of (A) persons homozygous for widow's peak, (B) persons heterozygous for widow's peak, and (C) persons lacking widow's peak?

Solution: Solve the problem using the Hardy-Weinberg formula.

$$p^2 + 2pq + q^2 = 1 \quad \text{Let p = the freq. of W, p=0.07}$$

$$\text{Let q = the freq. of w, q=0.93}$$

p + q = 1 so if the frequency for p is known, then q can be readily determined: q = 1 - p, q = 1 - .07 = .93

(A) p^2 = freq. of homozygous widow's peak (WW)

$$p^2 = (.07)^2 = 0.0049$$

(B) 2pq = freq. of heterozygous widow's peak (Ww)

$$2pq = 2(.07)(.93) = 0.1302$$

(C) q^2 = freq. of homozygotes for the recessive gene for no widow's peak.

$$q^2 = (.93)^2 = 0.8649$$

Albinism, a condition characterized by a lack of pigment in the skin, eyes and hair, occurs in certain populations with a frequency of 0.00005. Assuming albinism is determined by a single recessive gene, a (a) what is the probability of an albino resulting from a cross between an albino and an individual of a normal phenotype? (b) What proportion of albinos have phenotypically normal parents?

Solution: We can solve this problem with the same two equations used in the previous problems,

$$p + q = 1 \text{ and } p^2 + 2pq + q^2 = 1$$

when p = A and q = a.

(a) In order for a normal individual and an albino to produce an albino child, the normal parent must have the heterozygous genotype Aa. The proportion of heterozygous individuals is found in the following way:

$$\frac{\text{proportion of heterozygotes (Aa)}}{\text{proportion of normal phenotypes(Aa+AA)}} = \frac{2pq}{p^2+2pq}$$

Factoring out p gives:

$$\frac{2\not pq}{\not p(p+2q)} = \frac{2q}{p+2q}$$

Substituting in p = 1 - q gives:

$$\frac{2q}{1-q+2q} = \frac{2q}{1+q}$$

Since we are given that $q^2 = 0.00005$ we find q = 0.00707. Substituting these values into $\frac{2q}{1+q}$ we get:

$$\frac{2(0.00707)}{1+0.00707} = 0.014$$

Because q is so small, this is approximately $\frac{2q}{1}$ or: 2q = 0.014. Since half of the offspring from this cross will be albino, the probability of one resulting from this cross is:

$$1/2(0.014) = 0.007 \text{ or } 0.7\%$$

(b) The cross Aa x Aa must occur in order for two normal parents to have an albino. It occurs with the frequency

$$(2pq)^2 = (0.014)^2 = 0.000196$$

(p can be ignored since it is almost 1)

One-quarter of these matings will result in albinos, so

$$(\tfrac{1}{4})(0.000196) = 0.000049.$$

The proportion of all albinos that have normal parents is

$$\frac{\text{prop. of albinos w/normal parents}}{\text{prop. of all albinos}} = \frac{0.000049}{0.00005}$$

$$= 0.98$$

● **PROBLEM** 8-9

From 146 students tested for PTC tasting ability, 105 were tasters and 41 were non-tasters. Calculate the frequencies of tasters and non-tasters.

Solution: The ability to taste depends upon a dominant gene T. In the Hardy-Weinberg theorem, $p^2 + 2pq + q^2 = 1$, the percentage of non-tasters (tt) may be represented as q^2. Therefore:

$$q^2 = \frac{41}{146} = 0.28$$

$$q = \sqrt{.28} = 0.53 = \text{frequency of t}$$

We can find the frequency of T by substituting it for p in the equation

$$p + q = 1$$

$$p = 1 - q$$

$$p = 1 - 0.53 = 0.47 = \text{frequency of T.}$$

With the expression $p^2 + 2pq + q^2$, we can calculate the frequencies of TT and Tt tasters.

$$TT = p^2 = (0.47)^2 = 0.2209$$

$$Tt = 2pq = 2(0.47)(0.53) = 0.4982$$

282

$$\text{tt} \quad = \quad q^2 = (0.53)^2 \qquad = \quad 0.2809$$

We add these up, to check our calculations. They should add up to equal 1.

$$
\begin{array}{r}
0.2209 \\
0.4982 \\
\underline{0.2809} \\
1.0000
\end{array}
$$

● PROBLEM 8-10

In humans, the M, MN and N blood groups are determined by two codominant alleles: $\underline{L}^m$ and $\underline{L}^n$. In a population of 800 college students the following phenotypes were identified:

Blood Group	Number
M	392
MN	336
N	$\underline{72}$
	800

Determine the frequency of the $\underline{L}^m$ and $\underline{L}^n$ alleles.

Solution: Since both alleles can be identified in each individual in which they occur, the frequency of each can be calculated directly.

Let p = frequency of $\underline{L}^m$ and q = frequency of $\underline{L}^n$.

Then, $p = \dfrac{\text{total number of } \underline{L}^m \text{ alleles in population}}{\text{total number of genes in population}}$

and we have, $p = \dfrac{(392 \times 2) + 336}{800 \times 2} = \dfrac{1,120}{1,600} = .7$

283

Similarly, $q = \dfrac{\text{total number of } \underline{L}^n \text{ alleles in population}}{\text{total number of genes in population}}$

and we have, $q = \dfrac{(72 \times 2) + 336}{800 \times 2} = \dfrac{480}{1,600} = .3$

The frequency of allele S in an isolated population of 100 is 0.65. Immigrants with a frequency of S = 0.85 are introduced at a rate of one new immigrant per population per generation. Calculate the frequency of S after one generation of new immigrants.

Solution: The movement of immigrants into or out of isolated populations can have a marked effect on gene frequency. Since the gene frequency of the two populations is different, the equilibrium of the new population will shift accordingly after the migration.

The alteration in the gene frequency after one generation is given by the following relation:

$$q_1 - q_0 = m(q_m - q_0)$$

where m = the frequency of immigrations per generation

q_m = the frequency of gene S among the immigrant population

q_0 = the frequency of gene S among the original population

q_1 = the frequency of gene S in the combined population after one generation of immigration

$m = 1/100$

$q_m = 0.85$

$q_0 = 0.65$

Substituting into the equation, we get:

$$q_1 - 0.65 = 1/100(0.85 - 0.65)$$

$$q_1 - 0.65 = 0.002$$

$$q_1 = 0.652$$

The frequency of gene S after one generation is 0.652. The influx of immigrants who have a higher frequency of the gene has slightly increased the gene's frequency in the entire population.

● **PROBLEM** 8-12

A population of students taking a basic genetics class had their blood types classified in the ABO blood group system. The following numbers were recorded:

Phenotype	Number	Frequency
A	249	.2075
B	376	.3133
AB	77	.0642
O	498	.4150
	1,200	1.0000

Assuming this population of students is in genetic equilibrium, what are the frequencies of the three alleles $\underline{I}^A$, $\underline{I}^B$, and $\underline{i}$, respectively?

Solution: Since there are three alleles present in the population, we need to determine three gene frequencies. Let p = frequency of $\underline{I}^A$, q = frequency of $\underline{I}^B$ and r = frequency of $\underline{i}$. Having assumed that this population is in genetic equilibrium, we can solve directly for r, since r^2 is the frequency of the $\underline{ii}$ homozygotes, or type O. Thus, $r = \sqrt{r^2} = \sqrt{.4150} = .64$.

By algebraic manipulation we can show that

285

$p = \sqrt{1-}$ frequency of type B+frequency of type O, so

$p = 1- \sqrt{.3133+.4150} = 1 - .85 = .15$.

Similarly, we can show that

$$q = 1- \sqrt{A + O} = 1- \sqrt{.2075 + .4150}$$

$$= 1 - .70 = .21.$$

Since $p + q + r$ must sum to 1.0, we can check our answers and find that, indeed

$$p + q + r = 1.0.$$

● **PROBLEM** 8-13

Given a population in genetic equilibrium in which the initial gene frequency of d is 0.2; assume the rate of mutation (u) of D→d to be 4.1×10^{-5}, and the rate of back mutation (v) of d→D to be 2.5×10^{-7}.

a) If the above rates of mutation are introduced into the population, what will be the change in q (frequency of d) in the first generation?

b) Assuming that the above rates continue over time, what will be the value of q at mutational equilibrium?

Solution: a) If u is the rate of mutation from D to d, and p is the frequency of D, then there will be $(\overline{u})(p)$ new d genes after mutation. Similarly, if v is the rate of mutation from d to D, then there will be $(v)(q)$ d genes removed by back mutation. Thus, the new gene frequency, $q_1 = q_0 + up_0 - vq_0$, and the change of gene frequency Δq will be:

$$\Delta q = q_1 - q_0 = up_0 - vq_0$$

Therefore,

$$\Delta q = (.000041)(.8) - (.00000025)(.2) = .00003275.$$

b) At equilibrium, up = vq because $\Delta q = 0$.

Then, the gene frequency, $q_e = \dfrac{u}{u+v}$. By substituting in the values for u and v, we get:

$$q_e = \frac{0.000041}{0.00004125} = .9939$$

Assume a population of garden peas in genetic equilibrium in which the frequencies of the genes for full pods (F) and constricted pods (f) are .6 and .4, respectively. If this population is allowed only to reproduce by self-fertilization for three generations, what will be the distribution of the three genotypes by the third generation of self-fertilization?

Solution: If the population is in a state of genetic equilibrium initially, then the distribution of genotypes before self-fertilization is imposed will be: $(.6F + .4f)^2$ = .36FF + .48Ff + .16ff. Self-fertilization, which is the most severe form of inbreeding, will reduce the frequency of heterozygotes by one-half each generation, with the reduction being equally distributed between the two homozygotes.

Thus, the frequencies of these three genotypes will be:

generation 1 -- .48FF + .24Ff + .28ff

generation 2 -- .54FF + .12Ff + .34ff

generation 3 -- .57FF + .06Ff + .37ff

In Caucasians the incidence of cystic fibrosis is about 1 in 2,000 births; but, among nonwhites the incidence is about 1 in 250,000 births. What would be the rate of incidence among matings between Caucasians and nonwhites? If these offspring were to mate randomly among themselves, what incidence would be expected among their offspring?

Solution: Cystic fibrosis is a recessive inherited disease characterized by a defect in protein metabolism. This leads to degeneration of the pancreas and chronic lung infections leading to destruction of the lungs. Diagnosis is established by the discovery of an increased concentration of sodium in sweat, to levels above 88mmol/L. Since the disorder is autosomal recessive, both parents of an infected child must be heterozygous.

This problem is based on Wahlund's principle, which states that when mating occurs between populations, the frequency of homozygous genotypes is reduced.

Let the allele frequency of cystic fibrosis among Caucasians be q_1. The incidence among Caucasians is given as 1:2000.

$$q_1 = \sqrt{1/2000}$$

$$q_1 = 0.0224$$

Let the allele frequency among nonwhites be q_2. The incidence among nonwhites is 1:250,000

$$q_2 = \sqrt{1/250,000}$$

$$q_2 = 0.002$$

The expected frequency of the homozygous recessive condition which results from a mating between a Caucasian and a nonwhite is:

$$q_1 q_2 = (0.0224)(0.002)$$

$$= 4.48 \times 10^{-5}, \text{ about 1 in 22,000 births.}$$

The allele frequency of cystic fibrosis within the hybrid population is given by the formula

$$\bar{q} = (\tfrac{1}{2})[q_1(1-q_2) + q_2(1-q_1)] + q_1q_2$$
$$= \tfrac{1}{2}[0.0224(1-0.002)+0.002(1-0.0224)]+(0.0224 \times 0.002)$$

$$= 0.0122, \text{ or about 1 in 80 births.}$$

With random mating within the hybrid population, the frequency of homozygous recessives would be:

$$(\bar{q})^2 = (0.0122)^2$$

$$= 1.49 \times 10^{-4}, \text{ or about 1 in 6,700 births.}$$

● **PROBLEM** 8-16

Consider a population of garden peas in which the genes F for full pods and f for constricted pods are segregating. Assuming that gene frequencies for this population are found to be: p (frequency of F) = 0.7 and q (frequency of f) = 0.3, and that the population is in genetic equilibrium, what proportion of the progeny produced from matings of full-podded x full-podded will be constricted-podded?

Solution: Since the population is in genetic equilibrium, and therefore is undergoing random mating, there are three types of full x full matings:

(a) FF x FF which occurs at a frequency of p^4

(b) FF x Ff which occurs at a frequency of $4p^3q$

and (c) Ff x Ff which occurs at a frequency of $4p^2q^2$.

Of these, only the Ff x Ff matings will produce constricted-podded progeny at a frequency of p^2q^2. Thus the proportion of constricted-podded progeny from full x full matings will be:

$$\frac{p^2q^2}{p^4 + 4p^3q + 4p^2q^2}.$$

This can be simplified to:

$$\text{proportion ff progeny} = \left(\frac{q}{1+q}\right)^2.$$

Now by substituting in the value of q, we get the proportion of ff progeny $= \left(\frac{.3}{1.3}\right)^2 = .0532$.

The frequency of Tay-Sachs disease in the Jewish population of New York City is about 0.015 and approximately 0.0015 in non-Jewish individuals. Homozygotes die in infancy or early childhood. If the selection coefficient is 1 and the forward mutation rate is 1×10^{-6}, what is the equilibrium frequency of the Tay-Sachs gene in the Jewish population under the combined effects of mutation and selection?

Solution: Tay-Sachs disease is an autosomal recessive disease. Affected children lack the enzyme, N-acetylhexosaminidase which breaks down a ganglioside lipid. This ganglioside then accumulates in the ganglion cells of the cerebral cortex and other parts of the brain. Mental and motor deterioration followed by blindness and death before the age of three are the clinical consequences of this disease.

To solve this problem we need to use the formula

$$\Delta q_m = up - vq$$

where Δq_m is the rate of change in q due to mutation; q is the frequency of the mutating gene t in any one generation; p is the frequency of its mutating allele T; u is the rate of forward mutation; and v is the rate of back mutation. Now we must find the numerical values to substitute into the formula. We are given q = 0.015. Using the formula,

$$p + q = 1$$

$$p = 1 - q$$

and substituting, p = 1-0.015 = 0.985. So p = 0.985. We are also given u = 1×10^{-6}. The rate of back mutation, v, is effectively zero since Tay-Sachs disease is lethal very early in life. These values can be used in the formula to find Δq_m:

$$\Delta q_m = up - vq$$

$$\Delta q_m = (1 \times 10^{-6})(0.985) - (0)(0.015)$$

$$\Delta q_m = 9.85 \times 10^{-7}$$

This value is approximately equal to u, (1×10^{-6}) because $0.000000958 \cong 0.000001$. So $\Delta q_m \cong u$. This is the effect of mutation on the gene frequency; however, we must still find the effect of selection.

The rate of change of the frequency of a recessive gene under selection is given by the equation:

$$\Delta q_s = \frac{-sq_0^2 p}{1 - sq_0^2}$$

where s is the selection coefficient, which in this case is 1.

Substituting the values that we have into the equation:

$$\Delta q_s = \frac{-(0.015)^2(1)(0.985)}{1 - (1)(0.015)^2}$$

$$\Delta q_s = -2.22 \times 10^{-4}$$

This value is approximately equal to $-sq^2$ so $\Delta q_s \cong -sq^2$, since $-2.22 \times 10^{-4} \cong -(1)(2.25 \times 10^{-4})$. So we have $\Delta q_m \cong u$ and $\Delta q_s \cong -sq^2$. Since $\Delta q = \Delta q_s + \Delta q_m$, we can substitute u and $-sq^2$ for Δq_s and Δq_m to get $\Delta q = -sq^2 + u$. Since we are looking for the frequency at equilibrium where, by definition, $\Delta q = 0$, we have

$$u - sq^2 = 0$$

or

$$u = sq^2.$$

If we rewrite this to solve for q^2 we get:

$$q^2 = \frac{u}{s}$$

and therefore:

$$\hat{q} = \sqrt{\frac{u}{s}} \; .$$

Substituting our values of $u = 1 \times 10^{-6}$ and $s = 1$, we get:

$$\hat{q} = \sqrt{\frac{1 \times 10^{-6}}{1}}$$

$$\hat{q} = 1 \times 10^{-3}.$$

So with the combined effect of mutation and selection, the equilibrium frequency is 0.001. The frequency of Tay-Sachs births, q^2, in this group would be $(1 \times 10^{-3})^2$ or 1×10^{-6} instead of $(0.015)^2$ or 2.25×10^{-4}.

● **PROBLEM** 8-18

The frequency of the gene for sickle-cell anemia in American Blacks is less than that found in the people living in their ancestral home in Africa. What factors might account for this difference?

Solution: The sickle-cell disease is a homozygous recessive trait that usually results in death before reproductive age. In the heterozygous form only 1% of the red blood cells are sickle-shaped as compared to 50% in the homozygous form, so the sickle-cell gene is not harmful enough to cause death. Instead it is beneficial in certain environments because it gives the carrier an immunity to malaria. In Africa, malaria is a severe problem and the heterozygous individuals have a survival advantage over their fellow Africans. Therefore, the frequency of the sickle-cell gene has been kept fairly constant in the gene pool in Africa.

In America, where the incidence of malaria is insignificant, an individual carrying the sickle-cell gene has no survival advantage, and the sickle-cell allele is slowly being lost and diluted in the population. Those with the homozygous sickle-cell genotype usually die; hence, the frequency of the sickle-cell allele declines.

In addition, with more interracial marriages in America, the sickle-cell genes from blacks are being diluted by the normal genes from the non-black population. Thus, in the American black population, a trend is observed in which the frequency of the sickle-cell gene decreases gradually over generations.

A certain recessive gene (r) in a population has a frequency of 0.5. As a result of movement of the population to a new environment, homozygous recessive individuals (rr) are now selected against, with a loss of 80% of the homozygotes before maturity. Homozygous dominant (RR) and heterozygotes (Rr) are not affected. What is the frequency of the gene in the population after one generation? Has equilibrium in the new environment been reestablished?

Solution: Since there are only two alleles involved, and we know that the sum of their frequencies must be one, we can calculate the frequency of the dominant gene (R) in the population. Letting p equal the frequency of R, and q equal the frequency of r (which is known to be 0.5):

$$p + q = 1$$

$$p = 1 - q$$

$$p = 1 - 0.5$$

$$p = 0.5$$

We can now use the Hardy-Weinberg binomial expansion to determine the corresponding genotype frequencies after one generation.

$$(p+q)^2 = p^2 + 2\,pq + q^2$$

$$= (.5)^2 + 2(.5)(.5) + (.5)^2$$

$$= .25 + .50 + .25 \quad (=1),$$

293

where
$$p^2 = \text{frequency RR}$$

$$2\,pq = \text{frequency Rr}$$

$$q^2 = \text{frequency rr}$$

The frequency q^2, however, is only the initial frequency of recessive homozygotes in the offspring. 80% of these will be lost to the population before reproductive age. Thus, the number of rr individuals in the population will, in effect, be only 20% of what it originally was. The effect that this will have on actual gene frequencies can best be seen be first converting the frequencies to actual individual numbers. For convenience sake, let us assume an original population of 100. The original number of rr individuals is (.25)(100) or 25. Loss of 80% of these would give a final effective number of

$$25 - (.8)(25) = 25 - 20 = 5.$$

The new frequencies now are calculated for an effective total population of 100 - 20, or 80. The number of RR and Rr individuals, 25 and 50 respectively, remains unchanged. The new genotype frequencies are:

frequency RR = 25/80 = .313

frequency Rr = 50/80 = .625

frequency rr = 5/80 = $\dfrac{.062}{1.000}$

The allelic frequencies can be calculated using a new effective allelic population of 2(80) or 160 (two alleles/individual).

number R = 2 RR + Rr = 2(25) + 50 = 100

number r = 2 rr + Rr = 2(5) + 50 = $\dfrac{60}{160}$

frequency R = p = 100/160 = .625

frequency r = q = 60/160 = $\dfrac{.375}{1.000}$

Notice that the actual distribution of genotypes does <u>not</u> correspond to the binomial expansion of the gene frequencies, $(p+q)^2$ (i.e., .313 $\neq$ p, .625 $\neq$ 2 pq, .062 $\neq$ q^2). This is because our population is not in equilibrium, and the Hardy-Weinberg principle applies only to populations in equilibrium. Selection has upset the equilibrium in the population. Until the selection factor, whatever it is, is removed, the frequency of the recessive gene will continue to decrease as it is being removed from the population with each successive generation. We can see however, that it will never be entirely removed, due to the presence of heterozygotes in the population. Nonetheless, its frequency can be reduced to almost zero if the selection is strong enough, and if enough generations have gone by.

● **PROBLEM** 8-20

A gene C mutates to c with a frequency of 2×10^{-6} per generation. There are no other forces acting on these alleles and mating is random. How many generations are needed to increase the frequency of gene c from 2 percent to 3 percent?

Solution: Since we are told that the mating is random and that there are no other forces acting on the two alleles we do not have to worry about mutation and selection frequencies. We can use the formula

$$p_n = p_o(1-\mu)^n$$

where u is the rate of mutation from C to c; p_n is the frequency of C in the nth generation; p_o is the frequency of c initially. We are given $\mu = 2 \times 10^{-6}$. We need to find p_n and p_o. Remember that

$$p = 1 - q.$$

Our problem gives us the values of q_n and q_o which are the frequencies of c in the nth generation and initially. From these values ($q_n = 3\% = 0.03$ and $q_o = 2\% = 0.02$). We can find both p_n and p_o.

$p_n = 1 - q_n$	$p_o = 1 - q_o$
$p_n = 1 - 0.03$	$p_o = 1 - 0.02$
$p_n = 0.97$	$p_o = 0.98$

Substituting these values into the original equation:

$$p_n = p_o(1 - \mu)^n$$

$$0.97 = 0.98[1-(2 \times 10^{-6})]^n$$

To solve this we take the log of both sides and then manipulate the form of the equation by using the laws governing logarithms.

$$\log 0.97 = \log \left[0.98 \left[1-(2 \times 10^{-6})\right]^n\right]$$

$$\log 0.97 = \log 0.98 + n \log[1-(2 \times 10^{-6})]$$

$$\frac{\log 0.97 - \log 0.98}{\log[1-(2 \times 10^{-6})]} = n$$

$$5128 \text{ generations} = n$$

It will take 5128 generations in this population in order for the frequency of gene c to increase from 2% to 3%.

• **PROBLEM** 8-21

In a heavily polluted industrialized area in England about 87% of the moths of the species Biston betularia are melanic (dark colored). If the frequency of recessives is 0.13, what is the frequency of the dominant allele leading to melanism? What proportion of the dark colored moths are heterozygous?

Solution: In the Manchester area in England, dark moths are more common than light moths. The dark moths are much harder for birds to see on the soot-covered tree trunks. The light moths are more abundant in the rural areas of England where they are very well camouflaged on the lichen-covered tree trunks. The dark color is produced as a result of a single dominant mutation. If the allele for the dark color was represented as C, then the genotype of melanic moths would be either Cc or CC. The light phenotype has the genotype cc.

The Hardy-Weinberg principle tells us that

$$p + q = 1$$

where q is the frequency of the recessive allele and p is the frequency of the dominant allele. We are given that the frequency of the homozygous recessive (cc) is 0.13. This means

$$q^2 = 0.13$$
$$q = \sqrt{0.13} = 0.36$$

Therefore: p = 1 - q

p = 1 - 0.36

p = 0.64

Using the Hardy-Weinberg binomial expansion, we can find the frequencies of the dominant homozygotes and the heterozygotes.

$$p^2 + 2pq + q^2 = 1$$

CC   Cc   cc

$$CC = p^2 = (0.64)^2 = 0.41$$

$$Cc = 2pq = 2(0.64)(0.36) = 0.46$$

$$cc = q^2 = (0.36)^2 = 0.13$$

Since the observed percentage of melanic moths was 87%, the proportion that were heterozygous are:

$$\frac{\text{frequency heterozygous (Cc)}}{\text{frequency melanic (Cc + CC)}} = \frac{0.46}{0.87}$$

$$= 0.53 \text{ or } 53\%$$

Thus, 53% of the dark moths were heterozygous and (100 - 53) = 47% were homozygous.

● PROBLEM 8-22

Colorblindness is caused by a sex-linked recessive gene (d). A sample of 2000 individuals (1000 male and 1000 female) contained 90 colorblind males. What percentage of the women are phenotypically normal?

Solution: Since this gene is sex-linked we must consider the number of X chromosomes in the individuals. Males have one X chromosome and females have two, so we must take into account that females have twice as many X-linked genes as males. The genotype frequencies at equilibrium are therefore:

p+q for males who have two genotypic classes, D and d, and

$p^2 + 2pq + q^2$ for females who have three genotypic classes, DD, Dd and dd.

Ninety out of 1000 men were colorblind (d), so

$$p + q = 1$$

$$p + \frac{90}{1000} = 1$$

$$p = 1 - 0.09 = 0.91$$

Thus p = 0.91 and q = 0.09. If we assume that the population mates randomly, we can estimate the expected number of females who carry the trait:

$$p^2 + 2pq + q^2 = 1$$

$$(0.91)^2 + 2(0.91)(0.09) + (0.09)^2 = 1$$

$$0.83 + 0.16 + 0.01 = 1$$

So 83% of the females are DD, 16% are Dd, and 1% are dd.

Our total female population was 1000, so 830 are DD, 160 are Dd and 10 are dd and colorblind. The number of females who are phenotypically normal is 830 + 160 = 990 or 99%. So 99% of the females are phenotypically normal while only 91% of the males are.

● **PROBLEM** 8-23

For each of the following populations determine whether the population is in a state of genetic equilibrium. Assume that the sample present is a representative random sample:

Population	AA	Genotype frequency Aa	aa
I	.64	.32	.04
II	.36	.42	.22
III	.0361	.3078	.6561
IV	.050625	.348750	.600625

Solution: For a population to be in a state of genetic equilibrium, the genotype frequencies must be distributed in the following array:

$$p^2 \text{ AA} + 2pq \text{ Aa} + q^2 \text{ aa} = 1.0$$

where p = frequency of gene A

and q = frequency of gene a

We can find the gene frequency values for each population by the following identities:

p = frequency of AA + 1/2 (frequency of Aa) and

q = frequency of aa + 1/2 (frequency of Aa).

Then, by squaring the binomial, $(p \text{ A} + q \text{ a})^2$, we can generate p^2 AA + 2pqAa + q^2 aa for each population. If the values calculated are the same as those observed for our sample, then the population sampled is in genetic equilibrium.

Thus, the gene frequencies can be calculated for each population.

Population

I p=0.64 + 0.16   q=0.04 + 0.16
   p=0.80   q=0.20

II p=0.36 + 0.21   q=0.22 + 0.21
   p=0.57   q=0.43

III p=0.0361 + 0.1539   q=0.6561 + 0.1539
   p=0.19   q=0.81

IV p=0.050625 + 0.174375   q=0.600625 + 0.174375
   p=0.225   q=0.775

Now, when the binomial for each of the populations is squared, and compared to the values given in the problem, we see that all the populations are in genetic equilibrium except Population II.

Consider a population of garden pea plants in which the genes F for full pods and f for constricted pods are segregating. When a sample of 1,500 plants were classified, the following phenotypes were recorded: 1,365 full-podded plants and 135 constricted-podded plants. Assuming that the sample classified was representative of the population, and that the population was in a state of genetic equilibrium, what are the frequencies of the two alleles? How many of the full-podded plants are heterozygous?

Solution: There are two alleles segregating in the population so we must first establish their identities. Let p = frequency of F and q = frequency of f, and p + q = 1.0. Since we have assumed that this sample is representative and that the population is in a state of genetic equilibrium, we can predict that the three genotypes present are distributed as p^2FF + 2pqFf + q^2ff. Thus, the frequency of constricted-podded plants or q^2 is $\frac{135}{1,500}$ = .09, and since q = $\sqrt{q^2}$; q = $\sqrt{.09}$ = 0.3; p can now be determined simply as 1 - q. Thus, p = 1 - .3 = 0.7.

Having determined the values for p and q, we can now determine how many of the full-podded plants are heterozygous by the following:

$$2pq = 2(.7)(.3) \times 1,500 = 630$$

Thus, 630 out of 1,365 full-podded plants are heterozygous (Ff).

TWINS

In what ways are studies of twins useful in supplying information about the relative importance of inheritance and environment in the determination of a given trait?

Solution: Although both environment and heredity are involved in the development of any trait, a change in some aspect of the environment may alter one character relatively little as compared to its effect on another character. An individual's blood type, for example, seems fairly impervious to practically all environmental effects, while the phenotype of a diabetic can be radically changed by a mere alteration in diet. Moreover, not all characters are determined by simple genetic effects which have easily observable relationships with simple environmental changes. Some traits, such as intelligence in animals, are probably determined by complex genetic-environmental interactions, the results of which are then viewed as a single trait.

Performing studies using twins is one way of determining the relative contributions of genetic composition and environment to the expression of a given trait.

There are two kinds of twins; identical or monozygotic twins, which arise from a single fertilized egg, and fraternal or dizygotic twins, which result from the fertilization of two separate eggs. From this definition we can see that monozygotic twins are genetically the same in every respect, while dizygotic twins may differ genetically for any character. By comparing both kinds of twins with regard to a particular trait, we can evaluate the roles of environment and heredity on the development of that character. On the one hand we have genetically identical individuals of the same age and sex, raised in a single uterine environment; and on the other we have genetically dissimilar individuals of the same age, though not necessarily of the same sex, raised in a common uterine environment. Presumably the difference between these two kinds of twins is only in the extent of their genetic similarity.

Using twins for genetic studies, then, provides built-in controls for both the effect of environment and the effect of heredity on the expression of a given trait. For example, if phenotypic similarities for a particular character are greater among identical twins than among fraternal twins, we can ascribe this to the genetic similarity of the identical pair and the genetic dissimilarity of the fraternal pair. On the other hand, if both identical and fraternal pairs show the same extent of phenotypic differences for a particular character, we can assume that genetic similarity or dissimilarity plays less of a role than the differences which may occur in the post-uterine environment of the twins. As a concrete illustration of this, consider a pair of monozygotic twins reared in different postnatal environments and a pair of dizygotic twins reared in a common postnatal environment. If the monozygotic twins were found to exhibit a wide range of dissimilarities and the dizygotic twins a significant range of similarities, the importance of the environment as a phenotypic modifier of the genetic composition of an individual can readily be appreciated.

● PROBLEM 8-26

Eighty — three monozygotic twin pairs are examined for the presence of club feet. Fifty pairs do not show the trait at all; twenty pairs have one member with club feet; and thirteen pairs have both members affected. What is the frequency of concordance?

Solution: Concordant twins are alike with respect to a particular trait and discordant twins are different. Here, the concordant twins both have club feet. In the discordant pairs, one twin has club feet while the other does not. In identical twins - monozygotes - concordance varies with different traits. A high degree of concordance is due to the twins' genetic identity, to the similarity of their environments or to a combination of both of these factors.

In this problem we are asked to find the concordance frequency for the club foot trait. The frequency of concordance

$$= \frac{\text{number of pairs where both show trait}}{\text{number of pairs where at least one shows trait}}$$

$$= \frac{13}{20+13} = 0.39$$

So these twins are 39 percent concordant for the trait for club feet.

Assume that a trait has 60% penetrance. What would be the proportion of concordant to discordant pairs of twins?

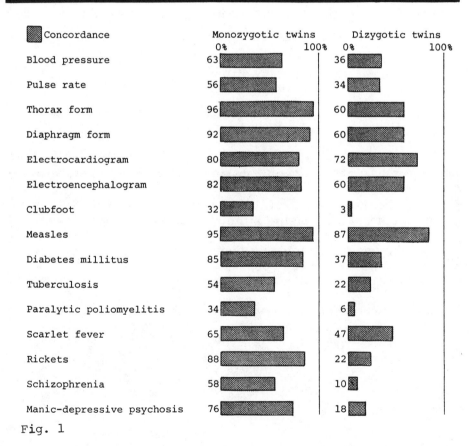

Fig. 1

Solution: Even identical twins can show variation in phenotype. This is due to the penetrance and expressivity of a gene. Penetrance is the proportion of individuals with the same genotype for a trait that show the expected mutant phenotype. Expressivity is the degree to which that mutant phenotype is expressed.

Twins that both show a certain phenotype are called concordant. Discordant twins are those that show different phenotypes for the trait. Figure 1 shows the concordance and discordance in twins for a variety of traits.

The penetrance is 60% or 0.6 in this problem. In identical twins, the trait would be expected to be present in both partners in $(0.6)^2 = 36$ percent. The percentage in which the trait is absent in both partners is $(100-60)^2 = (40\%)^2 = (0.4)^2 = 16\%$. The percentage in which the trait is present in only one partner is $2 \times 0.6 \times 0.4 = 48\%$. Therefore, the proportion of concordant to discordant pairs is $\frac{36+16}{48}$ or $\frac{52}{48}$ which is almost 1.1:1. If we calculate the ratio by only considering the expressed traits as concordant (both twins with normal phenotypes are excluded), we obtain a different ratio: $\frac{36}{48}$ or 0.75:1. Thus, depending on the assumption we make regarding concordance, we can obtain different values.

● **PROBLEM** 8-28

One thousand pairs of twins attend a twin convention in Minneapolis. Eight hundred pairs of these twins are of like sexes (male/male or female/female). The remaining two hundred pairs are of unlike sexes (male/female). What percentage of these twins is monozygotic and what percentage is dizygotic?

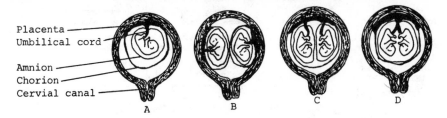

Placenta
Umbilical cord
Amnion
Chorion
Cervial canal

A   B   C   D

Twinning in man. (A) Human uterus with a single embyro. (B) Fraternal "twins"(from two eggs) with seperate chorions and placentas. (C) Identical twins (from one egg) with one placenta but with seperate amnions and yolk sacs (the latter are not shown). This results when two inner cell masses arise from one blastocyst. (D) Identical twins with one set of fetal membranes. This presumbly is the result of two embryonic axes forming from one inner cell mass.

Solution: Monozygotic twins arise from the same zygote and hence are identical genetically. Dizygotic, or fraternal twins, arise from two separate zygotes and are therefore as different as non-twin siblings. The only difference between fraternal twins and other siblings is that the twins share the same intrauterine environment.

To solve this problem, we must simply think logically - which may or may not be easy. First, realize that males and females are born with equal probability (1:1 ratio). So dizygotic twins stand a 50% chance of being of unlike sexes. Monozygotic twins, on the other hand, must be of the same sex. We know that 200 pairs of twins are of unlike sexes - these twins must be dizygotic. That is half of the dizygotic twins. The other half must be of like sex. (Remember that there is a 50% chance of being of unlike sex so there must be a corresponding 50% chance of being of like sex.) This gives us 200 extra pairs of dizygotic twins. Therefore, a total of 400 pairs of twins are dizygotic. This leaves 600 remaining pairs of twins as monzygotic. Dividing 400 dizygotes and 600 monozygotes by 1000 twins and then multiplying by 100% we have the answers. The twins at the Minneapolis twin convention are 60% monozygotic and 40% dizygotic.

● **PROBLEM** 8-29

Concordance for Down's syndrome in monozygotic twins is not 100 percent. Explain.

Solution: In about 11 percent of the cases where monozygotic twins have Down's syndrome, one of the twins is normal. This may be due to the loss of one of the three chromosome 21s by one of the two cells formed at the first cleavage. One of the cells would develop into a normal embryo with the proper two copies of each chromosome, and the other would develop into an embryo with three chromosome 21s. Another possibility is shown in the diagram. If somatic nondisjunction occurred at an early cell division of one of the twins, then that twin would develop Down's syndrome.

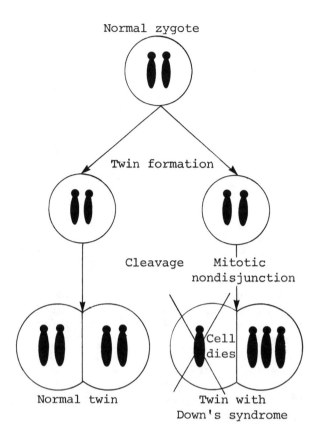

Normal zygote

Twin formation

Cleavage   Mitotic
            nondisjunction

Cell
dies

Normal twin   Twin with
               Down's syndrome

The average differences between the two members of identical twin pairs and nonidentical twins reared together and reared apart were found to be the following:

Difference in	Identical	Nonidentical	Identical (reared apart)
Height (cm)	1.7	4.4	1.8
Weight (lb)	4.1	10.0	9.9
Head length (mm)	2.9	6.2	2.20
Head width (mm)	2.8	4.2	2.85

How can these differences be explained?

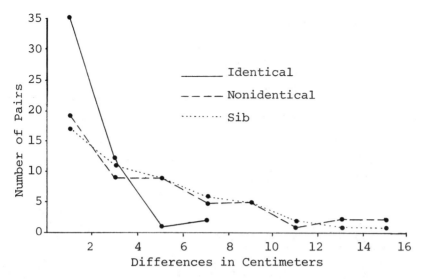

Fig. 1: Distribution of distances in standing height
of 50 identical twins, 52 nonidentical twins
and 52 pairs of siblings.

Solution: A glance at the table shows that identical twins
are more alike than nonidentical twins in regard to these
physical traits. Even when reared apart, the identical
twins have less differences in these characteristics. This
is understandable, since identical twins have identical
genomes. But why are there differences at all? Why aren't
identical twins truly identical?

Figure 1 shows graphically that there is more height
difference between nonidentical twins and siblings than
between identical twins - 35 out of 50 pairs of identical
twins (70%) had a height difference of 2 cm, whereas 17
out of 52 siblings (33%) and 19 out of 52 nonidentical
twins (37%) had such a small difference. The largest
difference between identical twins was 7 cm while there
were differences of up to 15 cm between siblings and
nonidentical twins. The variability is not due to genetic
factors alone. The variance of a population is given as
the sum of three components : genetic variability,
environmental variability and the variability due to the
interaction of these two factors.

$$V_{total} = V_{genetic} + V_{nongenetic} + V_{interaction}$$

Since identical twins are genetically identical, the genetic
component in the total variance can be ignored. Instead,
for identical twins, the nongenetic intrapair differences
and an interaction component are summed. The interaction
component is necessary because the environmental agents
that cause intrapair differences between twins of one
genotype may also affect another genotype.

$$V_{\text{total identical}} = V_{\text{nongenetic intrapair identical}}$$

$$+ V_{\text{interaction identical}}$$

Thus, identical twins have less variance than nonidentical twins because the nonidentical twins have more factors influencing variance.

PEDIGREE ANALYSIS

● **PROBLEM** 8-31

The pedigree of two families, the Browns and the Greens, is shown below. All of the members of the Green family have attached ear lobes. Only two members of the Brown family have attached ear lobes; the rest have free ear lobes. What is the mode of inheritance for the trait?

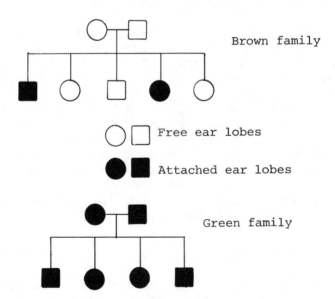

Brown family

○□ Free ear lobes

●■ Attached ear lobes

Green family

Solution: The pattern of inheritance shown is very characteristic for many human traits. Let us look at the pedigree to determine the mode of inheritance. When neither parent has attached ear lobes, only some of the children have the trait. However, when both parents have the trait, all of the children have it. Furthermore, both males and females are affected. This implies that the trait is not sex-linked, which would affect males more than females. To see whether the trait is dominant or recessive, we can perform the crosses that led to the children in each family. If the trait was dominant, Mr. and Mrs. Green would be either Aa or AA since they have attached ear lobes.

AA x AA	Aa x Aa	AA x Aa
AA AA AA AA	Aa Aa Aa aa	AA AA Aa Aa

The second cross is not consistent with the pedigree since it shows one child with a different phenotype (free ear lobes). But we cannot conclude anything from this because the first and the third crosses do agree with the pedigree. Let us look at the Brown family. If the allele for attached ear lobes is dominant, neither Mr. nor Mrs. Brown can have the allele. They must both be aa. Their cross would yield only aa (free ear lobe) children:

aa x aa

aa   aa   aa   aa

Thus, the allele for attached ear lobes cannot be dominant; it must be recessive. If crosses were performed with the attached allele as recessive to the free allele, the results would be consistent with the pedigree. Try it. Thus, the mode of inheritance is a recessive autosomal allele.

● PROBLEM 8-32

The pedigree chart shows how a trait is inherited through a single dominant gene. What is the probability of the trait appearing in the offspring if the following cousins marry: (a) 1 and 3; (b) 2 and 4?

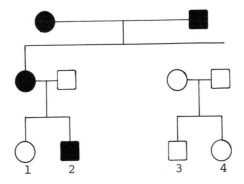

Solution: Since the trait is expressed through a single dominant gene we know that those individuals who do not show the trait must be homozygous recessive. We can determine the genotypes of the other individuals from this small amount of information. A diagram of the pedigree with the information that we know will help us to visualize the process:

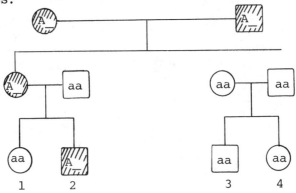

We must determine the genotypes of the individuals who have the trait. In order for individual 1 to arise from a union between a father with two recessive alleles and a mother with one dominant allele, the mother's second allele must be recessive. If it was dominant, an aa individual could not be produced. Now we can determine the genotype of individual 2 by performing the cross. The grandparents' genotypes can be determined in a similar manner. The genotypes are as follows:

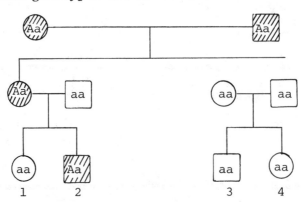

310

Now we are ready to find the results of the marriages.

(a) Cousins 1 and 3 are married.

$$aa \times aa$$
$$\downarrow$$
$$aa \; aa \; aa \; aa$$

None of their offspring will show the trait since neither parent has the dominant gene.

(b) If cousins 2 and 4 marry, the results are different because cousin 2 has the dominant gene.

$$Aa \times aa$$
$$\downarrow$$
$$Aa \; Aa \; aa \; aa$$

There is a 50 percent chance of their offspring having the trait.

● PROBLEM 8-33

Using the pedigree below, fill in the genotype of each individual. Assume that the trait is recessive and that an individual who marries into the family and does not exhibit a trait, does not carry the recessive gene for it.

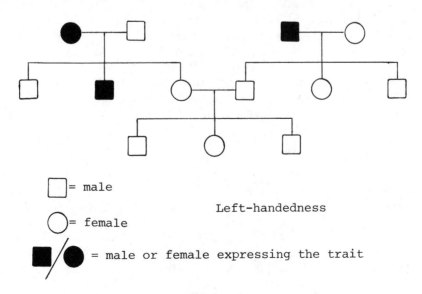

◻ = male

◯ = female

◼/● = male or female expressing the trait

Left-handedness

<u>Solution</u>: For simplicity and conciseness, we shall use the following system to refer to any one of the members in the pedigree:

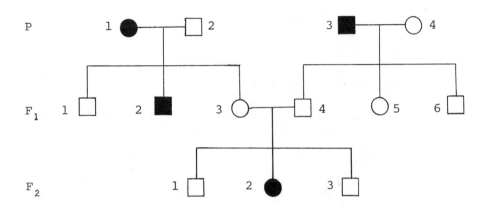

Let the allele for left-handedness be a and the allele for right-handedness be A. Consider P_1 (that is, the first member of the parental generation). Since she expresses the trait, her genotype is aa. To determine the genotype of P_2, we look at the progeny, F_1 (first generation). From the diagram, we see that $F_{1,2}$ is left-handed; hence his genetic make-up is aa. This means that he must have received a copy of a from each of his parents. Therefore we know that P_2 carries a copy of the recessive gene. But since P_2 is phenotypically normal, his genotype must be Aa. $F_{1,1}$ and $F_{1,3}$ are right-handed. Yet they must have received an a allele from P_1, since she has only a alleles to transmit. Therefore the genotype of $F_{1,1}$ and $F_{1,3}$ is Aa.

Consider the cross between P_3 and P_4. We know P_3 is aa (because he is left-handed) and P_4 can be AA or Aa (since she is right-handed). Since all the offspring are right-handed, it seems probable that P_4 is AA; however, we cannot be entirely certain of this, since both genotypes AA and Aa are compatible with the phenotypes of the offspring. We know, however, that $F_{1,4}$, $F_{1,5}$, and $F_{1,6}$ must all have the genotype Aa since they carry an a allele donated by P_3.

In the F_2 generation, we see that $F_{2,2}$ is left-handed, and therefore her genotype is aa. This is compatible with what we have determined to be the genotypes of the parents ($F_{1,3}$ and $F_{1,4}$) namely Aa. $F_{2,1}$ and $F_{2,3}$ are both right-handed, and are either AA or Aa. Since both parents are Aa either genotype is possible, though Aa is more probable.

312

The gene p causes phenylketonuria, a genetic disease in which the proper metabolism of phenylalanine is blocked. The gene p is recessive to its allele P for normal metabolism of phenylalanine. Circles represent females, squares represent males and solid figures represent victims of phenylketonuria.

(a) What are the probable genotypes of the grandparents, numbers 1 and 2?

(b) What is the probability that person 6 is a carrier?

(c) What is the probability that the child resulting from the marriage of cousins 4 and 5 will have phenylketonuria?

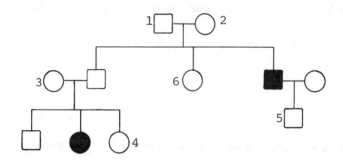

Solution: (a) If the parents are phenotypically normal but have a homozygous recessive child with phenylketonuria, they must both be heterozygous Pp. Each parent must have donated a recessive gene.

(b) A carrier is a person carrying a recessive gene in the heterozygous condition. The results of mating two carriers, Pp X Pp, would be expected to yield 1/4 PP, 1/2 Pp, 1/4 pp, or 3/4 normal and 1/4 with phenylketonuria. 2/4 of the 3/4 with normal phenotype would be carriers. Therefore 2/4 divided by 3/4 or 2/3 of the phenotypically normal children will be carriers. The probability is 2/3 that person 6 is a carrier.

(c) The probability is 2/3 that person 4 is a carrier because 2/3 of the phenotypically normal children of heterozygous parents will be carriers. Person 5 must be a carrier (P = 1) because he would have inherited a recessive gene from his father. The probability of heterozygous parents having a child with phenylketonuria is 1/4. This problem can be solved using the rule of probability for independent events. The probability of independent events occurring together is the product of their individual probabilities.

P of person 4 being a carrier		P of person 5 being a carrier		P of heterozygous parents having a recessive child	
2/3	x	1	x	1/4	= 1/6

● **PROBLEM 8-35**

Determine the chance of a male child being affected by the trait if:

(a) person V-3 marries person V-9.

(b) persons V-6 and IV-10 marry.

Solution: An examination of the pedigree shows that only males are affected by this trait. That implies that the trait is sex-linked; the allele for the gene is on the X chromosome. Since no females show the trait, the trait is probably the result of a recessive allele. Females must have that allele on both of their X chromosomes to express the trait, while males will express the trait when the recessive allele is on their single X chromosome. To find out what the progeny of a marriage will be like, we must know the parental genotypes. These can be found by first examining what we know. We know the genotypes of all of the males: those with the trait are $\underline{a}$ and those without the trait are $\underline{A}$. The genotypes of the females are found by deduction. Start at the top of the pedigree chart. The four children of parents I-1 and I-2 are all phenotypically normal. Since I-2 carries the trait $\underline{a}$ I-1 must be AA; otherwise, one of the daughters would have had the trait. From there we can establish the genotypes of the daughters. Similarly, we can write the entire pedigree chart by genotype:

314

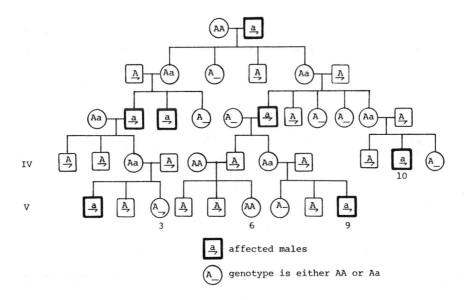

affected males

genotype is either AA or Aa

(a) If V-3 and V-9 were to have a child, the genotype of V-3 would determine the chances of that child carrying the trait. If V-3, the mother, was Aa, the cross would be:

$$Aa \text{ x } \underset{\rightarrow}{a}$$

$$Aa \text{ aa } \underset{\rightarrow}{A} \text{ } \underset{\rightarrow}{a}$$

Half of the children could be affected. The chance of an affected child being born would then be 1/2 x 1/2 or 1/4. Since the chance of a male child being born is 50%, or 1/2, the probability becomes 1/4 x 1/2 = 1/8. If the mother was AA, the cross would be the same as that described in (b).

(b) Neither the father nor the brothers of V-6 have the recessive allele, so her mother is probably AA. That would make V-6 also AA. If she married IV-10, their offspring would be:

$$AA \text{ x } \underset{\rightarrow}{a}$$

$$Aa \text{ Aa } \underset{\rightarrow}{A} \text{ } \underset{\rightarrow}{A}$$

None of the offspring show the recessive trait. None of the male children of this marriage would be affected by the sex-linked trait.

In the pedigree shown,

(a) if the woman (IV-2) marries a man showing the same trait as her brother and sister, what is the chance that her first child will be affected?

(b) if it is known that one person in 100 carries the defective gene, how would you answer the above question?

(c) what is the chance of an affected child being born to V-1 if she married a normal, unrelated man?

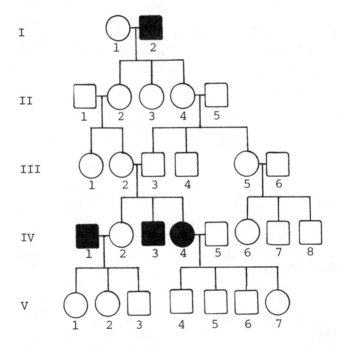

Solution: The pedigree shows a recessive trait since it is not necessary for the parents or even grandparents to show the trait. The trait is not sex-linked, since both males and females can be affected.

(a) We do not know whether or not IV-2 is a carrier of the recessive allele (a) since the trait will not be expressed when the genotype is heterozygous. Since both parents are normal and both the brother and the sister of IV-2 express the trait, both parents must be carriers (Aa). The genotypes of their children can be derived from a Mendelian monohybrid cross: Aa x Aa. The genotypes of the progeny would be in the ratio of 1AA:2Aa:1aa. Person IV-2 is not aa since she does not express the trait. The probability of her being a heterozygote are 2 out of 3 since the normal offspring occur, by chance, in a ratio of 1AA:2Aa. If her husband expressed the trait his genotype would be aa. The cross would be Aa x aa, if IV-2 was Aa. The chances of an affected child being born would be 1/2. If we multiply this by the probability that she is a carrier - 2/3 - we get the probability that her child will be homozygous recessive:

$$1/2 \times 2/3 = 1/3$$

We can do this because a probability is the product of the separate probabilities.

(b) The chance of the woman being a carrier are 2/3. Since the man is a carrier of two copies of the allele, the cross is Aa x aa and the chance of an affected birth is 1/2. To find the answer, we simply multiply the separate probabilities:

$$2/3 \times 1/2 \times 1/100 = 2/600 = 1/300$$

(c) If V-1 married a normal, unrelated male the chances of them having an affected child is low. Since her father is a carrier (Aa) she probably is Aa. A normal unrelated man would most likely have the genotype AA. Their cross would yield:

$$Aa \ x \ AA$$
$$\downarrow$$
$$AA \ AA \ Aa \ Aa$$

None of their children show the trait. This all depends on her partner not having the recessive allele. If he did, half of their children would show the recessive characteristic.

● **PROBLEM** 8-37

(a) If a normal woman outside the family marries V-4, what are the chances of a defective baby being born?

(b) If V-1 marries a normal man, can a defective child be born?

(c) What are the chances, at any birth, of a child

317

having the trait if V-1 marries a similarly afflicted person?

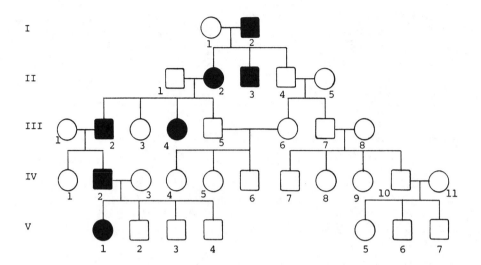

Solution: The trait shown in the pedigree is autosomal dominant. It is autosomal because it affects both males and females and it is dominant since whenever a parent is afflicted at least one child shows the trait. We can call the allele A and its recessive counterpart a. Since the trait is dominant, those individuals not showing the trait must be homozygous for the recessive allele. We can fill in a genotypic pedigree chart with this information and then determine the genotypes of the carriers (see Figure 2).

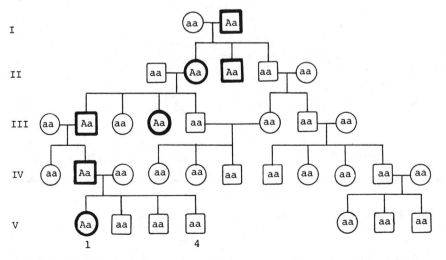

(a) If V-4 married a normal woman, the cross would be: aa x aa. All of the offspring would be homozygous recessive for the trait and hence be phenotypically normal.

(b) If V-1 married a normal man, however, she could give birth to a child with the trait since she carries the dominant allele:

Aa x aa

Aa Aa aa aa

There is a 50% chance that they would have a child with the trait.

(c) If V-1 married a man who was affected as she was, their cross would be Aa x Aa. Since the gene is dominant, the ratio of afflicted to normal children would be 3:1.

Aa x Aa

AA Aa Aa aa

This dominant trait occurs in each generation when one of the parents carries the allele.

● **PROBLEM** 8-38

The following is a pedigree for retinitis pigmentosa and cystinuria. Retinitis pigmentosa is an eye disease and cystinuria is a disease which shows high levels of cystine in the urine and is often accompanied by kidney stones.

(a) Are the traits due to dominant or recessive alleles?

(b) What are the genotypes of the parents?

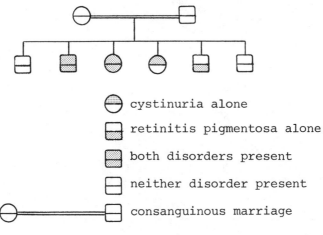

cystinuria alone

retinitis pigmentosa alone

both disorders present

neither disorder present

consanguinous marriage

Solution: (a) The pedigree chart shows that, although neither parent suffers from either disease, four out of six children suffer from at least one of the diseases. The affected children are both male and female. The inheritance of both disorders is therefore autosomal recessive.

The consanguinous marriage has a great deal to do with the inheritance of these diseases. Such parents are more likely to have inherited the same mutant gene from a common ancestor than are parents in nonconsanguinous marriages who have no common ancestor. The rarer the gene, the more unlikely are the chances that two unrelated people carry it. Generally, the rarer the gene the greater the frequency of consanguinity among the parents of the affected individuals.

(b) Since neither of the parents suffer from these two disorders, neither of them is homozygous. The parental genotypes must be AaBb since some of their progeny have one disease (aa), some have the other disease (bb), some have both (aabb) and some have neither (AaBb).

● PROBLEM 8-39

A man married twice. His two wives were sisters and also his first cousins. Of the nine offspring of one marriage, one was an albino, two of the three children of the other marriage were also albinos. Draw a pedigree chart and explain its implications.

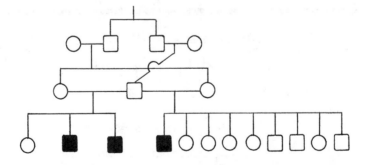

Solution: Albinism is a consequence of an inability to synthesize the pigment melanin. Melanin cannot be produced if the enzyme tyrosinase is defective or absent in an individual.

The man in this problem has married two of his cousins. Such consanguinous marriages often result in the appearance of rare deleterious conditions. The pedigree chart of this family indicates that albinism is caused by the homozygous state of a recessive allele since none of the parents expressed the characteristic.

Your pedigree chart may be slightly different from this one, due to the unspecified sexes of the children. Since albinism is the result of a faulty enzyme, a mutation in the gene that codes for the enzyme could cause such an abnormality. This mutation could be passed to succeeding generations in the heterozygous state. Only when two gametes, both with the abnormality, fuse would the trait be expressed. Otherwise, in the heterozygous state the allele's presence would be masked by the expression of the dominant allele. Consanguinous marriages increase the chances of two heterozygous gametes fusing to produce a homozygous individual. If both of the women and the man carry the allele for albinism in the heterozygous state (Aa), an albino child (aa) has a good chance of being born. The man could have married almost any other woman from the general population without too much risk of the birth of an albino child. The chances are good that another woman (from outside of the family) would not carry the mutant allele. So if the allele was passed to their children it would have done so in the heterozygous state. Thus, consanguinous marriages increase the probability that mutant alleles, if they exist in a family, will come together to form individuals homozygous for a mutant gene.

INBREEDING

• PROBLEM 8-40

The frequency of the gene for phenylketonuria (PKU), an enzyme deficiency disease which will produce irreversible and severe mental retardation in untreated infants, is about one per one hundred gametes (1/100). The risk of unrelated parents having an affected child is the square of this or 1/10,000. How much is the risk enhanced if the parents are cousins?

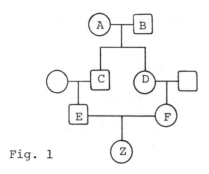

Fig. 1

Solution: A deleterious allele that arose because of a mutation in one individual is statistically very rare in the general population. Therefore, most individuals carrying the allele have it in the heterozygous, and hence unexpressed, form. The chances are very slim that two individuals from the general population who are heterozygous for the allele will meet. However, if members who are heterozygous inbreed, the chances of the homozygous condition occurring increase greatly. In fact, most pedigree data on inherited recessive traits come from families in which inbreeding has occurred.

To solve this problem we must first find the inbreeding coefficient, F, which is the probability that a child will be homozygous for a gene that derives from a common ancestor of his parents. This is written as:

$$F = \Sigma (\tfrac{1}{2})^n$$

where F is the inbreeding coefficient and n is the number of individuals that lead from the child to the ancestors and back. The exponent, n, does not include the child himself. The symbol Σ indicates that the values must be calculated for each common ancestor and added together. Once we have found the inbreeding coefficient, we can use the formula:

$$p^2(1-F) + pF = \text{proportion of homozygous recessives}$$

where p = frequency of the gene and
F = inbreeding coefficient.

Now, back to the beginning. We know that the parents are cousins, so their family tree may look something like that shown in Figure 1.

E and F are the cousins; Z is their child; C and D are brother and sister and one of the parents of E and F. A and B are the common ancestors. This tree can be written in the standard form called a path analysis (see Figure 2). In such a diagram, the arrows represent the transmission of gametes.

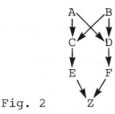

Fig. 2

If we follow the paths from Z back to each common ancestor we obtain the following routes: Z→E→C→A→D→E→F→Z and Z→E→C→B→D→F→Z. In both of these paths there are five individuals (excluding Z), so n = 5. We can find the inbreeding coefficient by:

$$F = \Sigma(\tfrac{1}{2})^5 \qquad \text{There are two paths, so}$$

$$F = (\tfrac{1}{2})^5 + (\tfrac{1}{2})^5$$

$$F = 1/32 + 1/32 = 1/16$$

The child has a one in sixteen chance of receiving the allele from both parents. To find how much the risk has been enhanced, we must find the proportion of individuals who would be homozygous for the trait when the inbreeding coefficient is 1/16.

Proportion of homozygous recessives

$$\text{in the population} = p^2(1-F) + pF$$

Here p = 1/100 and F = 1/16. Substituting, we get:

$$(1/100)^2(1 - 1/16) + (1/100)(1/16) = \frac{115}{160,000}$$

$$\simeq \frac{7}{10,000}$$

The proportion of homozygous individuals is now 7/10,000 instead of 1/10,000 so there is a risk seven times greater than initially. Thus, the consanguinous marriage of these two cousins has a higher chance of producing a child with phenylketonuria than if either of the cousins married outside of the family.

If the inbreeding coefficient of K is 1/4, C is 3/8, and that of all the others are zero, compute the inbreeding coefficient of individual I.

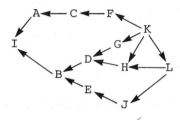

Solution: This path analysis has two ancestors that are common; K and L. The only inbreeding information that is important in this problem is when it involves a common ancestor. When a common ancestor is inbred we must use the formula:

$$F_I = \Sigma (\tfrac{1}{2})^n (1 + F_{ancestor})$$

Otherwise, if the ancestor is not inbred, we do not need the second factor since $F_{ancestor} = 0$:

$$F_I = \Sigma (\tfrac{1}{2})^n (1+0)$$

$$F_I = \Sigma (\tfrac{1}{2})^n$$

We now follow the paths from individual I through the common ancestors and back. The paths are, (with the common ancestor underlined in each case):

A C F $\underline{K}$ G D B	n = 7	$F_{ancestor}$ = 1/4
A C F $\underline{K}$ H D B	n = 7	$F_{ancestor}$ = 1/4
A C F K $\underline{L}$ J E B	n = 8	$F_{ancestor}$ = 0
A C F K $\underline{L}$ H D B	n = 8	$F_{ancestor}$ = 0

We can add up each contribution to get the total inbreeding coefficient of I.

$$F_I = \Sigma (\tfrac{1}{2})^n (1 + F_{ancestor})$$

$$F_I = (\tfrac{1}{2})^7 (1+\tfrac{1}{4}) + (\tfrac{1}{2})^7 (1+\tfrac{1}{4}) + (\tfrac{1}{2})^8 (1+0) + (\tfrac{1}{2})^8 (1+0)$$

$$F_I = 5/512 + 5/512 + 1/256 + 1/256$$

$$F_I = 14/512 = 0.027$$

Notice that the paths used never go through an individual twice and they always travel from offspring to parent and from parent to offspring on the return; the paths never zigzag.

The inbreeding coefficient of individual I is 0.027. This means that the chance of individual I being homozygous is 2.7%.

● **PROBLEM** 8-42

What is the inbreeding coefficient of individual Q assuming that none of the common ancestors is inbred?

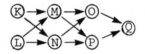

Solution: This pedigree shows two generations of brother-sister mating. There are four common ancestors and six paths altogether. The ancestors are underlined in the following paths:

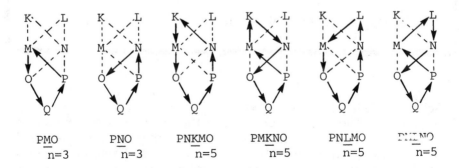

PMO	PNO	PNKMO	PMKNO	PNLMO	PMLNO
n=3	n=3	n=5	n=5	n=5	n=5

In each path, start at Q and follow the arrows to trace the path back to Q. Notice how none zigzag between generations. Since none of the ancestors are inbred, we can use the formula

$$F = \Sigma(\tfrac{1}{2})^n(1+F_{ancestor})$$

with $F_{ancestor} = 0$.

We simply have to add the probability of homozygosity due to each path:

$$F_Q = (\tfrac{1}{2})^3(1+0) + (\tfrac{1}{2})^3(1+0) + (\tfrac{1}{2})^5(1+0) + (\tfrac{1}{2})^5(1+0)$$
$$+ (\tfrac{1}{2})^5(1+0) + (\tfrac{1}{2})^5(1+0)$$
$$F_Q = (\tfrac{1}{2})^3 + (\tfrac{1}{2})^3 + (\tfrac{1}{2})^5 + (\tfrac{1}{2})^5 + (\tfrac{1}{2})^5 + (\tfrac{1}{2})^5$$
$$F_Q = 1/8 + 1/8 + 1/32 + 1/32 + 1/32 + 1/32$$
$$F_Q = \frac{12}{32} = \frac{3}{8}$$

Thus, the probability that Q is homozygous at a specified locus is 3/8.

POPULATIONS

● PROBLEM 8-43

How may the gene pool be altered?

Solution: The total genetic material of a given population is termed the gene pool. The Hardy-Weinberg principle tells us that the relative gene frequencies within the gene pool of a population will remain constant from generation to generation unless certain factors alter the equilibrium of gene frequencies in the gene pool. Such factors include mutation, natural selection, migration, random genetic drift and meiotic drive.

Mutations can change one allele to another, such as A to a. If they are recurrent or "one-way", the relative frequencies of the two alleles will be changed by an increase in the proportion of a at the expense of A. Owing to the low mutation rate of most genes, such direct change in allelic frequency alone probably does not cause significant change in the gene pool. More important is the fact that mutations are a source of new genes, and thus traits, within a population. Together with sexual reproduction, which creates new combinations of existing genes, mutations provide the variation which is the basis for the operation of natural selection.

Selection is the nonrandom differential retaining of favored genotypes. Unlike mutation, which operates directly on a gene to alter its frequency, selection indirectly alters a gene's frequency by acting on its carriers as a function of their ability to reproduce viable offspring. For example, if individuals carrying gene A are more successful in reproduction than individuals carrying gene B, the frequency of the former gene will tend to increase generation after generation at the expense of the latter. Any trait which gives an organism a better chance at survival in a given environment will increase that organism's ability to grow and reproduce, and it will increase the proportion of the gene for that trait in the gene pool. By the same token, any gene which confers a disadvantage to its carrier within its environment will decrease that organism's chance of survival to reproductive age and thus decrease the frequency of that gene in the gene pool. This is the principle underlying natural selection.

Migration acts both directly and indirectly to alter gene frequencies. Directly, a population may receive alleles through immigration of individuals from a nearby population. The effectiveness of immigration in changing allelic frequencies is dependent on two factors: the difference in gene frequencies between the two populations, and the proportion of migrant genes that are incorporated. Alternatively, there can be emigration of members from a population which, depending on the size of the emigration and whether or not it is selective, can result in a change in allelic frequencies in the gene pool.

Indirectly, migration acts as a source of variation, similar to mutation, upon which the forces of natural selection can operate. Migration can also enhance natural selection within a population by upsetting the equilibrium that may exist among the given genotypes in a population, concerning an advantage by sheer numbers to a given group. It can blur the effects of natural selection by replacing genes removed by selection.

Allelic frequencies may fluctuate purely by chance about their mean from generation to generation. This is termed random genetic drift. Its effect on the gene pool of a large population is negligible, but in a small effectively interbreeding population, chance alteration in Mendelian ratios can have a significant effect on gene frequencies and may lead to the fixation of one allele and the loss of another. For example, isolated communities within a given population have been found to have different frequencies for blood group alleles than the population as a whole. Chance fluctuations in allelic frequency presumably caused these changes.

Another factor that may alter allelic frequencies is meiotic drive. This is the term for preferential segregation of genes that may occur in meiosis. For example, if a particular chromosome is continually segregated to the polar body in female gametogenesis its genes would tend to be excluded from the gene pool since the polar bodies are nonfunctional and will disintegrate. There is significant evidence that, due to physical differences between certain homologous chromosome, preferential selection of one over the other often occurs at other than random proportions.

● **PROBLEM** 8-44

The gene frequency for the Rh allele among American whites is 0.028. Among American blacks, the frequency is 0.446. Among East African blacks, the frequency of the Rh allele is 0.630. Determine the degree of gene exchange (m) between the American whites and blacks.

Solution: This question involves two initial populations; American whites and African blacks. As slaves, the African blacks were brought to the American colonies about 300 years, or ten generations ago. The interbreeding between the American white population and the African population has led to a decrease in the frequency of the Rh allele in the contemporary American black population. The gene frequencies given in the problem, and the number of generations can be used to calculate the degree of gene exchange. We can use the relationship:

$$q_n - Q = (1-m)^n (q_o - Q) \quad \text{or}$$

$$(1-m)^n = \frac{q_n - Q}{q_o - Q}$$

where m is the degree of gene exchange, n is the number of generations, Q is the gene donor, q_n is the hybrid population and q_o is the original population. The white population can be considered the gene donor, Q, since it was so much larger than the incoming African population. Also, the African population was isolated from its original gene pool. So the African genes that were introduced into the American population are not prevalent enough to affect the gene frequency significantly. The American black population can then be considered as q_n and the African population as q_o. Using the formula and gene frequencies given in the problem, we can solve for m:

$$(1-m)^{10} = \frac{q_{10} - Q}{q_o - Q}$$

$$(1-m)^{10} = \frac{0.446 - 0.028}{0.630 - 0.028}$$

$$(1-m)^{10} = 0.694$$

$$\log(1-m)^{10} = \log 0.694$$

$$10 \log(1-m) = \log 0.694$$

$$\log(1-m) = \frac{\log 0.694}{10}$$

$$\log(1-m) = 1.98414$$

Taking the antilog of both sides gives:

$$1-m = 0.964$$

$$m = 0.036$$

This value of m means that, excluding all other causes of new gene formation (including mutation), 36 genes per 1000, or 3.6%, of the genes in the present day American black population were introduced from the white population each generation.

329

In a plant breeding experiment, cross-fertilization can cause a marked increase in the yield and height of the plants. Explain.

Solution: In cross-breeding experiments the progeny are very often more vigorous than the parents. This is called heterosis. Heterosis has been explained by two theories. The first is called the dominance hypothesis. This assumes that in the course of selecting for certain desirable traits the breeder has created strains with somewhat deleterious recessive genes in other places along the genome. The hybrid formed between two inbred strains would be heterozygous at these loci and hence would show vigor that the parents did not show.

The second hypothesis regarding heterosis is called the overdominance hypothesis. This theory says that the hybrid is more vigorous because it is more heterozygous. Heterozygotes may be more flexible than homozygotes since they have two different alleles for their heterozygous genes. The heterozygote may be better able to survive fluctuations in its environment since it has two versions of its heterozygous genes and hence, two versions of the gene products.

Heterosis has been used to increase crop yields and disease resistance in some plants such as corn and sorghum wheat.

What is polymorphism? What are some advantages of polymorphism?

Solution: A polymorphic locus has one or more alleles, in addition to the most common allele, present in more than one percent of the population. Polymorphism is extensive in natural populations. Its existence may offer flexibility of a species to a changing environment. An allele that was previously deleterious may, with the proper environmental climate, become beneficial. Alternatively, some mutant genes may be advantageous in the heterozygous state but deleterious in the homozygous state. Sickle-cell anemia, for instance, is a result of a mutant form of hemoglobin, HbS. In its heterozygous form, this trait offers a protection against malaria. In its homozygous form it is lethal.

Another hypothesis regarding the advantages of polymorphism in a population is that the allozymes (the slightly different enzyme products that arise from alleles at the same gene locus) may persist due to natural selection. For example, a population of isopod crustaceans, Asellus aquaticus, was found to have two allozymes for the enzyme that breaks down starch-amylase. One allozyme was better able to digest beech leaves and the other was better at digesting willow leaves. The pond where this population of isopods lived had a group of willows at one end and a group of beeches at the other. The isopods with the beech-digesting amylase lived near the beech trees and those with the willow-digesting allozyme lived nearer to the willow trees. This population was shown to interbreed, so it is not composed of separate populations with different allelic frequencies.

These examples show how polymorphism can be advantageous to different populations. Polymorphism, in these cases, enhances the survival of populations in potentially pernicious environments.

● **PROBLEM** 8-47

How are the effects of certain chemicals altered due to the genetic material of the individual?

Solution: The exact effect of drugs and chemicals on genetic material is difficult to assess. It is even more difficult to discover the reverse - the effects of the genetic material on the reaction of the chemical. But some individuals show a particular sensitivity to chemicals that may have a genetic basis.

Phenylthiocarbamide (PTC) is such a chemical. About 70 percent of those people tested could taste the chemical. The remaining 30 percent could not taste it at all. The inability to taste PTC has been found to be dependent on a single recessive allele. Those that can taste PTC describe its taste as sweet, salty or bitter. Thus, the gene determining PTC sensitivity has variable expressivity.

Another chemical which has genetically based effects is the drug primaquine. Primaquine is used to treat malaria. Sensitive people develop anemia caused by the hemolysis of the erythrocytes when administered the drug. The sensitive people lack the enzyme glucose-6-phosphate dehydrogenase (G6PD). This deficiency is inherited as an X-linked recessive gene. The exact correlation between G6PD and the fragility of the red blood cells is unknown.

People with the autosomal dominant disorder acute intermittent porphyria have severe reactions when given barbiturates or similar drugs. Porphyria is a disorder that is a result of the inability of the cells to convert porphyrins. Their concentrations increase in the liver and large amounts are excreted in the urine, giving it a port wine color. The attacks - abdominal pain and neurologic disturbances - are intermittent and may be brought about by barbiturates and estrogens.

These are just three examples of interactions between genetic material and chemicals. Since DNA itself is a molecule, it can be expected to interact with certain other chemicals. Whether the effects of such interactions are necessary, as in the case of enzymes such as the DNA polymerases, or harmful, as in the above three cases, depends on how the chemicals interact. How these substances affect DNA is not fully understood. Many more cases undoubtably exist.

SHORT ANSWER QUESTIONS FOR REVIEW

Choose the correct answer.

1. Factors which tend to change gene frequencies
    are (a) natural selection and mutation. (b)
    random mating. (c) migration and genetic drift.
    (d) both a and c.   d

2. Random mating, a condition required for
    maintaining genetic equilibrium is (a) often
    met. (b) rarely met because random
    reproduction means producing viable
    offspring 100% of the time. (c) always met
    because there is choice among members of the
    opposite sex. (d) none of the above   b

3. Gene frequencies will change if (a) one of the
    Hardy-Weinberg conditions isn't met. (b) none
    of the Hardy-Weinberg conditions are met. (c)
    two of the four conditions aren't met. (d)
    three of the four conditions aren't met.   a

4. In a population which cannot maintain genetic
    equilibrium (a) the number of lethal mutations
    increases. (b) the population evolves. (c) the
    gene frequencies change. (d) all of the above   d

5. The sickle-cell trait is very predominant
    in an African population of 1000 members.
    How many of these members would you expect
    to be homozygous for the normal allele AA?
    (a) 640 (b) 320 (c) 40 (d) 5   a

6. How many members would you expect to be
    heterozygous As in question 5? (a) 640 (b)
    320 (c) 40 (d) 5   b

7. How many members would you expect to be
    homozygous for the sickle-cell allele SS in
    question 5? (a) 640 (b) 320 (c) 40 (d) 5   c

8. The ability to taste the chemical phenylthio-
    carbamide is controlled by the dominant allele
    T. Tasters are T_ and non-tasters are tt.
    What is the frequency of the t allele in a
    population where 412 are tasters and 235 are
    non-tasters? (a) .70 (b) .60 (c) .50
    (d) .40   b

9. What fraction of the tasters in question 8

are heterozygous?   (a) .75 (b) .48 (c) .16
(d) .04

a

10.   Identical twins (monozygotic) having the same
      genotype for a given trait can show variation
      in the phenotype corresponding to that same
      genotype. This is due to (a) the environ-
      ment. (b) the penetrance and expressivity of
      that gene. (c) the concordance of the
      individuals. (d) none of the above

b

A single recessive gene, r, is largely responsible
for the development of red hair in humans. The
brown R_ allele is dominant. The pedigree below
represents the pattern in which red hair is
inherited. Answer questions 11 to 14 based on
this pedigree chart.

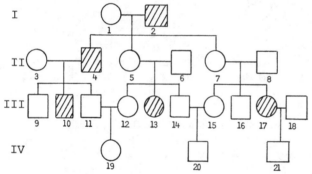

Key:

□ red haired male

○ red haired female

11.   What is the maximum probability of red hair
      appearing in children of the marriage between
      cousins III - 11 and III - 12? (a) 0 (b) 3/4
      (c) 1/4 (d) 1/8

d

12.   What is the probability of red hair appearing
      in children of a marriage between III - 12
      and III - 18? (a) 0 (b) 3/4 (c) 1/4 (d) 1/8

a

13.   What are the possible genotype and phenotype
      of individual III-9? (a) heterozygous Rr,
      brown hair (b) heterzygous Rr, red hair (c)
      homozygous RR, brown hair (d) homozygous
      rr, red hair

a

14. The genotype of the father, individual I-1
    is (a) RR (b) rr (c) Rr (d) cannot be
    determined.

    c

15. A metabolic disease of man, phenylketonuria
    is the result of a recessive gene. Its
    frequency is 1×10^{-4}. What is the probability
    that normal parents will produce a diseased
    child? (a) 10% (b) 5% (c) 1% (d) 0.01%

    d

16. Migration can change gene frequencies and
    alter selection by (a) introducing new genes
    to a population and stabilizing genotypes. (b)
    removing genes from a population thus
    decreasing the number of individuals with a
    given trait. (c) replacing genes removed by
    selection. (d) all of the above

    d

17. An advantage of a polymorphic trait is that
    it (a) allows separate species to coexist in a
    given territory. (b) produces variations in a
    trait. (c) confers greater vigor in the cross-
    bred progeny. (d) all of the above

    b

Fill in the blanks.

18. A population in equilibrium refers to a large
    _____ population in which _____ is random.

    inter-
    breeding
    mating

19. Self fertilization, the most severe form of
    inbreeding, reduces the frequency of _____
    by one half each generation.

    hetero-
    zygotes

20. Children affected with Tay-Sach's disease
    lack the enzyme _____.

    N-acetylhex-
    osaminidase

21. Twins which result from the fertilization of
    two separate eggs are _____.

    dizygotic

22. Fertilization of a single egg which later on
    separates into two zygotes results in _____
    twins.

    monozygotic

23. A _____ marriage is a union between two
    family members.

    consan-
    guinous

24. Consanguinous marriages increase the
    chances of heterozygous gametes fusing and

producing an individual _____ for a lethal
mutant gene.

homozygous

25. A is linebred to B as shown by the pedigree
below. The inbreeding coefficient is _____.

.25

26. The total genetic material of a given
population is termed the _____.

gene pool

27. _____ is the non-random differential
retention of favored genotypes.

Natural
selection

28. Any gene which confers a disadvantage to
its carrier within its environment will _____
that organism's chance for survival.

increase

29. Purely random fluctuations of allelic
frequencies are termed _____.

genetic
drift

30. Random genetic drift is only noticeable in
small _____ populations.

inbreeding

31. Mating of heterozygotes which yields a
progeny of greater vigor than the parents is
termed _____.

heterosis

32. _____ is the presence of three or more
alleles in a given locus .

Poly-
morphism

Determine whether the following statements are
tru or false.

33. The Hardy-Weinberg Law states that in an
equilibrium population individual genotypes
remain constant.

False

34. The Hardy-Weinberg Law predicts that an
individual's genotype will remain constant in
the following generations.

False

35. One condition for maintaining genetic
equilibrium is a large population size.

True

SHORT ANSWER QUESTIONS FOR REVIEW

36. Most populations are able to maintain a constant gene pool.

False

37. Migration in or out of an isolated population tends to shift its genetic equilibrium.

True

38. Concordant twins do not have similar traits.

False

39. Penetrance is the portion of a gene which dilutes another.

False

40. Generally, the rarer the gene, the greater the frequency of consanguinity among parents of individuals affect with a recessive condition.

True

41. Consanguinous marriages often result in the appearance of a rare deleterious trait.

True

42. The diagram below represents the linebreeding of individual A. This diagram indicates that the inbreeding coefficient of A is approximately .035.

True

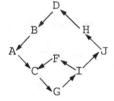

43. Inbreeding results in increased heterozygosity.

False

44. Mutations are part of the raw material upon which natural selection operates.

True

45. During oogenesis, chromosomes segregate in a non-random manner which helps to maintain equilibrium of allelic frequencies.

False

CHAPTER 9

GENETIC MATERIAL

DNA AND RNA

● **PROBLEM** 9-1

What is the nature of a "transforming agent"? What importance may this phenomenon have on our understanding of the chemical basis of inheritance?

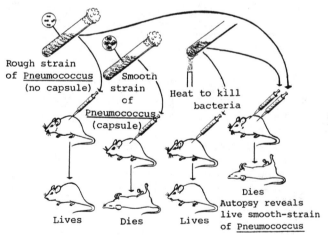

Rough strain of <u>Pneumococcus</u> (no capsule)

Smooth strain of <u>Pneumococcus</u> (capsule)

Heat to kill bacteria

Lives   Dies   Lives   Dies
Autopsy reveals live smooth-strain of <u>Pneumococcus</u>

The experiments of Fred Griffiths demonstrated the transfer of genetic information from dead, heat-killed bacteria to living bacteria of a different strain. Although neither the rough strain of <u>Pneumococcus</u> nor heat-killed smooth-strain pneumococci would kill a mouse, a combination of the two did. Autopsy of the dead mouse showed the presence of living, smooth-strain pneumococci.

Solution: The concept of transformation arises from the experiments performed by Griffith in 1928. It was observed that when injected into mice, some strains of pneumococcus bacteria caused pneumonia and usually death. Other strains of the bacteria were relatively harmless. The infective form always had a capsule (a complicated polysaccharide coating). The noninfective form did not have a virulent capsule. The encapsulated strain was called the "smooth strain" because the colonies looked smooth on a culture plate, and the harmless, unencapsulated strain was called the "rough strain" because of the rough appearance of its colonies.

In his famous experiment, Griffith injected one group of mice with the virulent smooth strain and another with the harmless rough strain. As expected, mice from the former group died while the latter group survived. Griffith then injected a third group of mice with the heat-killed smooth strain. This group lived, showing that bacteria killed by heat were no longer virulent. However, when a fourth group of mice was injected simultaneously with both the harmless rough strain and the heat-killed smooth bacteria, the mice died. The disease-causing organisms were of the smooth type bacteria. This process, by which something from the heat-killed bacteria converted rough bacteria into smooth bacteria, is known as transformation.

Griffith felt that protein from the dead bacteria might be the active transforming agent. But Griffith's interpretation of his experiment was later shown to be incorrect by Avery, Macleod, and McCarty in 1944. They made an extract from heat-killed smooth cells and purified the extract by removing any substance that did not cause transformation of rough bacteria into smoother bacteria. Eventually they determined that DNA was the essential transforming agent. Moreover, when this extracted DNA was added to other types of rough strains, the bacteria formed from transformation were always identical to the bacteria that donated the DNA. This indicated that hereditary information must be carried by DNA.

Transformation suggests that in bacteria genetic traits can be passed via DNA alone, from one bacterium to another.

• PROBLEM 9-2

What are the nitrogen-containing bases that are part of DNA and RNA? Draw the structures indicating which are purines and which are pyrimidines.

Purines

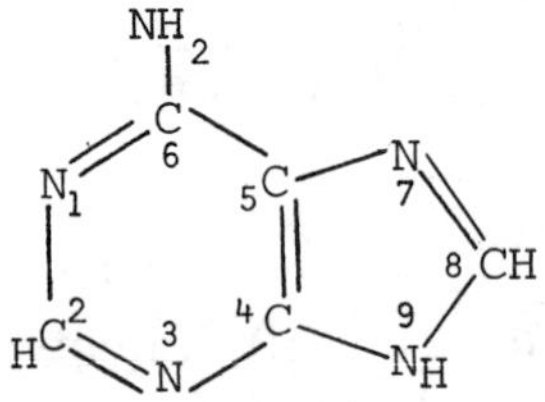

Adenine

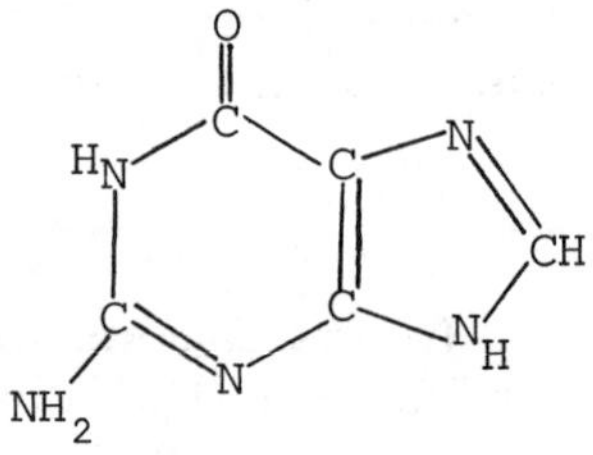

Guanine

Pyrimidines

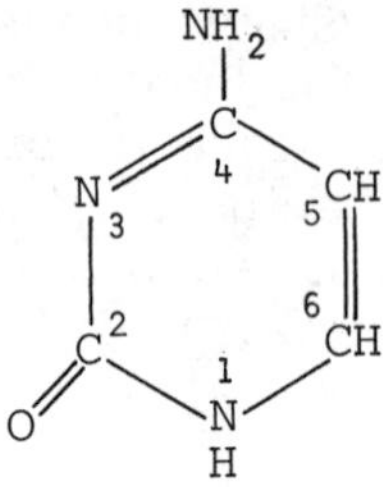

Cytosine

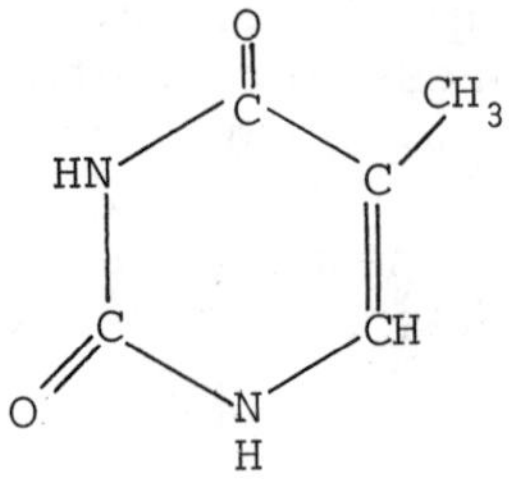

Thymine

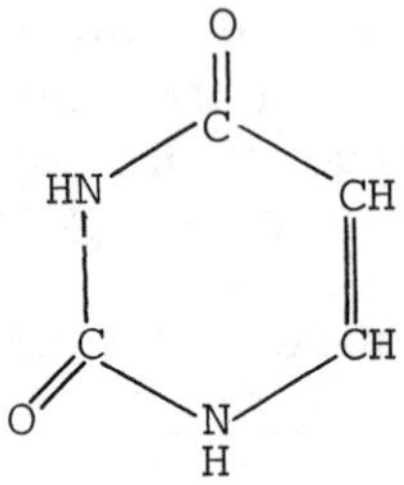

Uracil

Solution: DNA and RNA are made up of sugar moieties, phosphate groups and nitrogenous bases. It is the bases which encode the genetic information. DNA can contain the purines, adenine and guanine and the pyrimidines, cytosine and thymine. RNA contains uracil instead of thymine. Uracil is also a pyrimidine. Notice that purines contain two rings and pyrimidines have one ring.

• PROBLEM 9-3

Draw a diagram of a double-stranded piece of DNA with a sense strand sequence of A-G-T.

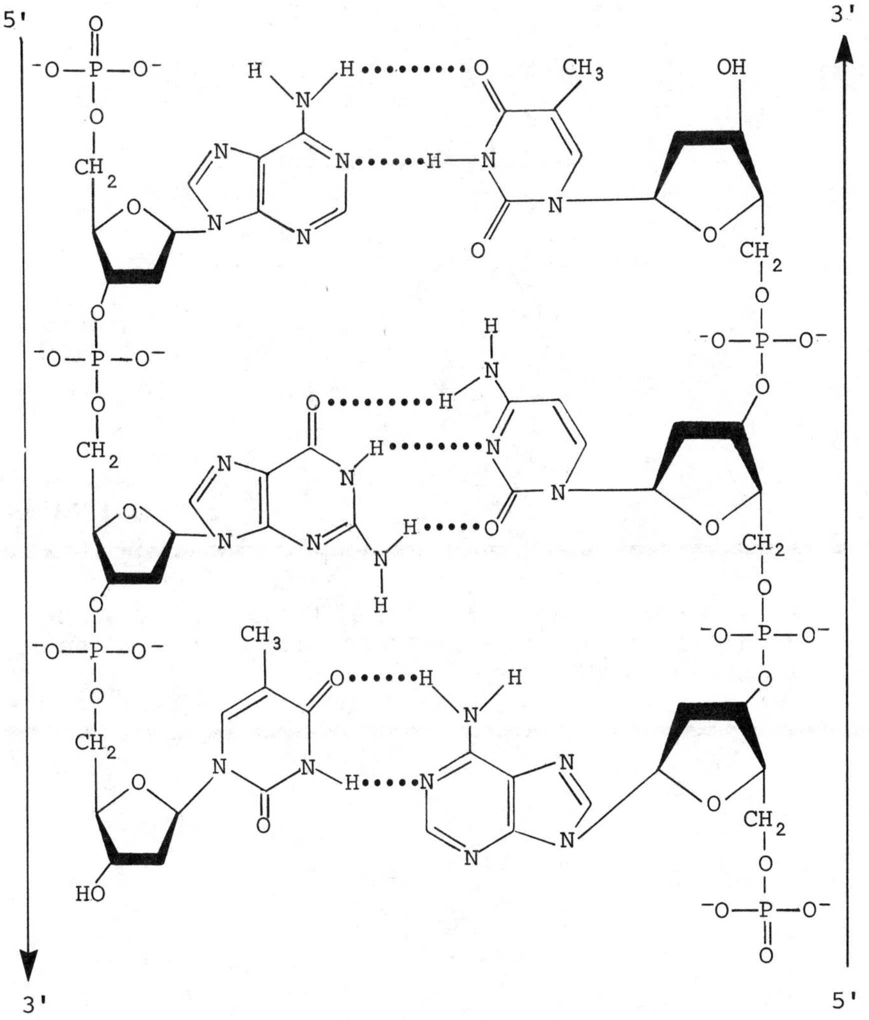

Fig. 1

Solution: Deoxyribonucleic acid is composed of two polynucleotide chains. Each chain is held together by 3'-5' phosphodiester bonds. The two chains are bound by hydrogen bonds and twisted into a helix. The backbone of the molecule is made of sugar moieties and phosphate groups. The bases are covalently bonded to this backbone.

The sense strand of a DNA molecule is that strand which codes for the mRNA and final protein product. It is read in the 5'-3' direction. The other chain - the antisense strand - is antiparallel and runs in the 3'-5' direction. Armed with this information, we can draw the molecule, see Figure 1.

This molecule can also be drawn schematically:

341

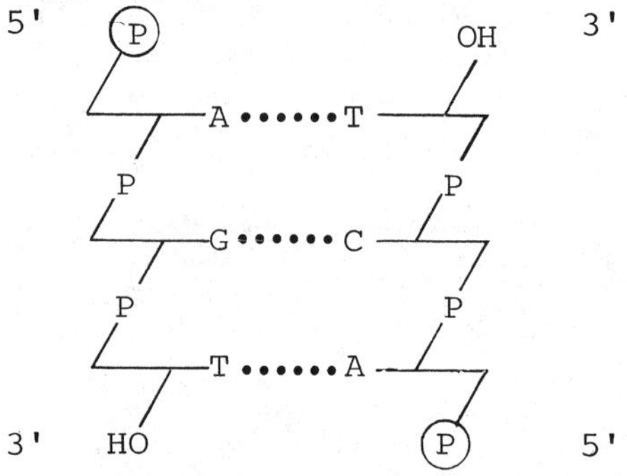

Fig. 2

• PROBLEM 9-4

Draw a molecular diagram of the mRNA that would be transcribed by the sequence ATA in the sense strand of a molecule of DNA.

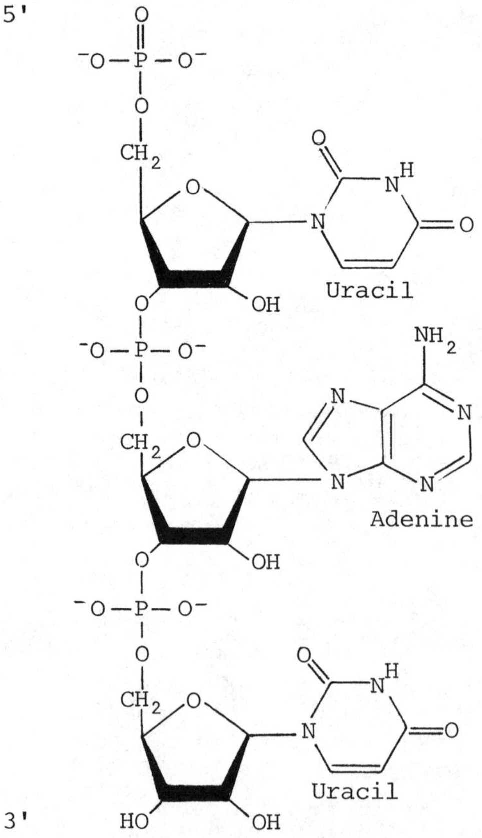

Solution: Ribonucleic acid (RNA) differs from DNA in three important ways: RNA contains the sugar ribose instead of deoxyribose; RNA has uracil instead of thymine; and RNA is single-stranded. RNA's backbone, like that of DNA, is held together by phosphodiester bonds. The mRNA molecule has the complementary sequence UAU as shown in the diagram.

● **PROBLEM** 9-5

RNA is readily hydrolized by alkali, but DNA is not. Why?

Solution: RNA and DNA have different chemical structures. RNA has uracil instead of thymine and it is single, rather than double-stranded. But most importantly for this problem, it has ribose as its sugar moiety. Ribose has two hydroxyl (-OH) groups while DNA's sugar, deoxyribose, has only one. This extra hydroxyl group is not bound up in the phosphodiester bond and is free to react (see Figure 1).

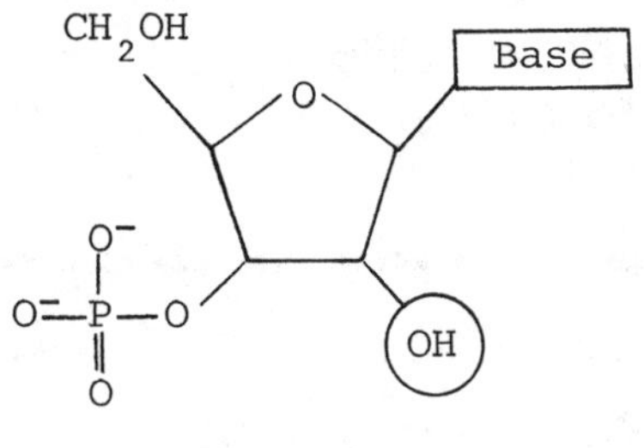

Fig. 1

When alkali is added to a solution containing RNA this hydroxyl group is ionized. It can then act as an intramolecular catalyst to cause the formation of a 2'-3' cyclic intermediate with the adjacent phosphate group. This reaction disrupts the phosphodiester bond, thus breaking the backbone of the molecule. Since DNA does not have this free hydroxyl group, it is not as readily disrupted by alkaline treatment.

A DNA molecule has 180 base pairs and is 20 percent adenine. How many cytosine nucleotides are present in this molecule of DNA?

Solution: In DNA, the complementary pairing between bases is always A-T (T-A) and G-C (C-G). Thus, if 20 percent of the nucleotides are adenine, then the total composition of A-T will be 40 percent, and the total composition of G-C will be 60 percent. The amount of cytosine will be 30 percent, or 108 nucleotides (360 x .30 = 108).

The A+G/T+C ratio in one strand of duplex DNA is 0.3.

a. What is the ratio in the complementary strand?

b. What is the ratio for the entire molecule?

c. If the A+T/C+G ratio is 0.3, what is the ratio in the complementary strand and in the entire molecule?

Solution: The GC content of DNA is used to characterize the molecule. Molecules with high GC content are more heat stable than molecules with a high AT content because guanine and cytosine are held together by three hydrogen bonds, while adenine and thymine are held together by two hydrogen bonds.

The molar concentration of purines A and G is equal to the molar concentration of pyrimidines T and C because one of each type makes up a base pair. Because of base pairing rules, A=T and G=C. The specific A-T and G-C content varies from species to species. But in any one species the ratio is constant.

a. The frequency of purines must equal the frequency of pyrimidines in the complementary strands.

So if:

$$\frac{A + G}{T + C} = \frac{0.3}{1} \text{ in one strand}$$

then the complementary strand must have a ratio of

$$\frac{A + G}{T + C} = \frac{1}{0.3} = 3.3$$

b. The ratio in the entire molecule = 1 because A = T and G = C.

c. The sum of A + T in one strand must equal the sum in the complementary strand. The same holds for G + C. So

$$\frac{A + T}{G + C} = 0.3 \text{ for each strand and for the entire molecule.}$$

● **PROBLEM 9-8**

The $\frac{A + T}{G + C}$ ratio of one of the strands of a DNA molecule is 0.2.

(a) What is the $\frac{A + T}{G + C}$ ratio in its complementary strand?

(b) If 0.2 referred to the $\frac{A + G}{T + C}$ ratio, what is the ratio in the complementary strand?

(c) What is the ratio of $\frac{A + G}{T + C}$ in double-stranded DNA in (a) and (b)?

Solution: We can solve this problem if we remember a few important facts about the double-stranded DNA molecule:

1. In complementary strands adenine pairs with thymine, so A = T.

2. In complementary strands cytosine pairs with guanine, or C = G.

3. A purine (A or G) always binds to a pyrimidine (T or C). A + G must equal T + C in the complementary strand.

4. The ratio $\frac{A + T}{G + C}$ is characteristic to a species. Most higher organisms have a high AT content while most bacteria have a high GC content.

Using this information we can answer the problem.

(a) We are given that the ratio of $\frac{A + T}{G + C} = 0.2$ in one strand. This means that 20 percent of the strand is composed of adenine and thymine. We can use facts 1, 2 and 4 above to see that the complementary strand must have the same amount of adenine and thymine and thus a ratio of 0.2.

(b) Here we are given that $\frac{A + G}{T + C} = 0.2$. Since adenine binds to thymine and guanine to cytosine, the amount of A + G in one strand should equal the amount of T + C in the other strand. So in the complementary strand, T + C = 0.2

$$\text{and} \quad \frac{A + G}{T + C} = \frac{1}{0.2} = 5$$

(c) The ratio in any double-stranded piece of DNA of $\frac{A+G}{T+C}$ will equal 1. This is because of the specific base pairing in the strands. The sum of the purines equals the sum of the pyrimidines so, A + G (purines) = T + C (pyrimidines). This ratio is then equal to 1.

● **PROBLEM 9-9**

Given the following sequence of nucleotides for a single strand of DNA:

5' ----A A A T C G A T T G C G C T A T C G----3'

Construct the complementary sequence that would be incorporated during replication to complete the double helix of DNA molecule.

Solution: Since there is specific complementary pairing between A-T or T-A and between G-C or C-G, the complementary sequence of nucleotides will be:

3'----T T T A G C T A A C G C G A T A G C ---5'

● PROBLEM 9-10

Given the following molecule of DNA:

strand 1---A A A T C G A T T G G C A C A---

strand 2---T T T A G C T A A C C G T G T---

Assuming that strand 1 will serve as the transcription template, construct the molecule of mRNA that will be transcribed.

Solution: Since RNA has U instead of T, the complementary pairing that will occur in transcription is A of DNA with U of RNA and T of DNA with A of RNA. Thus, the mRNA molecule that will be transcribed from the above DNA strand 1 will be:

---U U U A G C U A A C C G U G U---

● PROBLEM 9-11

Given the following DNA transcription template for an mRNA molecule:

----A A C G T A T T C A A C T C A----

what will be the polypeptide sequence if a transition mutation occurs to the G nucleotide? How will it differ from the normal polypeptide sequence?

Solution: First, we must determine what the normal polypeptide sequence will be. This we can do by constructing the mRNA molecule, which will be:

----U U G C A U A A G U U G A G U----

The normal polypeptide sequence will include the following amino acids:

----leu-his-lys-leu-ser----

Now a transition mutation for G would result in the substitiution of an A for the G, which would change the second codon for the mutant mRNA from CAU to UAU. This change would result in the substitution of the amino acid histidine (his) for tyrosine (tyr) in the polypeptide sequence.

● **PROBLEM** 9-12

Why and how do circular molecules of DNA become supertwisted?

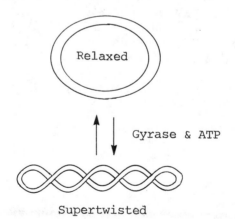

Solution: Circular molecules can become supertwisted by the action of gyrase along with ATP. Supertwisted DNA has a more compact shape than the untwisted (relaxed) DNA molecule so more DNA molecules can be packed into a small space. Supertwisting can also influence the degree of unwinding of the double helix; negative supertwisting can result in an unwinding of the double helix. This may aid in exposing the strands to the replication and transcription enzymes, thus allowing those processes to occur.

List the enzymes necessary for DNA replication in E.coli. What are the functions of each of these enzymes?

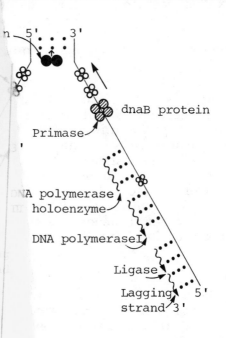

rep protein

SSB protein

dnaB protein

Primase

DNA polymerase III holoenzyme

DNA polymeraseI

Ligase

Lagging 5'
strand 3'

Fig. 1

Solution: Meselson and Stahl showed that each strand of the double-stranded DNA acts as a template for the synthesis of a new strand. Somehow the helix must be separated, held open and protected long enough for this replication to take place. Also, since DNA polymerase III works only in the 5' to 3' direction, other enzymes are needed to enable this to occur.

Figure 1 shows a schematic diagram of the replication process.

Replication is a very complex procedure. Many enzymes are needed for the process. These enzymes and their functions are listed in the table.

Protein	Role
1. dnaB protein	Enables primase to initiate
2. Primase	Synthesizes RNA primers
3. rep protein	Unwinds helix

349

4. SSB protein   Protects single-stranded regions

5. Gyrase   Helps unwind helix

6. DNA polymerase III holoenzyme   Synthesizes DNA

7. DNA polymerase I   Removes primer and fills in gaps

8. Ligase   Joins ends of DNA

These enzymes function in concert to replicate the DNA. Replication is initiated at a specific site. The rep protein and gyrase unwind the helix so that the replication enzymes can have the single-strand that they require. Since the single-strands of DNA are vulnerable to nuclease activity, single-strand binding (SSB) proteins are needed to stabilize the strands. Since DNA polymerase III can only synthesize DNA when there is a free 3'-OH group, a primer is needed to start the leading strand and each piece of the lagging strand.

The primer is RNA and it is synthesized by primase. The strands can now be elongated by DNA polymerase III holoenzyme which synthesizes only in the 5' to 3' direction. This is why one strand can be synthesized in one continuous piece while the complementary strand is synthesized in spurts as the helix unwinds. DNA polymerase I can remove the RNA primers and replace them with the appropriate DNA sequence encoded in the template strand. Finally, ligase can seal the remaining nicks between the bases by catalyzing the formation of phosphodiester bonds. The original DNA helix is now replicated and exists in two copies, each identical.

● **PROBLEM** 9-14

Would you expect the transfer RNA molecules and the messenger RNA molecules to be the same in the cells of a horse as in similar human cells? Give reasons for your answer in each case.

Solution: All tRNA and mRNA molecules are composed of the same chemical constituents, regardless of what species they come from. That is, they all contain the bases adenine, thymine, uracil and cytosine, ribose and phosphate (tRNA may have other bases in addition).

Observations from biochemical experiments aimed at elucidating the sequence and chemical composition of tRNA from different species have demonstrated that between species the different types of tRNA molecules have basically the same nucleotide sequence and the same three-dimensional configuration (cloverleaf-shaped). The reason for this lies in the fact that the function of tRNA is to transfer the amino acids to their correct positions specified by the mRNA. Since all organisms make use of the same 20 amino acids to make their proteins, the tRNA used to transfer these amino acids are basically the same for different species.

Unlike tRNA, mRNA molecules do not have a strict function. Their purpose is to provide the protein-synthesizing machinery with the information needed for protein production. The different mRNA molecules made by the cells of the same animal differ considerably in length. Different proteins are of different lengths and, therefore, there is a corresponding difference in lengths of the mRNA.

When we compare the mRNA from different species, such as man and horse, we have to bear in mind that there exist both equivalent and contrasting systems in the two species. Equivalent systems such as the Krebs cycle and electron transport system, which are almost universal among higher organisms utilize similar enzymes. The digestive system is an example of a contrasting system. The horse is a herbivore, whereas man is an omnivore. Because of the different modes of nutrition some very different enzymes are involved.

We know that enzymes, which are protein molecules, are the products of translation of mRNA. When translated, different mRNA molecules will give rise to different enzymes. Because horses and men rely on different enzymes - at least for digestion - we would infer that the mRNA from the two animals is different. However, we must not forget that both animals also use similar enzymes, as in Krebs cycle and electron transport system. Therefore they would also possess some similar, if not identical, mRNA.

In summary, we have determined that tRNA from cells of horse and man are basically the same, whereas the mRNA from the cells of these two animals would show much more difference.

351

GENES

Distinguish between a cistron, a muton, and a recon. Which of these is the largest and which is the smallest?

Solution: A cistron is defined as the genetic unit of biochemical function. One cistron corresponds to one functional unit (one gene coding for a polypeptide chain, protein, or enzyme) on a chromosome. A cistron can be defined by means of complementation tests. Complementation refers to the production of a normal phenotype through the combined activities of two chromosomes, each of which is incapable, due to a recessive mutation, of producing a normal phenotype. If two homologous chromosomes contain mutations in different cistrons, the normal gene of one can compensate for the mutated gene of the other and vice-versa when the two chromosomes are in combination with each other in the organism (see Figure 1). If each chromosome of the pair contains a mutation within the same cistron, neither can compensate for the other, and mutant phenotype will

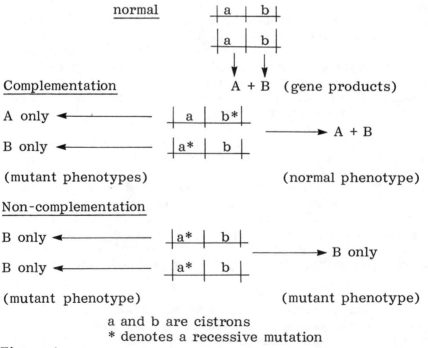

Figure 1

result. A cistron, thus, is the unit within which two chromosomes can have mutations and not complement each other when they occur in combination. It follows then that a cistron is the smallest unit capable of producing a gene product and is equivalent to a gene.

A muton is defined as the smallest unit which, if altered, gives rise to a mutant phenotype. A muton may thus be as small as a single nucleotide, since a change in a single nucleotide can cause a mutant phenotype (think, for example, of sickle-cell anemia). Of course, some single-point mutations may not result in a mutant phenotype. If a given codon were changed via a single base substitution, for example, from CCA to CCG, that codon would still specify proline, due to the degeneracy of the genetic code.

A recon is defined as the smallest unit that is interchangeable, but not divisible, by recombination. In other words, recons are the smallest units between which crossing over can occur. This is known to be equivalent to a single nucleotide. This is because the breakage point in crossing over is between any two given nucleotides. Given two crossovers it is thus possible for a single nucleotide to be exchanged (see Figure 2).

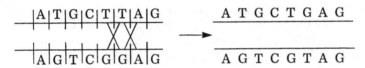

FIGURE 2. Double crossover between two strands of DNA, the base sequences of which are shown.

Since a cistron consists of a sequence of mutons or recons, it is the largest of the three. A recon may be as small as a single nucleotide, as may be a muton.

● PROBLEM 9-16

How can one estimate the total number of genes for a given organism?

Solution: Since genetic information is stored as DNA base sequences, the amount of DNA in a cell provides an initial basis for estimating the genetic information available to the cell. It is a well-established fact that chromosomes carry the genetic information for the ordering of amino acid sequences of the proteins that are made in the cell. Proteins consist of one or more polypeptide chains, which are composed of numerous amino acids. A given polypeptide chain is coded for by a specific gene with one gene carrying the information for only one polypeptide.

Genes are arranged in linear order on the chromosomes and are composed of a specific number and sequence of DNA base pairs. There is a direct correlation between the size of the gene (or the number of base pairs it contains) and the size of the protein it codes for (or the number of amino acids in that protein). A protein can consist of a few dozen to a few hundred amino acids, with 300-400 amino acids often used as the size for an "average" protein. Three mRNA bases are required to code for a single amino acid, and since mRNA is transcribed from only one of the two complementary DNA strands, this means that three DNA base pairs are needed to code for an amino acid. Thus, a very rough measure of the number of different proteins for which a cell might carry information is obtained by dividing the number of base pairs in its DNA by three, giving a theoretical number of amino acids in DNA. Dividing that number by the average number of amino acids per polypeptide gives a value for the possible number of polypeptides. If an estimate is made of the number of polypeptides the chromosomes can code for, then the number of genes found on the chromosomes can be estimated from the simple fact that one gene codes for one polypeptide.

In order for us to determine the total number of genes in an organism by this method, we must get a rather good estimate of the total number of DNA base pairs contained in the chromosomes. This is rather difficult to do with diploid organisms. In addition to the difficulty caused by the sheer number of chromosomes, large amounts of associated proteins known as histones, as well as other proteins, are found associated with the chromosomes. Moreover, the general structure of a diploid chromosome is, for the most part, not stretched out, but folded and convoluted into supercoils, further complicating the examination of the DNA. The chromosome structure of bacteria and viruses is simpler and better understood. Their chromosome is a pure DNA molecule, having no associated proteins, and is often circular in structure. Bacteria usually contain one DNA molecule per cell and the chromosome can be seen in rather good detail using an electron microscope. Owing to its simple chromosome structure then, let us estimate the total number of genes in the bacterium Escherichia coli.

In order to proceed we must first know the number

of base pairs in the chromosome of E. coli. This figure can be estimated either from the length of the DNA molecule, which has been found to be approximately 1000 μm or 1mm, or from the molecular weight, which is about 2×10^9 daltons. Each base pair has a molecular weight of approximately 660 daltons, and there are about 3000 base pairs per μm of DNA double helix molecule. Either way of determination (3000 base pairs/μm x 1000 μm or 2×10^9 daltons/660 daltons/base pair) indicates that there are approximately three million base pairs in the DNA molecule of E. coli. Dividing this by three, we can find out how many amino acids there are (recall that three DNA base pairs code for an amino acid). This gives us a value of about 1 million amino acids. Since the average protein contains about 400 amino acids, the chromosome of E. coli could possibly code for a maximum of 2500 proteins. (1,000,000/400)

This figure of 2500 genes may seem like an extremely large amount for one cell to contain. However, E. coli is a relatively complex organism. It is considered complex because it is relatively self-sufficient, living on a minimal medium of a glucose solution, from which it produces all other vitamins and nutrients necessary for life. This requires a great deal of enzyme and protein machinery, and thus a relatively large number of genes.

The mammalian cell, being more complex, should contain a larger number of genes than E. coli. We can determine how much DNA is present per mamalian cell. The amount is approximately 800 times that in E. coli. This number gives us an upper limit of the number of different genes. Thus, a mammalian cell would have 800 x 2500, or over two million genes.

Measurements of the amount of DNA present can be misleading, and we must be very cautious about relating DNA content directly to the number of different proteins that may be synthesized by a given cell and therefore, the number of genes in that cell. There is a definite lack of correspondence between DNA content and the number of genes. While in procaryotes and lower eucaryotes most DNA codes for amino acid sequences, the vast majority of DNA from multicellular organisms has no apparent genetic function. In Drosophila, only about 5% of the total DNA codes for amino acid gene products, while in humans even less DNA is so employed. There are a number of explanations for the presence of this "excess" DNA. There are multiple repetitive sequences of DNA, some of which are never transcribed, although their function is not clear. In Drosophila, about 25% of the DNA shows this kind of repetitive sequence, and in the higher eucaryotes, 10% to 20% of the DNA is repetitive. Some DNA might play structural roles, such as involvement in chromosome folding or pairing during meiosis. Other regions may have regulatory functions, acting as binding sites for repressor molecules or polymerases.

What experimental evidence indicates that genes control the amino acid sequences in proteins?

Solution: In 1953, the first amino acid sequence of a protein was completed. After six years, Frederick Sanger had succeeded in sequencing the amino acid sequence of a relatively small protein, insulin. He used different proteolytic enzymes to cleave the protein molecule into fragments that could be sequenced more easily than the large molecule. Many of the fragments had overlapping sequences, so the linear order of the whole insulin molecule could be pieced together. This showed that the amino acid sequence is what individualizes proteins. Insulin is insulin because of its specific amino acid sequence.

Vernon Ingram chose a well-studied inherited disorder, sickle-cell anemia. In 1957, he sequenced normal hemoglobin (HbA) and sickled hemoglobin (HbS). He compared the amino acid sequences and found a difference of one amino acid. This connected the abnormal amino acid sequence of a protein to an inherited, and hence, genetic disorder.

Ingram's discovery was proof that a mutation in a gene resulted in an abnormal amino acid sequence in a protein. But, as in almost all experimentation, he had to use techniques pioneered by others. The sequencing technique developed by Sanger was very important in the determination of a link between genes and amino acid sequences in proteins.

TRANSCRIPTION AND TRANSLATION

How does RNA polymerase transfer the genetic information from DNA to RNA?

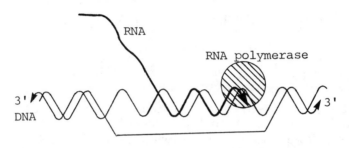

Fig. 1

Solution: To answer this question, we must examine the structure of an RNA polymerase. The RNA polymerase in E.coli is composed of a core enzyme which has three types of polypeptide subunits - β, β' and α. Each enzyme has two copies of the α subunit so the composition of the core enzyme is written $\beta\beta'\alpha_2$. This core enzyme can bind to DNA to transcribe RNA but does so unspecifically. Only when a polypeptide known as σ (sigma) associates with the core protein does the RNA polymerase, now called a holoenzyme (from the Greek holos meaning whole), bind specifically to the DNA's promoter region. Therefore σ is necessary for the proper initiation of transcription. Other auxiliary proteins are nusA protein and ρ(rho). These polypeptides associate with the core enzyme after σ has been released to ensure correct chain termination. They detect termination signals that are not recognized by the core enzyme alone.

This enzymatic system catalyzes the transcription of RNA from DNA. The RNA polymerase holoenzyme ($\beta\beta'\alpha_2\sigma$) binds to the promoter site of the DNA. This binding opens the helix at that point, exposing the hydrogen bonds and bases of the DNA. The holoenzyme then catalyzes the reactions that bring the complementary bases, ribose groups and phosphates together to create the RNA strand. The RNA polymerase adds one base at a time moving from the 3' to the 5' end of the DNA. The rate of the reactions is phenomenal: 40 to 50 nucleotides are added each second. Since the σ factor is no longer needed, it dissociates. This allows ρ and nusA to bind to the core enzyme. The elongation of the RNA strand continues until ρ and nusA detect a terminator region. These regions contain inverted repeats that can fold back on themselves to make structures called stem loops (see Fig. 2). When the termination factors sense a stem loop followed by a string of adenosine residues, the core enzyme dissociates from the DNA template. The termination factors dissociate and the core enzyme is free to begin another round of transcription.

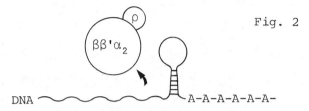

Fig. 2

Thus, one enzymatic system is used to catalyze the transcription of DNA to RNA. The fidelity of this process is much lower than the polymerization of DNA by DNA polymerase because RNA polymerase cannot proofread the product of its activity as DNA polymerase I can. But since many transcripts of a gene are produced, the lowered fidelity is not crucial.

● **PROBLEM** 9-19

What is the relationship between transcription and translation in the production of polypeptides?

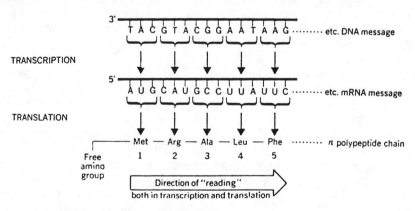

SCHEMATIC SHOWING THE RELATION BETWEEN TRANSCRIPTION AND TRANSLATION TO PRODUCE POLYPEPTIDES.

Solution: The genetic information that is stored in the nucleotide sequence of DNA is not directly used to make polypeptides. An RNA intermediate is used. This messenger RNA (mRNA) can be synthesized and degraded very rapidly. With the existence of this intermediate, the stable DNA acts simply as a blueprint of information, while the RNA can move away from the chromosome to the cytoplasm where the protein synthesizing machinery awaits. The actual protein producers are the RNAs: mRNA, rRNA and tRNA.

The formation of the mRNA from DNA is termed transcription. DNA-dependent RNA polymerase catalyzes the initiation and elongation of the RNA chain. The production of RNA is halted when the RNA polymerase reaches a string of thymine residues in an A-T rich region and an inverted repeat in a G-C rich region of the DNA. These sequences signal termination and the mRNA dissociates from the DNA template.

The genetic information can now move to the ribosomes in the cytoplasm in a form that the rRNA and the tRNA recognize. The codons in the mRNA are recognized by the anticodons of the tRNA molecules who transfer their amino acid to the growing polypeptide chain.

So, the relationship between transcription and translation is merely that of steps in the production of the final amino acid sequence of a polypeptide from the original nucleotide sequence of the chromosomal DNA.

● **PROBLEM** 9-20

How is protein synthesis initiated?

Solution: Messenger RNA molecules are translated to proteins at the ribosomes. At their 5' ends, the mRNAs have a leader sequence. This "cap" contains a methyl-guanosyl triphosphate group which binds to the small ribosomal subunit. In eukaryotes, the association of ribosome, mRNA and tRNA requires three protein factors called initiation factors - IF-1, IF-2 and IF-3. IF-3 is necessary for the binding of the ribosome to mRNA. Once bound, the other two initiation factors and the hydrolysis of GTP is required for the binding of the first codon of the mRNA to the small ribosome. When the initiation factors are released, the large ribosomal subunit attaches. The complete ribosome has two sites for tRNA molecules, the peptidyl (P) site and the aminoacyl (A) site. The mRNA codons are held near these spots so the tRNAs can bind. The initiation is complete and the machinery is poised for elongation of the polypeptide chain.

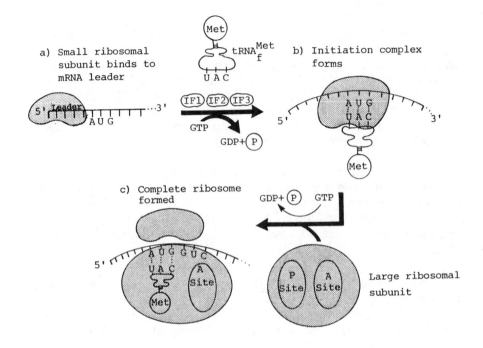

a) Small ribosomal subunit binds to mRNA leader

b) Initiation complex forms

c) Complete ribosome formed

Large ribosomal subunit

● **PROBLEM** 9-21

How is the peptide chain elongated during protein synthesis?

Solution: Peptide elongation is the next step in the synthesis of a polypeptide. The alignment of the initiator codon (AUG) with the P site leaves the A site aligned with the next codon. In E.coli, the association of the next mRNA codon with its tRNA anticodon requires the hydrolysis of GTP and the association of two protein elongation factors, EF-1 and EF-2. A displacement occurs to allow the peptide bond to form between the two amino acid residues. This reaction is catalyzed by peptidyl transferase. The next event, translocation, involves the movement of the tRNA from the A site to the P site and the movement of the whole ribosome three nucleotides. These simultaneous events result in the alignment of a new codon in the A site and the previous codon in the P site. This process is repeated until a termination signal is recognized.

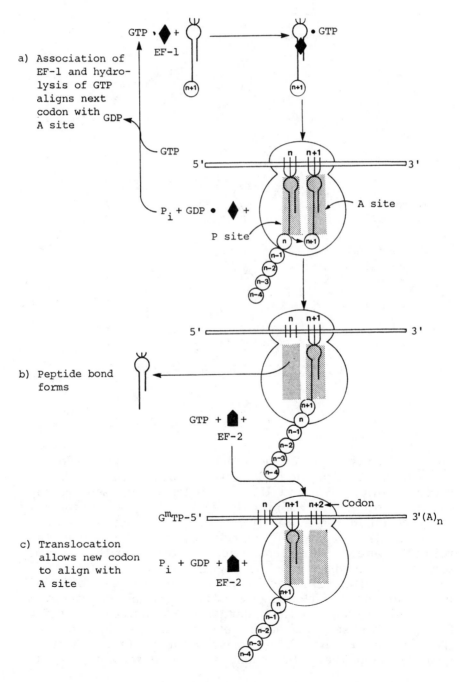

How is protein synthesis terminated?

a) Ribosome reaches   Termination
   terminator codon   (nonsense)
                             codon

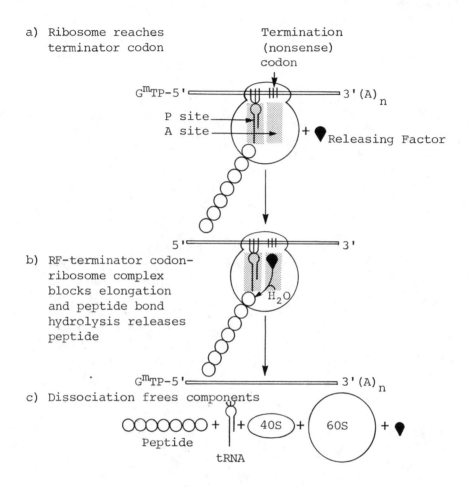

b) RF-terminator codon-
   ribosome complex
   blocks elongation
   and peptide bond
   hydrolysis releases
   peptide

c) Dissociation frees components

Peptide

tRNA

Solution: When a ribosome reaches a terminator codon in the mRNA, the peptide elongation halts. The terminator codons, UAA, UGA and UAG, are not recognized by any naturally occurring aminoacyl tRNAs. The terminator (or stop) codon in the A site prevents the further addition of amino acids to the polypeptide chain. There are two release factors in E.coli that interact with specific terminator codons: RF-1 recognizes UAA or UAG and RF-2 recognizes UAA or UGA. This interaction forms an RF-terminator codon-ribosome complex which clogs the A site and blocks further elongation. Another releasing factor hydrolyzes the bond between the peptide and the tRNA in the P site. This releases the protein and tRNA from the ribosome. The ribosome then dissociates into its two subunits, free to form new initiation complexes to begin another round of peptide synthesis.

Explain what difficulties would arise if messenger RNA molecules were not destroyed after they had produced some polypeptide chains.

Solution: Upon translation, mRNA molecules give rise to polypeptide chains. Normally, mRNA molecules are short-lived and are broken down by RNAase after a few translations. If an mRNA molecule were not destroyed, it would continue to synthesize its protein, and soon there would be an excess of this protein in the cell. This condition leads to some important implications for the cell.

The continual translation of mRNA into proteins would entail a serious depletion of the energy store in the cell. For example, before an amino acid can attach to a tRNA molecule, it has to be activated. Activation is brought about by the hydrolysis of one molecule of ATP. So for each amino acid in the polypeptide chain, one molecule of ATP molecules would be consumed and the energy supply in the cell would be depleted.

In addition, the cell would accumulate proteins that it may not need. This use of large amounts of energy to produce unneeded protein would be a wasteful process. Indeed the excessive accumulation of a protein may even be harmful to the cell or organism. For example, given the right environment, a protease such as pepsin, if present in more than sufficient amounts, will eat away the wall of the stomach, forming an ulcer.

The degradation of mRNA molecules allows a cell to control its metabolic activity. This control is important to the proper functioning of the cell.

Describe experimental evidence which indicates that it is not the kind of ribosomes but the kind of mRNA which determines the type of proteins which will be produced.

Solution: Most DNA is found in the nucleus. Transcription of this DNA gives rise to mRNA. If the nucleus is removed from a cell, the source of mRNA is removed. Such an enucleated cell can live for a short time, but growth and enzyme production will soon stop. For example, an enucleated ameoba (an ameoba with its nucleus removed) will crawl around for a time. It may engulf food but it will eventually be unable to digest it. Its growth stops and in time, the organism dies.

The above experimental observation can be explained in the following manner. The removal of the nucleus of the organism prevents further transcription of mRNA. The supply of digestive enzymes normally found in the organism becomes depleted because the source of mRNA is cut off and the translation of mRNA into enzyme cannot occur. Therefore, the engulfed food cannot be digested. This explanation shows that mRNA manufactured in the cell nucleus is essential for protein production in the cell.

In order to test what effect the type of mRNA has on the type of proteins produced, one can perform experiments where the nucleus of one species, producing certain types of mRNA, is introduced into an enucleated cell of a different species. For example, the nucleus of a mammalian reticulocyte, a cell that synthesizes hemoglobin, can be extracted and then introduced into an enucleated cell, such as an amphibian oocyte. This egg cell with a transplanted nucleus survives and produces mammalian hemoglobin instead of amphibian hemoglobin. This is good evidence showing that mRNA controls the type of proteins produced because the amphibian oocyte produces a mammalian protein even though its ribosomes are its own. The ribosomes, since they are cytoplasmic, are amphibian, but the protein product, like the nucleus and the mRNA, is mammalian. Thus, the ribosomes do not determine the type of protein that is produced; the mRNA molecules have control.

Mitosis is only one of four stages of the complete cell life cycle. List the other three and indicate the amount of RNA synthesis in each of the four stages. Explain why RNA output is greater in some stages than in others.

Solution: The length of the cell cycle under optimal conditions varies from 18 - 24 hours for most cells. Cell cycles are usually divided into four phases: M (mitosis), G_1 (period prior to DNA synthesis), S (period of DNA synthesis) and G_2 (period between DNA synthesis and mitosis). M is the shortest stage, usually lasting about one hour. There is no synthesis of either DNA or RNA in this stage. The absence of RNA synthesis may be the result of the tightly coiled and condensed nature of the DNA at this point, making it impossible to transcribe. Recall that for transcription to occur, DNA must first unfold.

During G_1, there is production of mRNA and the cell increases in size. Next, in the S phase, the DNA of the cell becomes doubled because the genes are duplicating. Duplicating genes cannot produce RNA, but since all the genes do not duplicate at once, there is still some output of RNA, although in reduced quantity. Finally, full output of RNA is resumed in G_2.

RNA production is greater in G_1 and G_2 because during these two stages the DNA is relaxed (uncondensed) and is not involved in duplication. The relaxed nature of the DNA favors RNA synthesis, which can only occur when the double-stranded DNA separates into two individual strands.

GENETIC CODE

Explain how the codon for phenylalanine was discovered.

Solution: It has been known for some time now that the genetic code is a triplet code - three bases in a messenger RNA molecule code for one amino acid. Each triplet is known as a codon and the entire set of codons comprising the RNA molecule constitute the genetic code for a polypeptide chain.

The translation of the genetic code resulted from recent research, the aim of which was to determine the exact sequence of the bases on the mRNA molecule which specifies a particular amino acid. An important breakthrough in this research came when a method of artificially synthesizing mRNA was developed. Ribose sugar, phosphate ions, and various bases, when combined under the proper conditions, result in the formation of a synthetic RNA molecule. By varying the kinds of bases used in producing this RNA, it has been possible to determine which base sequences result in which amino acids. The synthetic mRNA is placed with ribosomes, amino acids, ATP, and tRNA. The resulting polypeptide chain is analyzed for its component amino acids.

The codon for the amino acid phenylalanine was the first to be discovered using the above procedure. The only base used in the synthesis of the mRNA, was uracil, and therefore the molecule had a series of UUU codons. This mRNA was added to ribosomes, amino acids, ATP and tRNA, and the resulting polypeptide consisted only of phenylalanine. Thus, it was deduced that the codon UUU is the sequence of bases which causes phenylalanine to be placed in the polypeptide chain.

● **PROBLEM** 9-27

A wild-type mRNA and polypeptide sequence is:

mRNA: UAG UUUG <u>AUG</u> <u>GCC</u> <u>UCU</u> <u>UGC</u> <u>AAA</u> <u>GGC</u> <u>UAU</u>

<u>AGU</u> <u>AGU</u> <u>UAG</u>

polypeptide: met-ala-ser-cys-lys-gly-tyr-ser-ser STOP

What is the result, if at the arrow:

(a) one nucleotide, U, is deleted?

(b) one nucleotide, C, is inserted?

Refer to the genetic code given in Table 1.

THE GENETIC CODE (CODON ASSIGNMENTS IN MESSENGER RNA).*

First Nucleotide	Second Nucleotide				Third Nucleotide
	U	C	A	G	
	Phe	Ser	Tyr	Cys	U
U	Phe	Ser	Tyr	Cys	C
	Leu	Ser	CT	CT	A
	Leu	Ser	CT	Trp	G
	Leu	Pro	His	Arg	U
C	Leu	Pro	His	Arg	C
	Leu	Pro	Gln	Arg	A
	Leu	Pro	Gln	Arg	G
	Ile	Thr	Asn	Ser	U
A	Ile	Thr	Asn	Ser	C
	Ile	Thr	Lys	Arg	A
	Met(CI)	Thr	Lys	Arg	G
	Val	Ala	Asp	Gly	U
G	Val	Ala	Asp	Gly	C
	Val	Ala	Glu	Gly	A
	Val	Ala	Glu	Gly	G

*The terms first, second, and third nucleotide refer
to the individual nucleotides of a triplet codon.
U = uridine nucleotide; C = cytosine nucleotide;
A = adenine nucleotide; G = guanine nucleotide;
CI = chain initiator codon; CT = chain terminator
codon.

Table 1.

Solution: The addition or deletion of one nucleotide
results in a frameshift mutation. Since the reading frame is
three codons, such a change moves the frame. This
results in a severe alteration of the amino acid sequence
in the polypeptide. The frameshift not only introduces a
garbled sequence but may produce a premature terminator
codon which would interupt the synthesis of the remaining
message.

(a) When a uridine nucleotide is deleted at the arrow, the
altered mRNA would produce a new polypeptide sequence:

mRNA: UAG UUUG AUG GCC⁻¹CUU GCA AAG GCU AUA GUA GUU AG...

polypeptide: met - ala - leu - ala - lys - ala - thr - val - val - ser

garbled

(b) When a cytosine nucleotide is inserted at the same site another new sequence results:

(+1)

mRNA: UAG UUUG AUG GCC CUC UUG CAA AGG CUA UAG UAG UUAG...

polypeptide: met - ala - leu - leu - gly - arg - leu   STOP

garbled

What do the codons AUG, UAG, UAA and UGA code for?

Solution: These four codons are special since they can either signal the beginning or the end of a polypeptide chain. When strategically placed at the 5' end of the mRNA, AUG codes for methionine (which is formylated in prokaryotes but not in eukaryotes) and signals the start of protein synthesis. At other places in the mRNA, AUG codes for the amino acid methionine. The other codons, UAG, UAA and UGA, are terminator (or nonsense) codons. They code for no amino acids and signal the end of a polypeptide chain. They have been given the names amber (UAG), ochre (UAA), and opal (UGA).

The terminator codons occur naturally in a cell's mRNA to signal the termination of the polypeptide chain. However, mutations that change the reading frame or substitute wrong bases can create terminator codons in the middle of an mRNA chain. Such nonsense mutations result in the production of incomplete polypeptides. These polypeptides are not usable by the cell. The protein's activity can be restored if a second mutation, a suppressor mutation, occurred. A mutation in the anticodon region of a tRNA is a suppressor mutation. If the tRNA's codon became AUC, ACC or ACU, it would be complementary to the nonsense codons. Thus the tRNA could bind to the mRNA, donating its amino acid to the polypeptide chain. The resulting polypeptide will contain one wrong amino acid, but that usually does not affect its activity drastically. The protein will function more effectively than the incomplete fragment produced by the nonsense mutation.

Suppose the codons for amino acids consisted of only two bases rather than three. Would there be a sufficient number of codons for all twenty amino acids? Show how you obtain your answer.

Solution: There are two ways to approach this question. One way is to use a mathematical principle known as permutation and the other is to do it by common sense. The latter method will be discussed first.

In this question, we are told that a codon consists of two bases only. We know there are four different kinds of bases in DNA, namely adenine, guanine, cytosine and thymine. To get the total number of possible two-base codons, we will have to pick from the four bases and put them into two positions on the codon. For the first position, we can have any one of the four bases. That means there are four possible ways of filling the first position. For each of these four possible first positions, we again can put any one of the four bases into the second position. The only restriction we face is the number of different bases we have, which is four. So the total number of codons consisting of two bases is 4 x 4 or 16 codons.

The other way to solve this problem is to use permutation. The general formula used in permutation is $nPr = n^r$ where n is the total number of objects and r is the number of times changed (or permuted). nPr is read as "n permuted r times," and n^r as "n to the power of r." Applying this formula:

n is the number of different bases (that is, 4) and r is the number of bases in a codon (which is 2). Substituting in the numerical data, we have the total possible number of codons made up of 2 bases.

$$(n^r) = 4^2 = 16$$

In either case, we arrive at the same answer. There will be 16 different codons if each codon contains two bases. However, there are 20 different kinds of amino acids, thus 16 codons will be insufficient to code for all 20 amino acids.

If an mRNA molecule synthesized in the laboratory consists only of adenine and guanine in an approximate 2:1 ratio, what possible amino acids could be included in the polypeptide to be produced?

Solution: Since the only nucleotides present are adenine (A) and guanine (G), then only those amino acids coded for by codons possessing any combination of A and/or G will be present. There are four amino acids that fit such a requirement: lysine (lys), arginine (arg), glutamic acid (glu) and glycine (gly). Further, since the ratio of A:G is 2:1 in this molecule, it is likely that any numerical repetition of the combination of the following five codons will suffice:

AAA(lys),   AAG(lys),   AGA(arg),   GAA(glu)   and GGA(gly).

The amino acid tryptophan is coded for by a single triplet code. If only single base substitutions are allowed to occur, what amino acid substitutions would occur in mutants?

Solution: Refer to the genetic code in an earlier problem. We see that the codon specifying tryptophan is UGG. Replacing each codon sequentially, we will be able to determine the amino acids that will be incorporated instead of tryptophan in the mutants.

First, replace the first codon by A, G and C.

UGG ⟶ AGG

UGG ⟶ GGG

UGG ⟶ CGG

Now we find these codons in the table to see what amino acids (if any) they determine. Both AGG and CGG code for arginine. GGG codes for glycine.

At the second position, we do the same and obtain the following:

$$UGG \longrightarrow UAG \longrightarrow STOP$$

$$UGG \longrightarrow UUG \longrightarrow leucine$$

$$UGG \longrightarrow UCG \longrightarrow serine$$

At the third position of the original codon, substitutions will create:

$$UGG \longrightarrow UGA \longrightarrow STOP$$

$$UGG \longrightarrow UGC \longrightarrow cysteine$$

$$UGG \longrightarrow UGU \longrightarrow cysteine$$

Thus, single nucleotide substitutions can change the tryptophan codon to codons that specify arginine, glycine, leucine, serine or cysteine. The substitutions can also create nonsense codons in place of tryptophan. As discussed earlier, these codons would cause the premature termination of the polypeptide chain.

● **PROBLEM** 9-32

What are the effects of base substitutions on protein structure and function?

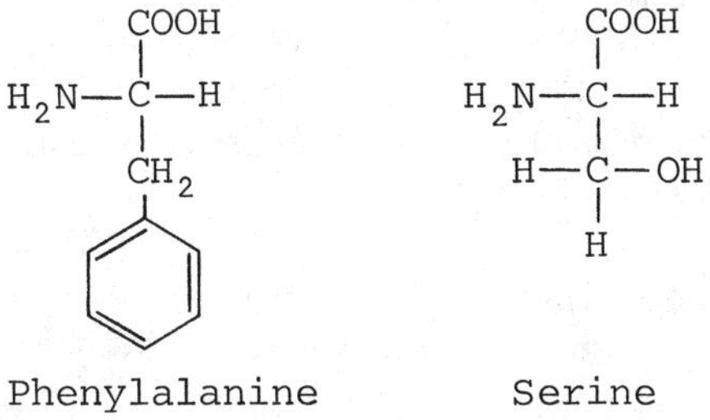

Phenylalanine   Serine

Fig. 1

Solution: Base substitutions alter codons. This results in a change in the amino acid sequence. If there is a single base substitution there will probably be a single amino acid change. Where this change takes place is important. The properties of each amino acid cause interactions that determine the three-dimensional (tertiary) conformation of the polypeptide chain. The amino acids react with each other and with their surroundings to form a shape which is the most energetically favorable. This shape is characteristic to each sequence of amino acids and dictates how the protein will function.

Amino acids have a similar structure. They consist of an amino group, a carboxyl group, a hydrogen atom and a distinctive side group, all bonded to a carbon atom. The side group, R, is what characterizes the individual amino acid. The properties of the side group determine whether the amino acid is hydrophobic (phenylalanine), hydrophilic (serine), basic (lysine), acidic (aspartate), small (glycine), bulky (arginine), capable of forming hydrogen bonds (threonine) or capable of forming disulfide bonds (cysteine).

The linear sequence of amino acids spontaneously folds into a three-dimensional shape because of the interactions among the amino acids and between the amino acids and their surroundings. The three-dimensional shape is what confers to the protein its function. The effect that an amino acid change has depends on the extent of the change and the position of the amino acid in the chain. Suppose a base pair substitution changes UUU to UCU. A glance at a table of the genetic code shows that this change results in the incorporation of serine instead of phenylalanine.

Their structures are obviously very different. Phenylalanine has a large hydrophobic side chain while serine has a smaller hydrophilic side chain. This is a very drastic change. If the amino acid's position in the chain is to become part of the active site in the final enzyme, the enzyme may not be able to recognize the proper substrate. This would render the enzyme nonfunctional. However, if the change is not in a critical position, the functioning of enzyme may not be drastically affected. The enzyme may suffer a decreased rate, but it is still a functional molecule.

The effect that a base substitution has, depends on the nature of the change. Some amino acids, such as valine and alanine, are very similar. A change substituting one for the other may not affect the protein's function at all.

COOH
|
H₂N—C—H
|
CH₃

Alanine

COOH
|
H₂N—C—H
|
CH₂
/   \
CH₃   CH₃

Valine

Fig. 2

Some base substitutions may have drastic effects on protein structure and function while others may have very little effect. Also, when numerous substitutions occur, the effects will be much more pronounced. Thus the effects of base substitutions vary according to their extent and their positioning.

● **PROBLEM** 9-33

Can the change of a single amino acid in a polypeptide drastically alter the function of the polypeptide? Hint: use the hemoglobin molecule to answer this.

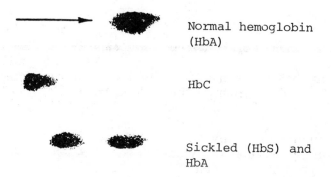

Normal hemoglobin (HbA)

HbC

Sickled (HbS) and HbA

Paper electrophoresis of hemoglobin specimens containing various types of hemoglobins. Negative molecules move fastest in direction of the arrow.

Fig. 1

Solution: The amino acid sequence of a protein is unique to each type of protein, much as skeletal structure typifies animal species. The amino acid sequence determines the types of interactions that can occur among them leading to the folded tertiary structure typical of each type of protein. Usually, the substitution of one amino acid for another causes no significant change in this structure. However, if the change occurs in an area important to the structure of the molecule and if the amino acids have different binding properties, the result could be a drastically altered molecule.

A single amino acid change in the β-chain of hemoglobin leads to the deformed shape of red blood cells seen in sickle-cell anemia. Glutamic acid, a polar, negatively charged amino acid, is replaced by valine, a neutral nonpolar amino acid. This lowers the total negative charge of the molecule, see Figure 1. It also reduces the solubility of deoxygenated hemoglobin S because the nonpolar valine is placed on the outside of the molecule. This area is "sticky" since it can interact with the sticky patch on another hemoglobin S molecule when both molecules are deoxygenated. Long aggregates which distort the red blood cell can be formed when there is a high concentration of deoxygenated hemoglobin S. The distorted blood cells get trapped in the small blood vessels. This impairs circulation, resulting in the damage of organs especially the kidneys and bone. Patients may go into shock during periods of high concentrations of sickled cells. Thus, the change of a single amino acid can have profound effects.

● PROBLEM 9-34

What is the minimum number of base substitutions that must be made to change the codons from:

(a) glutamic acid to lysine?
(b) leucine to alanine?
(c) phenylalanine to glycine?
(d) tryptophan to serine?
(e) valine to glutamic acid?

Solution: To answer these questions, we must use the genetic code from problem 9-27. Once the codons for both of the amino acids in question are known, we can find the minimum number of single nucleotide changes that will lead from one to the other.

(a) The codons for glutamic acid are GAA and GAG. Those for lysine are AAA and AAG. Only one base change is needed to go from GAA to AAA or from GAG to AAG.

(b) Leucine is coded for by CUU, CUC, CUA, CUG and alanine is specified by the codons GCU, GCC, GCA, and GCG. None of the leucine codons share two similar bases with any of the alanine codons. Therefore more than one base substitution is necessary. Two base changes would change:

CUU to GCU or CGA,

CUC to GCC or CGA,

CUA to CGA or GCG,

and   CUG to CGA or GCG.

Thus the minimum number of base substitutions needed to change leucine to alanine is two.

(c) Phenylalanine is coded for by UUU and UUC. Glycine is specified by GGU, GGC, GGA, GGG. Since UUC and GGC share a similar nucleotide, at least two bases must be changed to have glycine substituted for phenylalanine.

(d) Tryptophan is coded for by UGG and serine by UCU, UCC, UCA and UCG. UGG and UCG differ by only one base - so only one substitution is necessary to change a tryptophan codon to one specifying serine.

(e) Valine is coded by GUU, GUC, GUA and GUG. Glutamic acid is coded by GAA and GAG. Only one substitution is needed to go from:

GUA to GAA

and from

GUG to GAG.

This amino acid substitution is clinically important. The difference between HbS, the mutant hemoglobin responsible for sickle-cell anemia, and HbA, the wild-type hemoglobin, is simply the incorporation of a glutamic acid residue where a valine should be.

What is the wobble hypothesis?

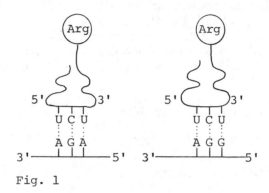

Fig. 1

Solution: Many amino acids are coded by more than one codon. Some examples of this degeneracy are UUU and UUC which code for phenylalanine, GAA and GAG which code for glutamate, and CUA, CUC, CUG and CUU which all code for leucine. The wobble hypothesis helps to explain this degeneracy.

Francis Crick developed the wobble hypothesis to explain some experimental evidence. Some experiments showed that highly purified tRNA species could recognize several different codons. Also, another anticodon base, inosine, was found. Inosine is similar to guanine and will normally pair with cytosine. Crick hypothesized that the base at the 5' end of the anticodon was not as rigidly fixed as the other two bases and it could hydrogen bond to several bases at the 3' end of the coding. The pairing is restricted to the combinations shown below:

Base in Anticodon	Base in Codon
G	U or C
C	G
A	U
U	A or G
I	A, U or C

An example of the pairing that is permitted by this hypothesis is shown in Figure 1.

What is the minimum number of tRNAs required to recognize all of the 61 sense codons without ambiguity?

Ala	Arg	Asp	Asn	Cys
GCU GCC } CGG	AGA AGG } UCU	GAC GAU } CUG	AAC AAU } UUG	UGC UGU } ACG
GCA GCG } CGU	CGA CGG } GCU			
	CGU CGC } GCG			
Glu	Gln	Gly	His	Ile
GAA GAG } CUU	CAA CAG } GUU	GGA GGG } CCU	CAC CAU } GUG	AUA-UAU
		GGC GGU } CCG		AUC AUU } UAG
Leu	Lys	Met	Phe	Pro
UUA UUG } AAU	AAA AAG } UUU	AUG-UAC	UUC UUU } AAG	CCA CCG } GGU
CUA CUG } GUA				CCU CCC } GGG
CUU CUC } GAG				
Ser	Thr	Trp	Tyr	Val
AGC AGU } UCG	ACA ACG } UGU	UGG-ACC	UAC UAU } AUG	GUA GUG } CAU
UCA UCG } AGU	ACU-UGA			GUC GUU } CAG
UCC UCU } AGG				

Table 1:   Codon}Anticodon

Solution: This problem is based on the wobble hypothesis. To answer the question, we need two sets of information. The first is a list of all of the mRNA codons and the amino acids that they specify. This can be obtained from a table of the genetic code. The second bit of information is the table given in the previous problem of the allowed pairings at the third codon base according to the wobble hypothesis. From this, we can make a list of all of the codons and the minimum number of anticodons that are needed to recognize them.

The anticodons were obtained by writing the first two complementary bases and then applying the wobble hypothesis to the third. For instance, the codons GCU and GCC both code for alanine. The first two complementary bases are C and G. The third anticodon base must be able to code for both U and C. By the wobble hypothesis, this is G. The anticodon is thus CGG. Since U and C in the third position can be coded by a single anticodon base and A and G can also be coded by a single anticodon base, the total of anticodons needed is not 64 or 20. The number of amino acids, 20, and the number of combinations with a three-letter code, 64, do not represent the minimum number of tRNAs needed. If we count up the anticodons from our list, we get 32. So a minimum of 32 types of tRNAs are needed to recognize all of the codons of the mRNA.

EXTRA PROBLEMS

The antisense (noncoding) strand of DNA is:

5' ATG GAT AAA GTT TTA AAC AGA GAG GAA TCT 3'

What is the:
(a) sense strand?
(b) mRNA transcribed?
(c) polypeptide chain that is translated?

Solution: We must simply write the complementary bases of the appropriate sequence for each question.

(a) The sense strand and the antisense strand of DNA make up the double-stranded helix. The sense strand is therefore complementary to the antisense strand. Its sequence is:

3' TAC CTA TTT CAA AAT TTG TCT CTC CTT AGA 5'

(b) The messenger RNA sequence is transcribed in the 5' to 3' direction from the sense strand of the DNA. So the sense strand is read in the 3' to 5' direction to allow the transcription to be 5' to 3'. Since this is mRNA, the residue thymine is replaced by uracil. The resulting mRNA is complementary to the sense strand.

5' AUG GAU AAA GUU UUA AAC AGA GAG GAA UCU 3'

(c) By using the table with the genetic code, the following polypeptide is produced from the mRNA:

H_2N-Met-Asp-Lys-Val-Leu-Asn-Arg-Glu-Glu-Ser-COOH.

● **PROBLEM** 9-38

If A, T, C, G and U represent adenine, thymine, cytosine, guanine and uracil, fill in the following blanks:

```
A G A _ _ _ _ _ _  ⎫
                   ⎬ DNA
_ _ _ A _ _ _ _ T  ⎭

A _ _ _ C A _ _ _    mRNA
‿‿‿ ‿‿‿ ‿‿‿
_ _ _ _  _ _ _ _  Ala   polypeptide
```

Solution: Using the base pairing rules and the genetic code, we can fill in all of these blanks. We know that in DNA, A pairs with T and G pairs with C. We also know that U replaces T in mRNA. We know that the genetic code consists of three nucleotides of the mRNA that specify amino acids. We even know that these mRNA codons are recognized by complementary sequences on the anticodon of the tRNA. We have more than enough knowledge to answer this question. We can also use the information given in the problem to find the completed sequences in a few steps.

1. Starting with the DNA, we can write the complementary bases for each chain of the duplex.

```
A G A T _ _ _ _ A  ⎫
                   ⎬ DNA
T C T A _ _ _ _ T  ⎭

A _ _ _ C A _ _ _    mRNA
‿‿‿ ‿‿‿ ‿‿‿
_ _ _ _  _ _ _ _  Ala   polypeptide
```

379

2. We can now move to the mRNA strand. Notice that the first nucleotide of the mRNA is complementary to the lower DNA strand. This DNA is therefore the sense strand which gives its information to the mRNA. We can fill in some of the blanks in the DNA strands from the information given in the mRNA. We can also fill in some of the mRNA from information on the DNA strands. However, we must remember to use U instead of T in the mRNA.

A G A T C A _ _ A
T C T A G T _ _ T } DNA

A G A U C A _ _ A   mRNA

_____ _____ Ala   polypeptide

3. Now, we need our table of the genetic code. We can find the first two amino acids of the sequence by finding the appropriate three letter codons in the table. We can also find the first two letters of the codon for alanine.

A G A T C A _ _ A
T C T A G T _ _ T } DNA

A G A U C A G C A   mRNA

Arg   Ser   Ala   polypeptide

4. We can finally fill in the remaining blanks with the complementary bases.

A G A T C A G C A
T C T A G T C G T } DNA

A G A U C A G C A   mRNA

Arg   Ser   Ala   polypeptide

This is the completed sequence.

Give the following molecule of DNA:

strand 1----A T G C G C T A C G G C A A T----

strand 2----T A C G C G A T G C C G T T A----

Determine the mRNA molecule, the tRNA anticodons, and the amino acid sequence that will be produced if strand 1 is the transcription template for the mRNA molecule.

Solution: Since the mRNA molecule is transcribed from DNA strand 1, and the complementary pairing that will occur is A with U and U with A, its nucleotide sequence will be:

----U A C G C G A U G C C G U U A----

In the translation process each of the appropriate tRNA anticodons will complementarily pair with its appropriate mRNA codon, thus, the sequence of anitcodons of the tRNA's will be:

----|A U G|C G C|U A C|G G C|A A U|----

Each of the mRNA codons specifies a particular amino acid and we can therefore identify for each of its appropriate amino acid from the mRNA Genetic Code as follows:

UAC codes for the amino acid tyrosine (tyr)

GCG codes for the amino acid alanine (ala)

AUG codes for the amino acid methionine (met)

CCG codes for the amino acid proline (pro)

and

UUA codes for the amino acid leucine (leu)

Thus, the amino acid (polypeptide) sequence produced will be:

---tyr-ala-met-pro-leu----.

The nucleotide sequence of a segment of DNA is:

3' TACAAATCTCATTGTATAGGA 5'

(a) What is the base sequence in the complementary strand?

(b) If transcription occurs from the 3' end of the strand, what is the mRNA base sequence?

(c) What are the amino acids represented by the sequence?

Solution: This problem calls for the complementary DNA and mRNA strands and the amino acid sequence. Again we use the base pairing rules and the genetic code.

(a) The two strands of a DNA helix are antiparallel. So when one strand runs in the 3' to 5' direction, the other runs in the 5' to 3' direction. Following the base pairing rules, the complementary strand is:

    5' ATGTTTAGAGTAACATATCCT 3'

(b) The transcription of the mRNA occurs in the 3' to 5' direction. This will only be allowed on the strand with the proper polarity. That strand is the one given in the problem. It is called the sense strand and complementary mRNA sequence is:

    5' AUGUUUAGAGUAACAUAUCCU 3'

(c) Using the three nucleotide genetic code, we obtain the following amino acid sequence from this strand of mRNA:

        met-phe-arg-val-thr-tyr-pro.

SHORT ANSWER QUESTIONS FOR REVIEW

Choose the correct answer.

1. Purines have a _____ chemical structure. (a)
    one ringed (b) two ringed (c) three ringed
    (d) straight chain

    b

2. DNA and RNA are composed of (a) a nitro-
    genous base, a 3-carbon sugar, and a
    phosphate group. (b) a nitrogenous base, a
    4-carbon sugar, and a phosphate group. (c)
    a nitrogenous base, a 5-carbon sugar, and a
    phosphate group. (d) a nitrogenous base, a
    6-carbon sugar, and a phosphate group.

    c

3. The mRNA that would be transcribed from the
    sequence GGC in a sense strand of DNA would
    be (a) AAT (b) TTG (c) UUG (d) CCG

    d

4. A DNA molecule with 200 base pairs that
    consists of guanine will contain _____ thymine
    nucleotides. (a) 40 (b) 80 (c) 120 (d) 160

    a

5. A strand of duplex DNA has a $\frac{A + T}{C + G}$ ratio of
    0.6. The ratio in the complementary strand
    would be (a) 1.33 (b) 1.45 (c) 1.67
    (d) 1.83

    c

6. The mRNA that would be transcribed from the
    DNA strand ---- GCGTCGAAAATT---- is (a)
    ----ATAUTACCCCUU---- (b) --TATUATGGGGUU--
    (c)--CGCAGGTTTTAA-- (d)----CGCAGGUUUUAA----

    d

7. Of the eight enzymes used during DNA
    replication, which enzyme is responsible for
    joining the ends of DNA? (a) gyrase (b)
    DNA polymerase I (c) ligase (d) SSB protein

    c

8. Which of the following is not an actual protein
    producer? (a) DNA (b) tRNA (c) mRNA
    (d) rRNA

    a

9. A cistron is (a) the smallest unit which, if
    altered, gives rise to a mutant phenotype. (b)
    the genetic unit of biochemical function. (c)
    the sole factor in genotypic determination. (d)
    the smallest unit that is interchangeable by
    recombination.

    b

To be covered
when testing
yourself

10. The complete ribosome has ___ spots for tRNA
molecules. (a) 4 (b) 3 (c) 2 (d) 1

c

11. The four stages in the cell cycle are (a)
mitosis, G, S_1, S_2. (b) mitosis, S_1, G, T. (c)
mitosis, meiosis, S, G. (d) mitosis, S, G_1, G_2.

d

12. The minimum number of base substitutions
necessary to change a sequence of codons
that represents phenylalanine to one that
represents valine is (a) 1 (b) 2 (c) 3 (d) 4

a

13. Which one of the following codons cannot
signal the beginning or end of a polypeptide
chain? (a) GAU (b) UAA (c) UGA (d) AUG

a

In questions 14 through 21, match the amino acid
on the left with its main property on the right.

14. phenylalanine   (a) hydrophilic   c
                     (b) bulky
15. serine   (c) hydrophobic   a
                     (d) small
16. lysine   (e) can form disulfide   f
                          bonds
17. aspartate   (f) basic   h
                     (g) can form hydrogen
18. glycine   bonds   d
                     (h) acidic
19. arginine   b

20. threonine   g

21. cysteine   e

Fill in the blanks.

22. The structures of RNA and DNA are helped
to remain constant by the presence of _____
bonds.

phospho-
diester

23. The complimentary sequence of the DNA
strand 3'----GCGTCGAAAATT----5' is _____.

5'----CGCAGCTT
       TTAA----3'

24. To allow for a circular DNA molecule to become
supertwisted, _____ and ATP must be
present.

gyrase

SHORT ANSWER QUESTIONS FOR REVIEW

25. Sanger's work with insulin helped to prove
    that _____ control the amino acid sequence
    in proteins.

    genes

26. _____ is the formation of mRNA from DNA.

    Trans-
    cription

27. Two separate, specific _____ are responsible
    for the initiation and termination of protein
    synthesis.

    codons

28. Most of the DNA in a cell is found in the ____.

    nucleus

29. The _____ hypothesis helps to explain why
    many amino acids are coded by more than one
    codon.

    wobble

30. The amino acid sequence described by
    the mRNA sequence AAA AGU CUA GUU is
    _____.

    lysine-
    serine-
    leucine-
    valine

Determine whether the following statements are
true or false.

31. The passing of genetic information from one
    bacterium to another via DNA only is an
    example of transformation.

    True

32. Thymine and cytosine are two examples of
    pyrimidines.

    True

33. DNA is readily hydrolized by alkali.

    False

34. The sum of the bases thymine and adenine in
    a strand of DNA never equals the sum in the
    complementary strand.

    False

35. A transition mutation alone in a DNA strand
    can result in the formation of a new amino
    acid.

    True

36. During the replication of chromosomes, DNA
    polymerase III holoenzyme is the enzyme
    responsible for synthesizing DNA.

    True

37. The tRNA from the cells of cows is similar to
    that from human cells.

    True

SHORT ANSWER QUESTIONS FOR REVIEW

38. Given the total number of base pairs in a chromosome of an organism, and a basic knowledge of genetics, the number of genes present on the chromosomes can be determined.

    True

39. RNA polymerase helps to transfer the genetic information from DNA to RNA.

    True

40. Three or more factors are responsible for elongation of the peptide chain during protein synthesis.

    False

41. mRNA molecules are short lived and are broken down after only a few translations.

    True

42. A single base substitution on a chromosome can cause a sequence to stop rather than just alter the amino acids produced.

    True

43. The sense strand of DNA is never complementary to the anti-sense strand.

    False

CHAPTER 10

BACTERIAL AND VIRAL GENETICS

BACTERIAL GENETICS

GENE TRANSFER AND CONJUGATION

● **PROBLEM** 10-1

How are genes transferred in bacteria?

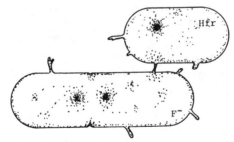

Fig. 1: Conjugation between two E. coli
cells.

Solution: Bacteria, unlike eukaryotic organisms, can only pass genes in a one-way transfer; there is no reciprocal exchange of genetic information. Thus, in bacteria the genetic information travels from a donor to a recipient cell. There are three main ways this can occur: conjugation, transformation and transduction.

Conjugation involves the transmission of the genetic

material through a specialized sex pilus, see Figures 1
and 2. Bacterial cells which can make a pilus are said to
have the F factor. The F factor contains at least 15 genes
which include those that control the F pili. F^+cells will
only establish contact with cells without the F factor (F^-).
The F pilus probably serves as a channel between the two
cells. Usually only a single copy of the F factor is
transferred.

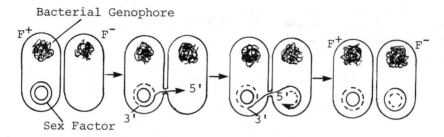

Fig. 2: Transfer of the sex factor from an F^+ donor
to an F^- recipient by conjugation. Dotted
lines indicate replication of the sex factor.

Transformation, Figure 3, is the process in which
genes enter the recipient in fragments. Certain strains of
bacteria, <u>Streptococcus pneumoniae</u> and <u>Bacillus subtilis</u>,
undergo transformation readily. Other strains, such as
<u>E.coli</u>, have to be made competent by special laboratory
conditions. Once the single-stranded pieces of DNA have
been pulled into a cell, they can incorporate themselves
into homologous regions of the host chromosome.

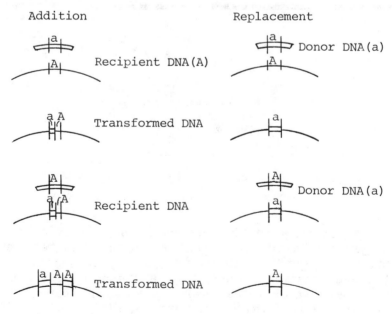

Fig. 3: Two explanations of transformation in
Pneumococcus.

Transduction, Figure 4, is the process in which a bacteriophage picks up some genes from one bacteria and carries the information to another bacteria. In the recipient bacteria, the DNA fragment may become incorporated as in transformation.

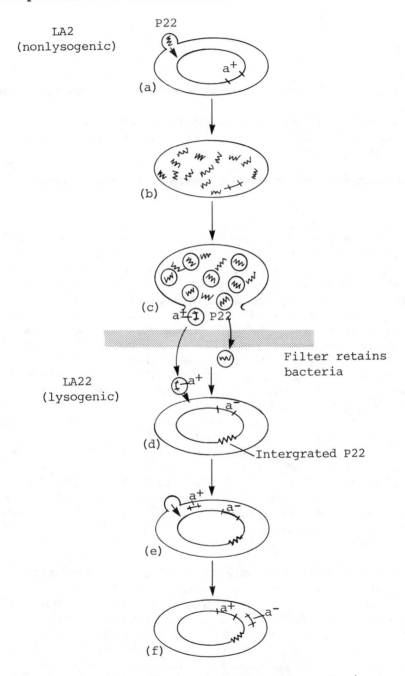

Fig. 4: Transduction in Salmonella. Strain is nonlysogenic and is lysed by phage P22. Strain LA22 is lysogenic and allows integration of P22 into its genome.

Thus, there are several ways that bacterial genes can move from one bacterium to another. These are methods of introducing variety in haploid organisms that cannot induce variety through the means employed by diploid organisms.

● **PROBLEM** 10-2

A male bacterium conjugates with a female bacterium. After conjugation, the female becomes a male. Account for this "sex change".

Solution: Conjugation occurs between bacterial cells of different mating types. Maleness in bacteria is determined by the presence of a small, extra piece of DNA, the sex factor, which can replicate itself and exist autonomously (independent of the larger chromosome) in the cytoplasm. Male bacteria having the sex factor, also known as the F factor, are termed F^+ if the sex factor exists extrachromosomally. F^+ bacteria can only conjugate with F^- the female counterparts, which do not possess the F factor. Genes on the F factor determine the formation of hairlike projections on the surface of the F^+ bacterium, called F or sex pili. The pili form cytoplasmic bridges through which genetic material is transferred and aids the male bacterium in adhering to the female during conjugation. During conjugation of an F^+ with an F^- bacterium, the DNA that is the most likely to be transferred to the female is the F factor. Prior to transfer, the F factor undergoes replication. The female thus becomes a male by receiving one copy of the F factor, and the male retains its sex by holding on to the other copy. The DNA of the male chromosome is very rarely transferred in this type of conjugation.

If this were the only type of genetic exchange in conjugation, all bacteria would become males and conjugation would cease. However, in F^+ bacterial cultures, a few bacteria can be isolated which have the F factor incorporated into their chromosomes. These male bacteria that conjugate with F^- cells are called Hfr (high frequency of recombination) bacteria. They do not transfer the F factor to the female cells during conjugation, but they frequently transfer portions of their chromosomes. This process is unidirectional, and no genetic material from the F^- cell is transferred to the Hfr cell.

390

There are genes on the <u>E. coli</u> chromosome which determine amino acid synthesis. For one particular strain of <u>E. coli</u>, how can one determine the order of genes for the synthesis of threonine (thr$^+$), methionine (met$^+$), histidine (his$^+$) and arginine (arg$^+$)"? Use your knowledge of conjugation.

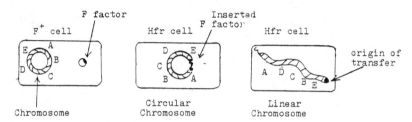

Figure 1. Insertion of F factor into chromosome.

<u>Solution</u>: To become an Hfr bacterial cell, the F factor must become integrated into the chromosome. When an Hfr cell and an F$^-$ cell begin conjugation the F factor portion of the circular Hfr chromosome initiates synthesis of a linear chromosome. This linear chromosome carries a fragment of F factor on both its ends, with one end acting as the origin for the transfer of the chromosome. Since the other end of the chromosome contains the remaining portion of the F factor, and since the whole chromosome rarely gets transferred, the F$^-$ cell usually does not receive a complete F factor to become F$^+$. In a particular Hfr strain, the F factor inserts at the same place on the chromosome, so that the origin of transfer is at the same site in all bacteria of this strain.

During conjugation, the origin is the first part to travel through the conjugation tube and enter the F$^-$ cell. Usually the conjugating cells separate before the complete transfer of the chromosome. The part that enters the F-cell acquires new traits that are determined by the newly transferred Hfr genes.

To determine the order of the genes on the chromosome of a particular Hfr strain one can use the interrupted mating technique. We must first acquire an F$^-$ strain that is auxotrophic (demonstrating a nutritional requirement) for the four amino acids but is resistant to streptomycin, an antibiotic which kills <u>E. coli</u>. The F$^-$ genotype in consideration would be as follows: thr$^-$, met$^-$, his$^-$, arg$^-$, str$^+$. The Hfr strain must be

391

prototrophic (can synthesize the amino acids in question) and be sensitive to streptomycin. It is also necessary that in the Hfr strain selected, the gene for streptomycin sensitivity be located far from the origin of transfer of the linear chromosome to avoid its transfer. The Hfr genotype would be thr$^+$, met$^+$, his$^+$, arg$^+$, str$^-$. The reason for selecting streptomycin sensitive and resistant strains will be made evident later.

The two cultures of F$^-$ and Hfr cells are then mixed and incubated. At specific time intervals (e.g. every ten minutes), samples are removed from the conjugating mixture and agitated in a blender. This separates the conjugating bacteria to prevent genetic transfer. Since the linear Hfr chromosome always enters the F$^-$ cell in a regular sequence, we can order the genes according to the length of time it took for the Hfr cells to transfer the genes to the F$^-$ cells. For example, in the first ten minutes, only the thr$^+$ gene might be transferred. In the first fifty minutes both the thr$^+$ and his$^+$ genes get transferred. The arg$^+$ gene after 60 minutes. The genes can then be located sequentially on the chromosome by noting their time of transfer. For this particular Hfr strain, the chromosome map is as follows:

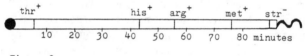

Figure 2.

In order to find out which gene is transferred after a certain period of time, the bacterial mixture is plated on four special media:

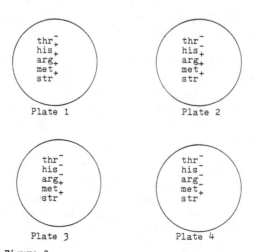

Figure 3.
- denotes the absence of that substance;
+ denotes the presence of the corresponding substances.

392

The sample produced after ten minutes will only grow on plate I since the only gene transferred is the thr$^+$ gene. It cannot grow on the others since it is still auxotrophic for the other three amino acids. The sample after the fifty minute time interval would grow on both plates I and II. We thus know that the his$^+$ gene follows the thr$^+$ gene. The reason why all the plates contain streptomycin is that any Hfr bacteria remaining in the sample placed on the special media plates will be killed. Although F$^-$ cells are streptomycin resistant, the only F$^-$ cells that will grow on the special plates are those that have conjugated with Hfr cells and have received and incorporated the genes for determining amino acid synthesis. The streptomycin thus acts as a control to allow only newly-made recombinants to live. Another relevant point is that in an actual experiment, more media plates with different combinations of amino acid supplements would be required. For example, Plate I, which selected for thr$^+$, should also check for his$^+$, or for arg$^+$, or for met$^+$, since we would not know which gene is really first.

● PROBLEM 10-4

What happens when Hfr cells are mixed with an excess of F$^-$ cells?

Solution: The F (or fertility) factor is an episome. An episome is a bacterial genetic factor that can exist either as an autonomous circular element in the cytoplasm or as an integrated part of the chromosome. When autonomous, it replicates independently of the bacterial chromosome. When integrated, the F factor is replicated along with the bacterial chromosome. Cells that have the F factor (F$^+$) can act as donors by giving a copy of the F factor to recipient cells who lack the factor (F$^-$). Hfr, which stands for high frequency of recombination, are F$^+$ cells which have the F factor integrated into their chromosome. When a suspension of Hfr cells is mixed with an excess of F$^-$ cells, all of the Hfr cells attach to an F$^-$ cell and begin conjugation. Since the F factor is part of the main chromosome, chromosomal DNA gets transferred to the F$^-$ cell (see Figure 1). The transfer is interrupted by the spontaneous breakage of the DNA molecule at random times. Usually the chromosome is broken before the F factor crosses to the F$^-$ cells. The result of an Hfr x F$^-$

cross usually is not an F⁺ cell. By using bacterial cells with phenotypic markers, linkage maps can be constructed by varying the time of conjugation termination.

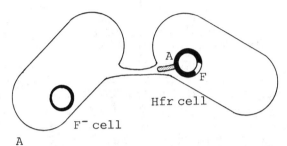

A
Linear chromosome is synthesized and moves from Hfr cell to F⁻ cell.

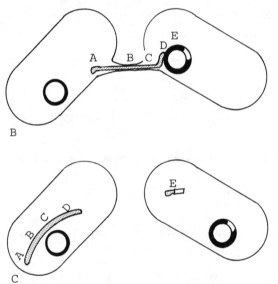

B

C
Conjugation stops before the entire chromosome has moved across; hence F factor usually remains in Hfr cell.

Fig. 1

● **PROBLEM 10-5**

How do bacteria develop drug resistance?

Solution: Most antibiotic resistant bacteria result from genetic changes and subsequent selection. The genetic changes may be due to chromosomal mutations or to the introduction of extra chromosomal elements.

Spontaneous mutations in a bacterial chromosome can cause antibiotic resistance in several forms. The mutation may make the cell impermeable to the drug by changing the shape of the receptor molecule. The mutation may create an enzyme that inactivates the drug once it enters the cell. The mutation may make the drug's intercellular targets resistant to the drug. Streptomycin, which inhibits the binding of formyl-methionyl tRNA to the ribosomes, may be blocked if the ribosome was changed so that the interaction was prevented.

Antibiotic resistance may also arise extrachromosomally. Conjugal plasmids, such as R plasmids, contain genes which mediate their genetic transmission. R plasmids carry genes conferring antibiotic resistance. Thus, R^+ cells can pass the genes for resistance to R^- cells by conjugation.

Once a bacterial cell strain has become resistant to an antibiotic, the presence of that antibiotic in the environment favors the cells that contain the resistance element. Cells without the resistance will be killed by the antibiotic; those that have the resistance will flourish.

● PROBLEM 10-6

How does the antibiotic streptomycin work?

Solution: Streptomycin is a highly basic trisaccharide that inhibits protein synthesis in prokaryotes. Streptomycin interferes with the binding of formylmethionyl tRNA to the ribosomes and thus prevents the proper initiation of protein synthesis. Streptomycin interacts with a single protein in the 50S ribosomal subunit of sensitive bacteria. It also leads to a misreading of the mRNA. The effect that this antibiotic has depends on whether the cell is resistant (mutant) or sensitive (wild-type). Figures 1 and 2 show some of the results in sensitive and resistant E. coli cells.

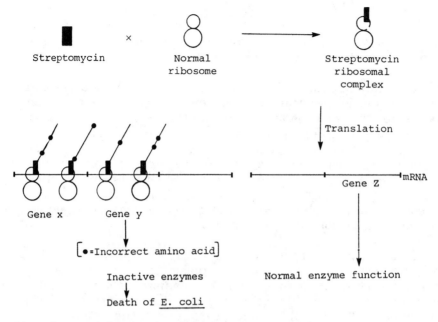

Fig. 1 Sensitive to streptomycin

Figure 1 shows the extensive misreading that occurs as a result of the binding of streptomycin to normal ribosomes. This causes insertion of incorrect amino acids into the polypeptide chain. These peptides are inactive and cause the cells to die.

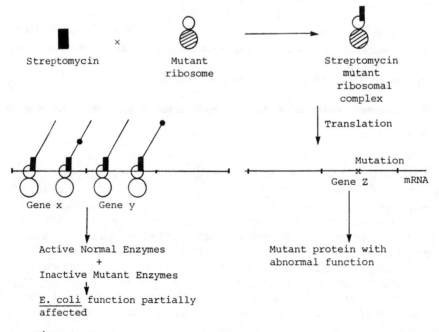

Fig. 2 Resistant to streptomycin

Figure 2 illustrates the action of streptomycin on resistant cells. These cells have a mutation in one subunit of their ribosome which partially wards off the ill effects of the antibiotic. Misreading still occurs, but not as extensively as in the first case. The E. coli cells still have abnormalities but can survive.

● **PROBLEM** 10-7

In Japan, the frequency of the R-governed multiple drug-resistant strain of Shigella, which causes dysentery, rose from 0.2% in 1953 to 58% in 1965. Also, 84% of the E. coli and 90% of Proteus collected from affected hospital patients showed similar resistance. How could such an increase happen?

Solution: All three strains contain an R plasmid in this example. R plasmids carry genes for conjugal transfer and genes for antibiotic resistance. The antibiotic genes are contained within larger units called transposons. Transposons are short segments of DNA which cannot self-replicate. They persist by inserting into a chromosome or plasmid and being replicated along with the host DNA. They can hop (transpose) from one plasmid to another or from one site on the plasmid to another site on the same plasmid. R plasmids can pick up additional transposons, so they can acquire resistance to more antibiotics.

R plasmids can be transmitted from cell to cell and even from cells of one species to those of another. Thus, if nonpathogenic bacterial strains, such as E. coli and Proteus, obtain an R plasmid they can spread to other bacteria, their own kind as well as infectious pathogenic strains such as Shigella. Normally the R factor is passed at a very low frequency. However, the indiscriminate use of antibiotics in medicine and agriculture has selected for drug-resistant enterobacteria (bacteria which live in the intestinal tract and aid the digestion). These bacteria can then pass their resistance to potentially harmful strains. The use of antibiotics should be moderated to prevent the spread of resistant pathogenic bacteria.

How is a bacterial zygote different from a eukaryotic zygote?

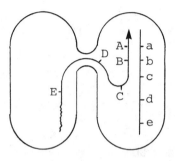 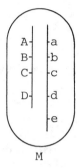

Fig. 1: A merozygote (M) formed by the transfer of genes A,B,C and D from one bacterium to another by conjugation.

Solution: A eukaryotic zygote is formed by the fusion of two haploid gametes. True cell fusion does not take place in bacteria and the genetic exchange is not reciprocal as in eukaryotes. Instead, one cell donates some if its genetic information to a recipient cell. The recipient is temporarily diploid for the genes that have been transferred. Such cells are partial zygotes or merozygotes. The genes then incorporate into the cell's chromosome. Any extraneous fragments of DNA are lost from the cell line in subsequent divisions. The clones are once again haploid.

Genetic variation occurs in bacteria as a result of mutations. This would seem to be the only process giving rise to variation, for bacteria reproduce through binary fission. Design an experiment to support the existence of another process that results in variation.

Solution: It was originally thought that all bacterial cells arose from other cells by binary fission, which is the simple division of a parent bacterium. The two daughter cells are genetically identical because the parental chromosome is simply replicated, with each cell getting a copy. Any genetic variation was thought to occur solely from mutations. However, it can be shown that genetic variation also results from a mating process in which genetic information is exchanged.

One can show this recombination of genetic traits by using two mutant strains of E. coli which lack the ability to synthesize two amino acids. One mutant strain is unable to synthesize amino acids A and B, while the other strain is unable to synthesize amino acids C and D. Both these mutant strains can be grown only on nutrient media, which contains all essential amino acids. When both strains are plated together on a selective medium lacking all four amino acids in question, some colonies of prototrophic cells appear which can synthesize all four amino acids (A, B, C, and D). These prototrophs are a result of recombination. When the two strains are plated on separate minimal medium plates, no recombination can occur, and no prototrophic colonies appear.

These results may be proposed to be actually a spontaneous reversion of the mutations back to the wild-type (normal prototroph) rather than recombination. If a single mutation reverts to wild-type at a frequency of 10^{-6} mutations per cell per generation, two mutations would simultaneously revert at a frequency of $10^{-6} \times 10^{-6}$ = 10^{-12} mutations per cell per generation. If one plates about 10^9 bacteria, no mutational revertants for both deficiencies should occur. Recombination occurs at a frequency of 10^{-7}, and thus if 10^9 bacteria are plated, prototrophic colonies should be found.

This recombination of traits from the two parent mutant strains is brought about through a process called conjugation. During conjugation, two bacterial cells lie close to one another and a cytoplasmic bridge forms between them. Parts of one bacterium's chromosome are transferred through this tube to the recipient bacterium. The transferred chromosomal piece may or may not get incorporated into the recipient bacterium's chromosome.

The following Hfr strains of <u>E. coli</u> donate the markers shown in the order given.

Hfr strain	Marker order
1	TLPAM
2	SGHMA
3	RIXSG
4	RTLPA

All of these Hfr strains were obtained from the same F$^+$ strain. What was the order of the markers on the E. coli F$^+$ chromosome?

Solution: This problem involves the mapping technique that utilizes bacterial conjugation to find the order of chromosomal markers. The markers occur in different combinations in the donors because the conjugation was disrupted at different times. Since the genetic information is transmitted linearly, the order is not changed. To find the order in the complete circular chromosome, we simply have to fit the fragments together by examining the overlapping areas.

TLPAM

    AMHGS

        GSXIR

           RTLPAM

Notice that the first and the last fragments overlap. This is because the chromosome is circular. The complete map of these markers is:

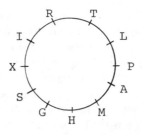

TRANSFORMATION

What is transformation?

Solution: Transformation is a means by which genetic information is passed in bacterial cells. The recipient cell takes up the DNA that has been released by the donor cell. This occurs naturally in some species; however, it is usually performed as part of an experimental procedure. The DNA is extracted from the donor cell and mixed with recipient cells. Hemophilus influenzae and Bacillus subtilis are naturally competent; they are capable of taking up high molecular weight DNA from the medium. Competent cells have a surface protein called competence factor, which binds DNA to the cell surface. Other cells, such as E.coli, cannot readily undergo transformation. They will only pick up extracellular DNA under special laboratory conditions. The cells must have mutations that stop exonuclease I and V activity. The cells must be treated with high $CaCl_2$ concentrations to make their membranes permeable to the DNA. The donor DNA must be present in very high concentrations.

The DNA that is picked up by the recipient cell must be double-stranded. As it enters the cell, an intracellular DNAase degrades one of the strands. This hydrolysis provides the energy needed to pull the rest of the DNA into the cell. Once inside the cell, the now single-stranded DNA can insert into homologous regions of the recipient's chromosome. When the donor DNA and recipient DNA have genetic mutations that act as markers, genetic linkage can be established through transformation experiments.

● PROBLEM 10-12

The results of a transformation experiment are given below. The organism used was Bacillus subtilis, which has natural competence.

Experiment	Donor DNA	Recipient DNA	Transformant classes trp	tyr	Number	%
1	trp$^+$tyr$^-$	trp$^-$tyr$^-$	A +	-	190	42.4
			B -	+	256	57.1
	trp$^-$tyr$^+$		C +	+	2	0.4
2	trp$^+$tyr$^+$	trp$^-$tyr$^-$	D +	-	196	22.0
			E -	+	328	36.8
			F +	+	367	41.2

(a) Are the trp and tyr genes linked?

(b) If they are linked, what is the map distance between them?

Solution: Bacillus subtilis is a naturally competent organism and is readily transformed by a donor's DNA. Transformation results in a changed phenotype when crossing over occurs between the donor DNA and the homologous region of the recipient DNA. The recipient cells in this experiment are grown on selective media: minimal + tryptophan to find trp$^-$tyr$^+$ transformants, minimal + tyrosine to find trp$^+$tyr$^-$ transformants and minimal to find trp$^+$tyr$^+$ cells.

(a) To find if these genes are linked, we must analyze the data. In experiment 1 two pieces of DNA were used to transform a double mutant cell. The transformants that gained the ability to synthesize one of the amino acids did so by the recombination of one of the donor DNA fragments. C, the double transformant class, trp$^+$tyr$^+$, was transformed as a result of two fragments of DNA. The frequency of this occurance was very low, 0.4%. In experiment 2 a wild-type DNA was used to transform the same mutant recipient. The single transformants were again due to the recombination of one fragment. The double transformant, F, showed a very high frequency, 41.2%. If the genes were not linked, this frequency would have been comparable to that of experiment 1. That the difference is so large suggests linkage.

(b) To calculate the map distance between the two linked genes we have to know the number of recombinations that occurred between them. We cannot use transformant classes A or B in our calculations because the recombination could have occurred between the two markers or outside them.

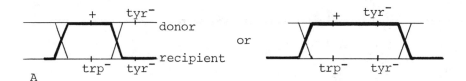

A

or

Transformant class C cannot be used for similar reasons. Classes D and E could only result as a recombination between trp and tyr.

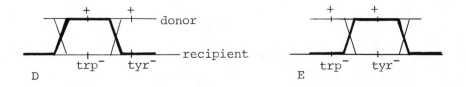

D

E

Transformant class F is a result of a recombination outside of the two markers.

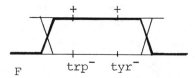

F

We can use the values obtained from classes D, E and F to find the map distance. The distance between the markers is the percentage of recombination between them:

$$\frac{D+E}{D+E+F} = \frac{196+328}{196+328+367} = \frac{524}{893} = 0.587 = 58.7\%$$

This is equivalent to 58.7 map units. The distance between the linked genes tyr and trp in Bacillus subtilis is 58.7 map units.

TRANSDUCTION

What is transduction?

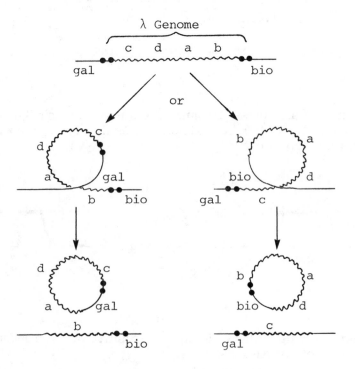

Fig. 1: Specialized transducing phages
produced by the improper excision
of λ from the bacterial genome.

Solution: Transduction is a phage-mediated transfer of genetic material between two bacteria. There are three types of transduction: generalized, specialized, and f-mediated.

Generalized transduction occurs when a piece of bacterial chromosome becomes incorporated in a phage head and is transferred to a recipient bacteria. It can become incorporated in the recipient by recombination at the homologous region of the chromosomal DNA. The bacterial DNA becomes incorporated at the end of the phage's lytic cycle. The phages that can accomplish this are not as selective towards the DNA fragments that they incorporate as those which cannot transduce. But the incorporation of bacterial DNA is not always so simple. For example, in phage P22 a gene can recognize particular signals in the Salmonella chromosome. The gene is responsible for cutting up the DNA into sizes appropriate for the head protein. The signals that the gene recognizes may be certain base sequences and, as a result, certain Salmonella markers are transduced more frequently than others.

Specialized transduction, Figure 1, results in restricted parts of the bacterial chromosome being incorporated into the phage particle. This happens when the original transducing particle is produced by a faulty outlooping of the prophage. The phage thus formed is defective since some of its genes remain in the bacteria replaced by some of the bacterial genes.

F-mediated sexduction is the third form of transduction. An F element that contains extra bacterial genes is called an F' element. By conjugation, the F' element can be transferred to a bacterial cell that is mutant in the extra genes on the F' element. Cells are then selected for those that have the F element integrated next to where a phage has integrated. When the prophage is induced, the phage that results will probably contain the genes from the F element. This virus is then used as the vector to transfer the bacterial genes to another bacterial cell.

These viral-mediated gene transfer mechanisms have been exploited by geneticists to map bacterial chromosomes. Very detailed maps that are continuously being revised are the result.

● **PROBLEM 10-14**

A gal^+/gal^- cell is produced by an abortive transduction. Will it grow in a medium in which galactose is the sole carbon source?

Solution: Abortive transductants are cells in which the transduced chromosome fragment does not incorporate into the recipient chromosome through recombination. This may occur when the donor phage comes from a mutant cell which is functionally different than the recipient. Since the fragment contains the genes that are selected for, its presence is essential for a cell's survival. The fragment is not replicated with the rest of the genome because it has not been incorporated. It is passed in unilinear form to one cell at each division. The one cell that has the fragment's genes is prototrophic in the selective media. The cells without it can only undergo a few divisions. A very small colony results from the limited growth of the sibling cells.

Thus, in the gal^+/gal^- abortive, only the cell with the fragment will produce the galactose-fermenting enzyme. The other cells will be able to use the excess enzyme. Limited growth will continue until the demand for enzyme is greater than the production ability of the one cell. The resulting colony is minute.

● PROBLEM 10-15

A bacterial strain is unable to synthesize the amino acids methionine and histidine and is also unable to ferment arabinose. It is transduced by a phage with the wild-type genome, met^+ his^+ ara^+. Recombinants are selected for by growth on plates supplemented with histidine. The colonies that grew on his^+ plates were placed on plates containing arabinose. A total of 320 colonies grew on histidine supplemented plates and 150 of these could also ferment arabinose. What is the amount of recombination between met and ara?

Fig. 1

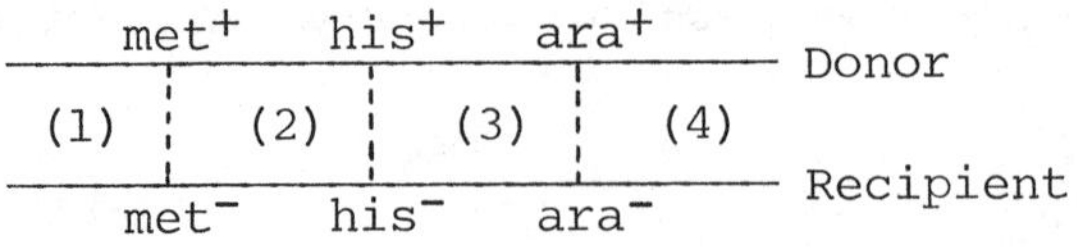

Solution: Transduction is the process whereby bacterial DNA is transferred from one cell to another via a phage vector. The phenotype of the recipient bacteria will be altered to that of the donor if recombination occurs between the incoming and the native DNA. Figure 1 shows how the homologous areas of DNA could line up and where crossing over could occur.

Crossing-over in the different regions produces different recombinants. Since the original plates were supplemented with histidine, both his$^+$ and his$^-$ cells will be able to grow; crossing-over in regions (2) and (3) are thus not accounted for in the selected colonies. Crossing-over in regions (1) and either (2) or (3) produce prototrophic mutants (met$^+$ara$^-$) that can grow on unsupplemented medium. The frequency with which recombination occurs between met and ara can be found by dividing the number of met$^+$ara$^-$ prototrophs by the total number of recombinants.

$$\text{recombination ratio} = \frac{\text{\# of met}^+\text{ara}^-}{\text{\# of met}^+\text{ara}^+}$$

$$= \frac{320-150}{320}$$

$$= 0.531 \text{ or } 53.1\%$$

● **PROBLEM** 10-16

Phage P1 incorporates the genes leu$^+$thr$^+$azi^r from E.coli. Transducing P1 phage are then used to infect E.coli cells with the markers leu$^-$thr$^-$azi^s. The cells are placed on media that will select for one or two of the genetic markers. For each experiment, the frequency of the unselected markers is as follows:

Experiment	Selected marker(s)	Unselected marker(s)
1	leu$^+$	50% azi^r 2% thr$^+$
2	thr$^+$	3% leu$^+$ 0% azi^r
3	leu$^+$, thr$^+$	0% azi^r

What is the sequence of the three genes?

Solution: The frequency with which unselected markers occur is a reflection of how closely linked they are to the selected traits. If the recipient cells are placed on a minimal medium free of azide but supplemented with threonine, then the selected marker is leucine since only leu$^+$ recombinants will grow. Thr and azi are the unselected markers because, in the presence of threonine, the genetic marker could be thr$^+$ or thr$^-$; in the absence of azide the genetic marker could be azi^r or azi^s. Thus, specific markers can be selected for. The unselected markers will appear only if they are sufficiently close to the selected marker.

From experiment 1 we see that azide resistance occurs in 50% of the cases that leu$^+$ is selected for. We conclude that azi and leu are close. Since threonine independence occurs in 2% of the cases when leu$^+$ is selected for, the leu and thr loci must be farther apart. There are two possible models that account for these results:

<table>
<tr><td>leu azi</td><td>thr</td></tr>
</table>

and

<table>
<tr><td>azi leu</td><td>thr</td></tr>
</table>

From experiment 2, by similar reasoning, we can conclude that leu is closer to thr than azi is. This is because 3% of the time leu$^+$ and thr$^+$ are transduced together but thr$^+$ and azi$^+$ are never cotransduced. This supports the sequence:

<table>
<tr><td>azi leu</td><td>thr</td></tr>
</table>

Experiment 3 is consistent with this sequence since the thr$^+$leu$^+$ fragment never carries azide resistance.

These experiments also imply something about the size of the transducing fragment. The length of DNA between the thr and leu markers must be close to the limit because they are only cotransduced 2-3% of the time. The additional outside marker, azi, is never cotransduced with the other outside marker, thr. Thus, the maximum size of the transducing fragment is from the thr locus to somewhere between the azi and leu loci.

● PROBLEM 10-17

Three E.coli strains are given to you as a birthday present. They are:

1. $\dfrac{F'leu^+pro-1}{leu^+pro-1}$ (partially diploid for the two genes)

2. F⁻ leu pro-2Z (lysogenic for the generalized transducing phage Z)

2. F^- leu pro-2Z (lysogenic for the generalized transducing phage Z)

3. F^- leu⁺pro-1 (an F^- derivative of strain 1, having lost F)

The strains either synthesize leucine (leu⁺) or do not and require it as a nutritional supplement (leu). All of the strains require proline.

(a) How could you determine whether pro-1 and pro-2 were alleles of the same gene?

(b) Suppose pro-1 and pro-2 are allelic, and the leu locus is cotransduced with the pro locus. If you used phage Z to transduce genes from strain 3 to strain 2, how would you determine the order of the leu, pro-1 and pro-2 markers?

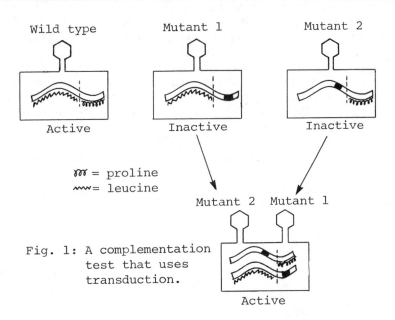

Wild type   Mutant 1   Mutant 2

Active   Inactive   Inactive

𝔀 = proline
〜 = leucine

Mutant 2   Mutant 1

Fig. 1: A complementation test that uses transduction.

Active

Solution: This problem asks you to draw on your knowledge of bacterial genetics to devise the outlines of experiments that would prove certain facts. First, we must look at what we are asked to find; then we can find ways of answering the questions.

(a) Here we are asked to find if two markers are alleles of the same gene. To do this, we have to perform a genetic cross between strains that have one or the other of the markers. Since strains 2 and 3 are both F⁻, no exchange of genetic material could occur. However, an exchange through conjugation could occur between strains

1 and 2. Strain 1 contains the F-element. The prime (F')
denotes the fact that some chromosomal genes have been
picked up by the F-element. Because the markers that we
are concerned with are responsible for the auxotrophic or
prototrophic state of the cells, we can use a
complementation test. A complementation test helps to
characterize different mutants. We mix strains 1 and 2
and allow them to conjugate. We then plate the cells onto
minimal medium. Any cells with the genotype of strain 1
will die because they require proline as a nutrient. Strain
2 cells will also die because they require proline but also
because they need leucine. The new strain of cells
produced by the conjugation may survive on the minimal

medium. Their genotype would be partially diploid

$$\frac{F' \, leu^+ pro\text{-}1}{leu^- pro\text{-}2} \, .$$

If pro-1 and pro-2 are not alleles, the partial diploid will
be able to survive on the minimal plates because it has
two sets of genes that complement each other. The
$F^+ leu^+ pro\text{-}1$ genome provides leucine and proline
independence because it has a wild-type pro-2 gene. The
leu⁻pro-2 genetic sequence has a mutation in pro-2 but
presumably a wild-type and pro-2 are separate genes. If
they were alleles of the same gene, the partial diploids
would not be viable and no colonies would grow on
minimal media. If they were allelic, the partial diploids
would contain two mutant alleles of the same gene and no
complementation would occur. Figure 1 shows an
alternative method of performing a complementation test.
The results are similar.

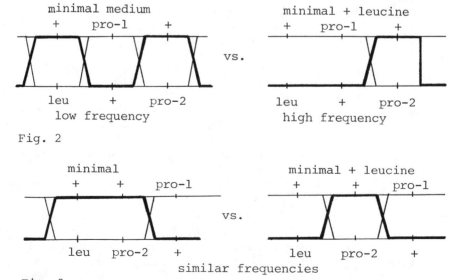

vs.

minimal medium
+   pro-1   +

leu   +   pro-2
low frequency

minimal + leucine
+   pro-1   +

leu   +   pro-2
high frequency

Fig. 2

minimal
+   +   pro-1

leu   pro-2   +

vs.

minimal + leucine
+   +   pro-1

leu   pro-2   +

similar frequencies

Fig. 3

(b) We follow the instructions given in the problem and then plate the phage infected strain 2 onto selective media. If we infect strain 3 with phage Z, we obtain phage with strain 3's mutant genome, F^-leu^+pro-1. The phage that is produced when the bacteria lyse can be taken and mixed with strain 2. Strain 2, however, is lysogenic for the phage, so it will incorporate the DNA of the phage. Strain 2 will then have strain 3's genetic information homologously incorporated into its genome. It will have the ability to synthesize leucine if it can cross over with the homologous section of DNA to incorporate the wild-type <u>leu</u> locus into its genome. By examinimg the frequency of leucine requiring recombinants on minimum + leucine media, we can determine the order of the loci. Strain 2's genome woukd be partially diploid for the three

mutant genes: $\dfrac{leu^+pro\text{-}1pro\text{-}2^+}{leu\ pro\text{-}1^+pro\text{-}2}$. The order, either leu-

pro-1-pro-2 or leu-pro-2-pro-1, could be found by the frequencies obtained in an actual experiment, of the types of recombinants that grow, see Figures 2 and 3.

VIRAL GENETICS

● **PROBLEM** 10-18

What are the two types of bacteriophage infection?

<u>Solution</u>: Bacteriophage are viral particles that infect bacteria. The bacteriophage, or phage, like all viruses, cannot self-replicate. They are made of nucleic acid surrounded by a coat of protein. Their nucleic acid contains genes for the construction of new viruses but they have little or none of the necessary machinery, such as ribosomes and enzymes. They must use the apparatus of their host if they are to replicate.

Once a phage infects a cell it can follow one of two paths; lysis or lysogeny. Some phages are restricted to the lytic cycle. The lytic cycle causes the release of many viral particles and the death of the host cell. The phages

T2, T4, T3 and T7 can only conduct infection through the lytic cycle. The lysogenic cycle does not lead to the immediate death of the host cell. Temperate phages can undergo either lysis or lysogeny depending on the conditions.

The lytic cycle begins when the phage makes contact with the host cell and injects its nucleic acid into the cell. In the case of T2 infection of E.coli, three sets of genes are expressed. They are the early gene that inhibits E.coli RNA synthesis; the DNA metabolism gene products which are enzymes that replicate the phage chromosome; nuclei that degrade the bacterial chromosome so the nucleotides are free for use by the phages; and the late gene products which include the phage proteins necessary to package the newly synthesized chromosomes into mature phage particles. One of the last gene products is lysozyme which digests the bacterial cell wall releasing as many as 250 phage particles. These viruses are free to find their own hosts to begin the cycle all over again.

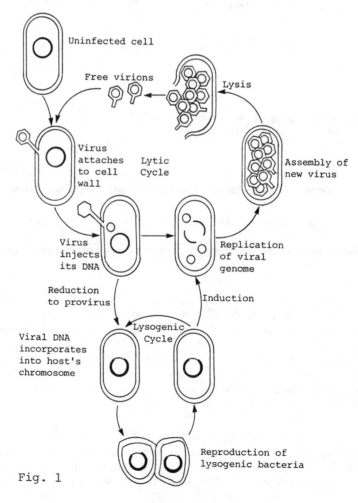

Fig. 1

The lysogenic infection cycle, Figure 1, occurs in temperate phages such as λ and φ 80. These phages can eventually lyse their host by following the lytic cycle. Under certain conditions the infection of a bacterial cell by a temperate phage does not cause lysis. The viral chromosome dictates the synthesis of a repressor molecule that inhibits the expression of the lytic genes. The chromosome inserts into a special region of the host chromosome where it is replicated along with the bacterial chromosome for many generations. The phage in this state is called a prophage. The viral genome, once incorporated, may produce phenotypic changes in the bacterial cell. For instance, the diphtheria bacteria, Corynebacterium diphtheriae, can produce the toxin that causes the disease only when it carries a certain prophage. The viral genes also give the bacteria immunity to further infection by the same type of virus. A drop in the level of the repressor molecules releases the viral producing genes from repression, thus initiating the lytic cycle. This can be induced experimentally by irradiation with ultraviolet light or by the exposure to certain chemicals such as nitrogen mustard or organic peroxides.

Bacteriophage, although relatively simple physically, have very effective means for reproducing even without their own equipment. Nature has once again designed very elegant solutions to problematic situations.

● **PROBLEM** 10-19

If DNAse is added to a bacterial cell then the DNA is hydrolyzed. The cell cannot make any more proteins and it eventually dies. If DNAse is added to certain viruses, they continue to produce new proteins. Explain.

Solution: By means of electron microscopy and x-ray diffraction studies, we have discovered much about the structure and composition of viruses. The infective ability of viruses is due to their nucleic acid composition. An individual virus contains either DNA or RNA but not both as is true for cells. Therefore, the virus proposed in the question contains RNA since it is not affected by DNAse. The RNA replicates, forming a complementary RNA strand which acts as messenger RNA in order to code for the synthesis of new viral proteins. To produce new viral

RNA, the viral RNA first synthesizes a complementary strand and thus becomes double-stranded. The double-stranded RNA serves as a template for synthesis of new viral RNA. The virus could have been tobacco mosaic virus, influenza virus or poliomyelitis virus. These are all viruses which contain single-stranded RNA as their genetic material. There are at least two groups of RNA viruses in which the RNA is normally double-stranded, and assumes a double-helical form. DNA viruses, such as the smallpox virus, SV 40 (a tumor-inducing virus), and certain bacterial viruses, such as bacteriophages T_2, T_4, and T_6, contain double-stranded DNA. Yet there are some bacteriophages which have a single-stranded DNA molecule. It does not matter whether the genetic information is contained in DNA or RNA, or if it exists as a single strand or as a double helix. For viruses, the important point is that the genetic message is present as a sequence of nucleotide bases.

● **PROBLEM** 10-20

Using a virus, how can one transform E.coli bacteria unable to utilize galactose (gal-mutants) into those that can utilize galactose (gal$^+$).

Solution: E. coli are usually able to utilize galactose, a monosaccharide, as a carbon and energy source. However, mutations arise which affect an enzyme necessary for galactose utilization. These E. coli mutants are unable to utilize this sugar and are called gal⁻mutants. To transform some of these gal⁻mutants into the wild-type, gal$^+$, one can use a lysogenic virus·such as the λ (lambda) bacteriophage.

One can infect a culture of prototrophic E. coli (gal$^+$) with the lysogenic phages. The viruses will inject their DNA into the bacterial cells. In the host the viral DNA molecule changes from a linear structure to a circular one. At a specific attachment site on the bacterial chromosome the viral DNA pairs with the bacterial chromosome and integrates into it after recombination. The viral DNA, now called a prophage, remains incorporated within the E. coli chromosome until conditions are favorable for the excision of the prophage and its induction to a vegetative virus which replicates and lyses the cell.

The gene necessary for galactose utilization is very near the incorporated prophage. In the case of the λ phage its proximity to the bacterial gal+ gene allows rare errors to occur in which excision of the prophage includes the gal+ gene. The λ prophage may coil in such a way that the recombination event leading to excision of the circular viral DNA includes the gal gene. To remain approximately the same size, the circular viral DNA leaves behind some if its own genes, which were replaced by the substituted bacterial region. Since it now lacks some necessary genes, the virus, now called a transducing particle or λ gal, is considered to be defective. These transducing particles can lyse the bacterial cell, but they cannot establish a lysogenic relationship with, or cause lysis of, subsequent bacterial cells. The excision of the prophage which has the incorporated gal+ gene can be illustrated as shown in fig. 1.

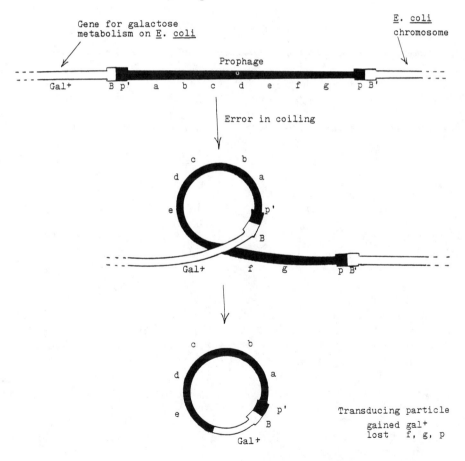

One can then harvest these transducing particles and add them to a culture of gal⁻ E. coli mutants. These phages attach to the mutant bacteria and inject their DNA

(containing the gal⁺ gene). The gal⁺region of the viral
DNA may then recombine with the gal⁻ region of the
bacterial chromosome. The gal⁺ gene may be incorporated
into the <u>E. coli</u> through the recombination process,
transforming them to the wild- type, which are able to
utilize galactose. The whole viral DNA rarely becomes
incorporated, since the transducing phage lacks a
complete genome. The viral chromosome, containing the
gal⁻ gene, cannot be inserted into the bacterial
chromosome and so is lost.

This process by which a virus transfers genes from
one bacterial cell to another is called transduction. In
specialized transduction, as opposed to generalized
transduction, only one gene is transferred. Transduction
thus serves as a mechanism for recombination in bacteria.

● PROBLEM 10-21

What is viral complementation? How does complementation
differ from recombination?

Solution: The principle of complementation is used to
determine whether bacteriophage have mutations in
separate genes or whether the mutations are allelic.
Suppose we have two strains of phage particles, one with
the genotype Ab (mutant for the B protein) and the other
with the genotype aB (mutant for the A protein). When
these phage infect the same bacterial cell, their nucleic
acid is injected into the cell. The protein synthesizing
apparatus of the bacteria cell proceeds to synthesize the
proteins encoded in both sets of nucleic acid. The nucleic
acid from each of the cells has the instructions for
making mutant and wild-type proteins. Strain Ab's nucleic
acid is capable of producing wild-type A protein along
with mutant b. Strain aB's genome codes for wild-type B
protein along with mutant A protein. Viral particles will
be assembled because wild-type proteins are available.
However, the genomes of the new phage particles will still
be mutant. Some viruses will be Ab while the rest will be
aB. Because complementation could occur, the mutations
reside on different genes. If they were alleles of the same
gene, no complementation could occur since both sets of
nucleic acid contained some form of mutation in the same
gene. No phage would be produced since no wild-type
form of the necessary structural protein was produced.

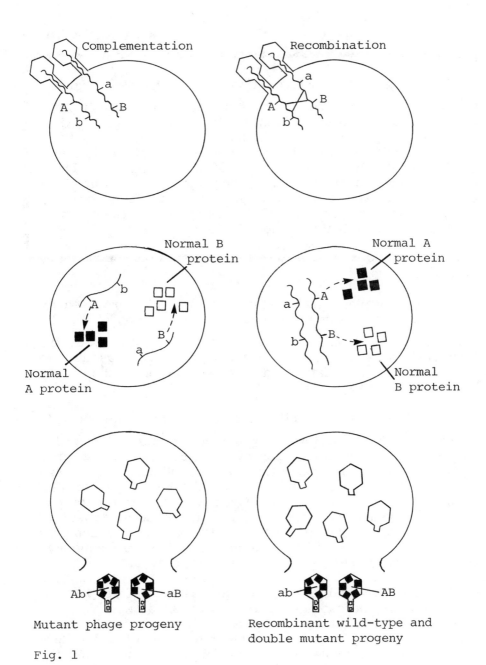

Complementation

Recombination

Normal B
protein

Normal A
protein

Normal
A protein

Normal
B protein

Ab — aB

ab — AB

Mutant phage progeny

Recombinant wild-type and
double mutant progeny

Fig. 1

Figure 1 shows the difference between complementation and recombination. In complementation, phage particles with mutant genomes are produced. In recombination, the genotype changes because of crossing over. Complementation can also occur during recombination to produce phenotypically normal phage. But, as a result of the recombination, some phage have wild-type genomes while others are now genotypically doubly mutant.

T_4 phage that carry mutations in the genomic region called rII can cause the lysis of strain B of E.coli but not of E.coli strain K. A plate of E.coli strain B is infected by two types of mutant phage simultaneously. The resulting lysate is divided in half. Half is diluted $1:10^7$ and plated onto a lawn of E.coli strain B. The other half is diluted $1:10^5$ and plated on strain K. Four plaques are found on K and 40 are found on B. Determine the amount of recombination between the two mutations in this region of the T_4 genome.

Solution: Complementation tests such as this were used by Seymour Benzer when he mapped the rII region of T_4. He did numerous tests between mutants and found the recombination frequencies between them. He was able to determine the relative distances between the many mutations on this basis.

Mutations in the rII region of T_4 are unable to lyse E.coli K. Therefore, any plaques found on K are due to some type of recombination event between the two phages. This recombination event allows one phage genome to become wild-type and hence to acquire the ability to cause the lysis of E.coli K. Since two mutations are involved, we can assume that both types of recombination are produced with equal frequencies. Therefore, in the calculation of recombination frequency, we must multiply the number of wild-type by 2.

One more adjustment is necessary before we can calculate the percentage of recombination between the two mutants. The dilutions made to the lysate were different. This difference must be taken into account since less phage are available for bacterial infection when the diluation is high. A dilution of $1:10^7$ is one hundred times more dilute than a dilution of $1:10^5$. If the dilutions had been the same, one hundred times more plaques would have formed since one hundred times more phage particles would have been present to lyse the bacteria. Thus, we must multiply the number of plaques of the $1:10^7$ dilution by 100 to bring the dilutions into accord. To find the percent of recombination, we use the following:

$$\% \text{ recombination} = \frac{\text{number of recombinants}}{2 \times (\text{wild-type+recombinants})} \times 100\%$$

Only recombinants can grow on strain K, this value goes in the numerator. On strain B, wild-type mutants and recombinants can grow, this value belongs in the denominator. We must also remember to multiply the number of plaques on strain B by 100 to equalize the dilutions. Plugging the appropriate numbers into their proper places, we can find the percent recombination:

$$\% \text{ recombination} = \frac{4}{2 \text{x} (40 \text{x} 100)} \text{ x } 100\% = 0.2\%.$$

Thus, the recombination frequency observed between the two mutations on the rII region is about 0.2%. This means that 0.2% of the time these markers can undergo recombination. They must be reasonably close since the frequency is so low. However, Benzer was able to resolve frequencies as low as 0.02% which corresponded to a distance of 2 to 3 nucleotides. So the two mutations of our problem are about 20 to 30 nucleotides apart.

● **PROBLEM 10-23**

Five point mutations (a through e) were tested for recombination with seven deletion mutants. What is the order of the mutations on this deletion map? The symbol + = recombination and 0 = no recombination.

		deletions						
		1	2	3	4	5	6	7
	a	0	+	0	0	+	+	0
	b	+	+	+	0	+	0	0
point muta- tions	c	+	+	+	+	0	0	0
	d	0	+	+	0	+	0	0
	e	+	0	0	0	+	+	0

Solution: Two homologous sets of genes exist in this problem. One set, presumably from a strain of phage, has a series of point mutations. The other set has a series of deletions. If these strains are combined systematically, data regarding the amount of recombination that occurs, as evidenced by phenotypic changes, can be used to generate a map of the point mutations.

A deletion chromosome lacks some nucleotides for a stretch of bases. The deleted piece is not there to recombine with the homologous piece of DNA. So mutations, such as the point mutations in our problem, will be able to recombine and be expresed only if they are outside of the homologue's deletion. If they lie within the deletion, they will have no partner with which to recombine, so no recombination will occur.

To find the order of the five point mutations we have to see which can be expressed with the various deletions. First, notice that deletion 7 does not allow any recombination. It must cover all of the point mutations. It does not help us in our quest to map the mutations. Next, deletion 4 only allows recombination at c. Since the deletion is in one piece, c must be at the end of our sequence:

c ∿∿∿∿∿∿

Similarly mutation e is the only mutation that cannot recombine with deletion 2. The mutation e must also be at an end.

c ∿∿∿∿∿ e

Deletion 3 covers a and e. We know where e is so we can place a next to it.

c ∿∿∿∿ae

Deletion 1 covers a and a. We know where a is and since the deletion is continuous, d is next to a.

c ∿∿∿dae

That leaves only one place left for b, but we can use another deletion to make sure. Deletion 6 does not allow recombination at b, c, or d. Looking at our sequence, we see that b must be between c and d. The complete sequence is

cbdae.

Once we have the sequence we check it to make sure that all of the data fits. If it does, we have successfully mapped a series of mutations.

The following are the results from two-point crosses and three-point crosses in the bacteriophage lambda (λ).

(a) Construct the genetic map for all five genes: co_1; mi; s; c; co_2.

(b) What are the map distances?

	Parents		Progeny				% Recombinants
1.	co_1+ x +mi	6341 co_1+	7580 +mi	372 ++	412 co_1mi		5.3
2.	co_1mi x ++	111 co_1+	86 +mi	1800 ++	1576 co_1mi		5.5
3.	s+ x +co_1	7101 s+	5851 +co_1	145 ++	169 sco_1		2.4
4.	sco_1 x ++	46 s+	53 +co_1	1615 ++	1774 sco_1		2.8
5.	s+ x +mi	647 s+	502 +mi	65 ++	56 smi		9.5
6.	smi x ++	1024 s+	1155 +mi	13083 ++	13253 smi		7.6
7.	s+ x +c	808 s+	566 +c	19 ++	20 sc		2.8
8.	c+ x +mi	1213 c+	1205 +mi	84 ++	75 cmi		6.2
9.	c+ x +co_1	6000 c+	6000 +co_1	14 ++	-cco_1[a]		0.1
10.	co_2+ x +mi	1477 co_2+	1949 +mi	109 ++	131 co_2mi		6.6

Table 1: Two-factor crosses involving lambda.

Parents	+++	scomi	s++	+comi	sco+	++mi	s+mi	+co+	Total
1. sco$_1$mi x +++	975	924	30	32	61	51	5	13	2091
2. s+mi x +co$_1$+	38	23	273	318	112	121	6389	5050	12324
3. c++ x +co$_1$mi	8	(-)[a]	(-)	(-)	(-)	1	(-)	(-)	6600
4. co$_2$++ x +cmi	28	(-)	(-)	(-)	(-)	13	(-)	(-)	5800
	A	B	C	D	E	F	G	H	

Mutation?

Table 2: Three-point cross with lambda.

Solution: A two-point or three-point cross in bacteriophage is carried out by simultaneously infecting bacteria with phage that differ at two or three genetic loci respectively.

We can draw several conclusions from the ten two-point crosses shown in Table 1. In the cross (co_1+) x (+mi), the percentage of recombination is 5.3 and in the cross (co_1mi) x (++) the percentage is 5.5. The average distance between these two markers is therefore 5.4. Similarly, the third and fourth crosses show that the co_1-s distance is about 2.6 map units. From the fifth and sixth crosses the distance between s and mi is about 8.5. We can reason that the endpoints are s and mi and that co_1 is in the middle:

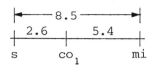

Relative to s and mi, c is very close to co_1. The c-co_1 distance is only 0.1 map unit, placing them very close together. The s-c distance is 2.8 and the mi-c distance is 6.2. But we do not know whether the sequence is

$$s\text{-}co_1\text{-}c\text{-}mi \quad \text{or} \quad s\text{-}c\text{-}co_1\text{-}mi.$$

We also don't know where co_2 fits in. We know that the co_2-mi distance is 6.6 but we don't know whether it is on the left or the right of mi. We need to use the three-point cross to map any further.

Table 2 shows that classes G and H are double-crossovers in cross 1, since they have the lowest frequencies. This suggests that the middle gene is co_1 in the sequence s-co_1-mi, which we already know. Classes A and B of cross 2 are the double-crossovers confirming the s-co_1-mi sequence. In cross 3, we assume that class A is the only double-crossover since class F is probably the result of a spontaneous mutation. This gives us the fact that co_1 is in the middle of c and mi. Class F of cross 4 is the double-crossover giving co_2-c-mi. We can combine our data to complete the map.

s-co_1-mi

c-co_1-mi

co_2-c-mi

Integrating this:

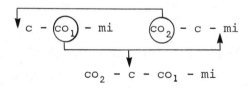

From the two-point cross analysis we know that s is on the left of co_2. The final sequence is:

The central dogma of biochemical genetics is the basic relationship between DNA, RNA, and protein. DNA serves as a template for both its own replication and for the synthesis of RNA, and RNA serves as a template for protein synthesis. How do viruses provide an exception to this flow scheme for genetic information?

Solution: The central dogma of biochemical genetics can be summarized in the following diagram

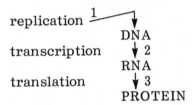

Arrow 1 signifies that DNA is the template for its self-replication. Arrow 2 signifies that all cellular RNA molecules are made on DNA templates. All amino acid sequences in proteins are determined by RNA templates (arrow 3). However, in the viral infection of a cell, RNA sometimes acts as a template for DNA, providing an exception to the unidirectionality of the scheme involving replication, transcription and translation. The agents involved are certain RNA viruses. For example, an RNA tumor virus undergoes a life cycle in which it becomes a prophage integrated into the DNA of a host chromosome. But how can a single-stranded RNA molecule become incorporated into the double-helical structure of the host DNA? It actually does not.

An RNA tumor virus first absorbs to the surface of susceptible host cell, then penetrates the cell by a pinocytotic (engulfment) process, so that the whole virus particle is within the host cell. There, the particle loses its protein coat (probably by the action of cellular proteolytic enyzmes). In the cytoplasm, the RNA molecule becomes transcribed into a complementary DNA strand. The enzyme mediating this reaction is called reverse transcriptase and is only found in viruses. (Thus, cells do not have the capacity to transcribe DNA from an RNA template; a virus is not a true cell.) Cellular DNA polymerase then converts the virally produced single stranded DNA into a double-stranded molecule. This viral DNA forms a circle and then integrates into the host chromosome, where it is transcribed into RNA needed for new viral RNA and also for viral-specific protein synthesis. The RNA molecules and protein coats assemble, and these newly made RNA tumor viruses are enveloped by sections of the cell's outer membrane and detach from the cell surface to infect other cells. The release of the new virions does not require the lysis of the host cell and is accomplished by an evagination of the outer membrane. Other cells are infected through the fusion of the envelope and the potential host cell's outer membrane, thereby releasing the virus particle into the cytoplasm. Unlike the λ phage infection of an E.coli cell, the RNA tumor virus does not necessarily interfere with normal cellular processes and cause death.

The mechanism of the action of reverse transcriptase is somewhat like other DNA polymerases. It synthesizes DNA in the 5' to 3' direction and needs a primer. The primer is a noncovalently bound tRNA molecule that was picked up by the RNA viral genome from the host during the previous round of replication. Since retroviruses have single-stranded linear RNA genomes, they encouter a problem during replication: the newly formed RNA molecules are incomplete because, when the primer was degraded, there was no complement to act as a template strand. The solution to this problem is that there are initially two molecules of RNA, hydrogen bonded to each other near their 5' ends. Each of these molecules has an identical sequence of the 5' and 3' ends:

5' ABCDE ----WXYZABC 3'

When new RNA strands are replicated they form concatamers because the single-stranded tails are complementary to each other.

```
        3' 5'
       a|  |A
       b|  |B
       c|  |C
       x|  |X
       y|  |Y
           |Z
       a|  |A
       b|  |B
       c|
       d|  |D
       e|  |E
       f|  |F
       a|  |A
       b|  |B
        3' 5'
```

The gaps can be filled since the 3' end of one duplex forms as a primer to fill in the missing nucleotides at the

5' end of the adjoining molecule.

Thus, the enzyme reverse transcriptase of RNA viruses provides the basis for the single known exception to the standard relationship between DNA, RNA and proteins by catalyzing the transcription of DNA from RNA.

● **PROBLEM** 10-26

Explain how Herpes viruses infect eukaryotic cells.

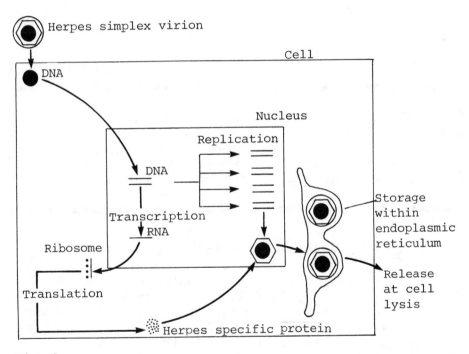

Fig. 1

Solution: Herpes virus has double-stranded DNA in a core enclosed by an icosahedral (twenty-sided) protein coat. It is a complex virus type and many of the functions of the genes are not known. However, some Herpes viruses have been associated with cancer in lab animals.

The Herpes virus group is broadly divided into three groups: alpha, beta and gamma. Herpes simplex type 2, an alpha herpes virus, is associated with cervical carcinoma. Epidemiologic studies have demonstrated that in most geographic areas, patients with cervical cancer have a high frequency of type 2 antibodies. Whether the virus initiates the cancer process is not known. Epstein-Barr virus, a gamma herpes virus, is associated with Burkitt's lymphoma.

Herpes viruses induce the lytic cycle in permissive cells. As shown in the diagram, the viral DNA moves into the nucleus, is transcribed to RNA and eventually replicated into many copies. A Herpes-specific repressor keeps the complete viral particles in a nonfunctional state. A cell containing such a virus will show no effect. A cancerous state may be produced when incomplete genomes are integrated into the host's genome. When the Herpes genome is integrated, it is not under the influence of the repressor and can transform the host cell into a cancerous one.

● **PROBLEM 10-27**

If antibodies can be brought into contact with a virus before it attaches itself to the host cell, the virus will be inactivated. Once infection has occurred, the production of interferon may protect the host from extensive tissue destruction. Explain.

Solution: Many human diseases have a viral etiology (cause). Among the more common viral diseases are smallpox, chicken pox, mumps, measles, yellow fever, influenza, rabies, poliomyelitis, viral pneumonia, fever blisters (cold sores), and the common cold. Although most viral infections do not respond to treatment with many of the drugs effective against bacterial infection, many are preventable by means of vaccines.

Buildup of an adequate supply of antibodies requires some time. During this period, extensive viral infection may occur. Most recoveries from viral diseases occur before full development of the immune response (production of antibodies). A factor that is important in the recovery from a viral infection is interferon. Interferon is a protein produced by virus-infected cells, which spreads to uninfected cells and makes them more resistant to viral infection. Thus, extensive viral production and resultant tissue damage are prevented.

Upon infection, the host cell is induced to synthesize interferon, which is then released into the extracellular fluid and affects the surrounding cells. It is thought that the interferon does not directly confer viral resistance to the uninfected cell, but induces formation of "interferon" ribosomes. These ribosomes bind cellular mRNA normally, but do not bind viral mRNA effectively. This prevents synthesis of viral proteins which are essential for viral production. The interferon acts as a mediator or messenger from infected cells to uninfected cells, enabling the uninfected cells to synthesize products which prevent viral multiplication. Since interferon ultimately acts in the cytoplasm of the uninfected cell, viruses can enter the cell but cannot replicate and cause infection.

Interferon produced by a cell infected with a particular virus can prevent healthy cells from becoming infected by almost all other types of viruses. Interferon is therefore not virus-specific. However, interferon produced by one host species is not effective if administered to a different species. It is therefore host species specific. Since interferon produced by birds and other mammals cannot be used in treating human beings, it is difficult to obtain large enough quantities of interferon to provide effective chemotherapy for viral diseases. (Human donors cannot provide the needed amount of interferon.)

Interferon is a more rapid response to viral infection than antibody response. Interferon production is initiated within hours after viral infection, reaching a maximum after two days. Within three or four days, interferon production declines as antibodies are produced.

Prevention of viral infection by interferon production must be distinguished from another phenomenon - viral interference. Viral interference is observed when an initial viral infection prevents a secondary infection of the same cell by a different virus. The initial virus somehow prevents reproduction of the second virus or inactivates receptors on the cell membrane (there are specific sites for viral attachment). It may also stimulate production of an inhibitor of the second virus. Viral interference does not prevent uninfected cells from becoming infected. Vaccination involves administration of an attenuated (weakened) strain of virus, which cannot produce the disease, but which stimulates antibody production and thus prevents infection by the pathogenic virus.

What is an oncogene?

Solution: Cancerous cells differ physiologically from noncancerous cells: they have a different shape, a higher rate of sugar transport, membrane differences, uncontrolled growth, and a high degree of anaerobic respiration. Oncogenes (from the Greek word onkos which means mass or tumor) may cause cells to become cancerous.

Oncogenes were first found in viruses. The src gene is the oncogene of the Rous sarcoma virus. Analysis has shown that this single gene is capable of transforming cells to a cancerous state. The src gene codes for a tyrosine kinase. This enzyme catalyzes the phosphorylation of tyrosine whereas most kinases phosphorylate serine or threonine. Phosphorylation of proteins is a means by which the activities of growing cells are governed. The viral src gene thus codes for a protein that affects the growth of cells. This may induce secondary effects that lead to tumors and cancer.

Genes related to the src gene have been found in fruit flies, fish, birds and mammals, including humans. The gene is not there as a result of a viral infection; it is a part of each cell's genome. It is active in normal cells. It produces a tyrosine kinase which is almost indistinguishable from the viral protein. These cellular genes are called proto-oncogenes because there are a number of molecular mechanisms that can change them into oncogenes. The mechanisms include mutations, chromosomal rearrangements and gene amplification. Most virologists agree that the viral oncogene was copied from these cellular genes. How or why this happened is unknown. Evidence indicates that the copying continues to this day.

There are two hypotheses that have been proposed to explain the drastic differences in effects of viral oncogenes and cellular proto-oncogenes:

1. The mutational hypothesis states that cellular genes differ from viral oncogenes in subtle ways due to mutations that occurred when the genes were copied into the viral genome.

2. The dosage hypothesis proposes that viral oncogenes act by overburdening cells with too much of an essential protein. There is some experimental evidence for this proposal.

Cellular proto-oncogenes may be part of a delicate balance that regulates the growth and development of normal cells. If this balance is upset, the cell may be converted to a cancerous state. Viruses (although no viruses have been definitely implicated in producing human cancers) and some chemicals may interact with the proto-oncogene to disturb the balance and induce cancer. The treatment of cancer is complex because the disease's mechanisms have been enigmatic. Recently, further complications have been introduced in the treatment of cancer because the mechanism that makes the cell cancerous is no different from the mechanism at work in normal, healthy cells. Further understanding of the genetics of cancer should aid in the quest for a cure.

SHORT ANSWER QUESTIONS FOR REVIEW

Choose the correct answer.

1. Which of the following choices is not a way
   bacteria can donate genetic material? (a)
   transformation (b) transduction (c) meiosis
   (d) conjugation

   c

2. An episome can exist (a) as an integrated
   part of a chromosome. (b) as an autonomous
   cytoplasmic structure. (c) extracellularly in
   fluid. (d) a and b

   d

3. R plasmids carry (a) genes for antibiotic
   resistance. (b) only mutant genes. (c) only
   phenotypic information. (d) a and b

   a

4. Merozygotes are (a) never diploids. (b) always
   diploids. (c) temporarily partial diploids. (d)
   temporarily full diploids.

   c

5. In transformation (a) the recipient gains a full
   strand of DNA. (b) the recipient gains the
   DNA in fragments. (c) the newly obtained DNA
   is transcribed, then lysed. (d) DNA is
   transferred both ways.

   b

6. Specialized transduction (a) has only
   restricted parts of the bacterial chromosome
   incorporated into the phage. (b) varies
   according to the size of the chromosome.
   (c) does not occur in human cells. (d)
   can only occur in gametes.

   a

7. Bacteriophages are (a) viral particles in
   general. (b) viral particles that infect bacteria.
   (c) bacteria in general. (d) bacteria that infect
   viruses.

   b

8. As a result of the lysogenic cycle _____
   is (are) formed. (a) four infected daughter
   cells (b) three infected daughter cells (c)
   two infected daughter cells (d) one infected
   daughter cell

   c

9. Viruses contain (a) RNA only. (b) DNA only.
   (c) both RNA and DNA. (d) either RNA or
   DNA.

   d

10. Interferon (a) inhibits the lytic cycle. (b) makes the cell more susceptible to infection. (c) makes the cell more resistant to viral infection. (d) lyses the DNA of the host cells.

c

11. Vaccinations involve the administration of weakened forms of certain viruses. The vaccinated organism will then become more resistant to these viruses. This is an example of (a) viral interference. (b) interferon mediated viral resistance. (c) a retroactive virus. (d) preventive viral resistance.

a

12. In which of the following ways can a mutation cause an organism to be resistant to an anti-biotic? (a) by changing the shape of the receptor molecule (b) by creating an enzyme that inactivates the drug (c) by acting on the drug's intracellular targets (d) a,b and c

d

13. The following zygote $\dfrac{rstu}{PQRSTU}$ was just formed by the conjugation of two bacteria This is an example of a _____ (a) homo-zygote. (b) merozygote. (c) total haploid. (d) total diploid.

b

Fill in the blanks.

14. During conjugation, genetic material is transmitted through a _____.

sex pilus

15. An Hfr cell has the F factor _____ into each chromosome.

integrated

16. Most antibiotic resistant bacteria result from _____ changes.

genetic

17. Streptomycin inhibits _____ in prokaryotes.

protein synthesis

18. In abortive transduction, the transduced fragment does not incorporate into the recipient chromosome through _____.

recombina-tion

19. Complementation determines whether or not mutations are _____.

allelic

SHORT ANSWER QUESTIONS FOR REVIEW

20. In viral infections only, _____ may act as a template for DNA.

RNA

21. Herpes virus has a double stranded DNA molecule in a core enclosed by a(n) _____ . protein coat.

icosohedral
or
20 sided

22. Herpes virus induces the _____ in permissive cells.

lytic cycle

23. Interferon production declines as _____ are produced.

antibodies

24. Oncogenes may cause cells to become _____ .

cancerous

25. Oncogenes were first observed in _____ .

viruses

26. Streptomycin inhibits the binding of _____ tRNA to the ribosomes.

formyl-
methionyl

Decide whether the following statements are true or false.

27. During transformation, genes enter the recipient in fragments.

True

28. After conjugation, a female baterium can become a male.

True

29. Spontaneous mutations in a bacterial chromosome cannot cause antibiotic resistance.

False

30. R plasmids can pick up additional transposons.

True

31. True cell fusion takes place in bacteria.

False

32. The only way to get genetic variance is as a result of mutations.

False

33. Transduction is phage mediated.

True

34. Phages cannot self replicate.

True

35. The lysogenic cycle leads to the immediate deterioration of the host cell.

False

36. Lysogenic phages can cause beneficial mutations.

True

432

SHORT ANSWER QUESTIONS FOR REVIEW

37. A cancerous state may be produced when incomplete genomes are incorporated into the host's genome.

True

38. Few human diseases have a viral cause.

False

39. Interferon is not virus specific.

True

40. The fertility factor (F) is an episome.

True

41. Transposons can self replicate.

False

42. An increased use of antibiotics would prevent the spread of resistant pathogenic bacteria.

False

CHAPTER 11

BIOCHEMISTRY AND REGULATION

BIOCHEMICAL GENETICS

● **PROBLEM** 11-1

What is the genetic basis of albinism?

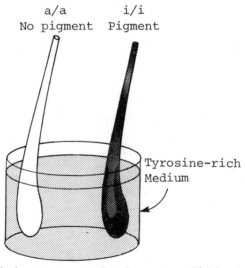

Fig. 1 Albinism can result from two different mutant recessive genes. Gene *a* fails to code for the enzyme necessary to convert tyrosine products into melanin; gene *i* prevents normal absorption of tyrosine. When hair, including roots, is cultured in tyrosine-rich medium, the homozygous *a/a* still fails to produce pigment but homozygous *i/i* does produce pigment.

Solution: Albinism is characterized by a failure to form the black pigment melanin. Normally melanin is formed from the product of the hydroxylation of tyrosine. This product, 3,4-dihydroxyphenylalanine, or dopa, is converted to melanin in a series of reactions by the enzyme complex tyrosinase. These reactions occur in melanocytes. Albinos have the normal number of melanocytes in their skin, but tyrosinase activity is not evident.

There are a number of genes that are involved in determining the amount of pigment deposited in the skin, hair and eye cells. This accounts for the great variability in human coloring. However, only one gene locus is involved in the production of melanin. A person who is homozygous for the recessive allele of this gene, which codes for the enzyme that converts tyrosine to dopa, cannot produce melanin.

Albinism can be caused by another genetic factor. Melanin production is dependent on the presence of tyrosine in a cell. A person who is homozygous for an allele at a different loci, will not have membranes permeable to tyrosine. People with this type of albinism have a small amount of melanin due to the breakdown of phenylalanine to tyrosine that occurs inside the cell. A test for this type of albinism is shown in Figure 1.

● **PROBLEM 11-2**

How does the measurement of enzymatic activity help to detect galactosemia?

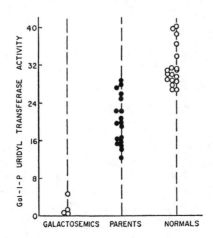

Fig. 1

Solution: Galactosemia is an inherited disorder in which dietary galactose accumulates because its metabolism is blocked. The absence of the enzyme galactose 1-phosphate uridyl transferase blocks the metabolism of galactose. This enzyme is usually present in such large amounts that a 50 percent reduction does not produce clinical symptoms. Heterozygotes have between 60 and 70 percent of the enzymatic activity and thus show no symptoms, see Figure 1. Homozygotes, however, produce no enzyme and usually fail to thrive. When milk is consumed, the affected infants vomit or have diarrhea. Many are mentally retarded. The absence of galactose 1-phosphate uridyl transferase in the red blood cells is a definitive test for the disease.

This disease can be treated with a diet that excludes galactose. Almost all of the clinical symptoms, except for the mental retardation, regress with a galactose-free diet.

● **PROBLEM** 11-3

Tay-Sachs disease is an inborn error of metabolism. How can heterozygotes be detected?

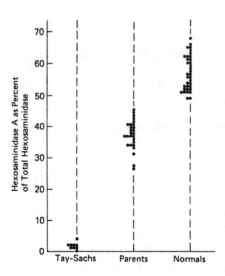

Fig. 1 The detection of heterozygotes for the recessive allele causing Tay-Sachs disease. The percentage of hexosaminidase A is very low in affected children, and lower in their parents (who must be heterozygotes) than in normal individuals.

Solution: Tay-Sachs disease is a recessive disease in which the nervous system degenerates. Most affected individuals do not live past age three. Homozygous recessives do not produce the enzyme β-N-acetylhexosaminidase. This enzyme is responsible for the removal of the terminal sugar of one type of lipid. This ganglioside, as it is called, accumulates in the cerebral cortex causing striking pathological changes.

The absence of the enzyme can be detected prenatally by amniocentesis. Heterozygous parents can be detected since the enyzme is only present in 50 percent of the normal amount.

● **PROBLEM 11-4**

What is the genetic basis for phenylketonuria (PKU)? When are heterozygotes for PKU more likely to have abnormalities?

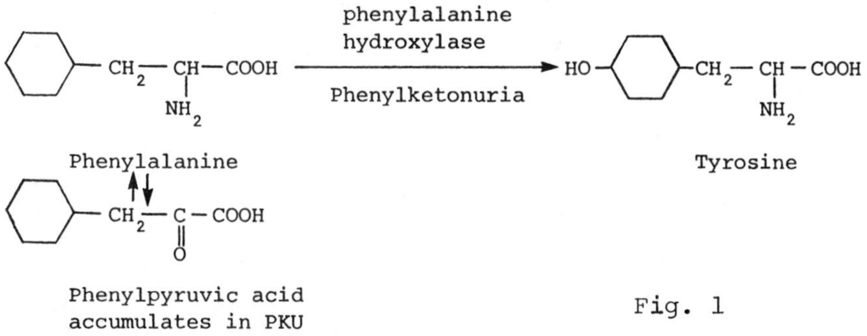

Fig. 1

Solution: Phenylketonuria is an inborn error of metabolism. Untreated individuals almost always become severly mentally retarded. These individuals have decreased brain weight, defective myelination of their nerves and hyperactive reflexes. Their life expectancy is only about thirty years.

This disease is caused by the absence or deficiency of phenylalanine hydroxylase. This enzyme converts phenylalanine to tyrosine. In homozygous individuals, phenylalanine accumulates in all body fluids. Up to a gram a day of phenylalanine may be secreted in the urine. The phenylalanine can be metabolized in phenylketonurics in ways that are quantitatively insignificant in normal people. The transamination of phenylalanine to phenylpyruvic acid is the most evident effect, (Figure 1).

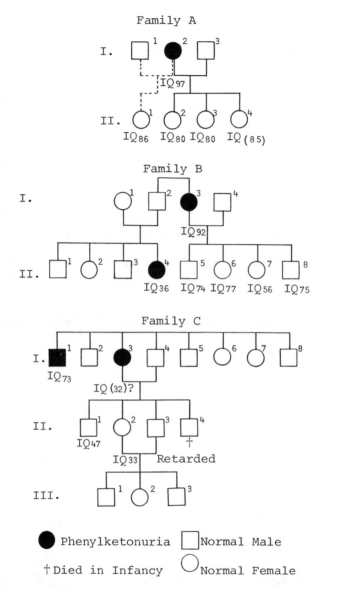

Fig. 2: Three families in which the mother was
      homozygous and all children (heterozygous)
      suffered as a result.

Normally, heterozygotes do not show the disorder. One normal allele is sufficient to produce enough enzyme to metabolize the phenylalanine to tyrosine. However, if the mother of heterozygotes is homozygous, they may have severe mental deficiencies. Figure 2 shows a pedigree of three families with homozygous mothers.

• PROBLEM 11-5

When a person eats food containing phenylalanine or tyrosine, his urine turns black when exposed to air. Explain.

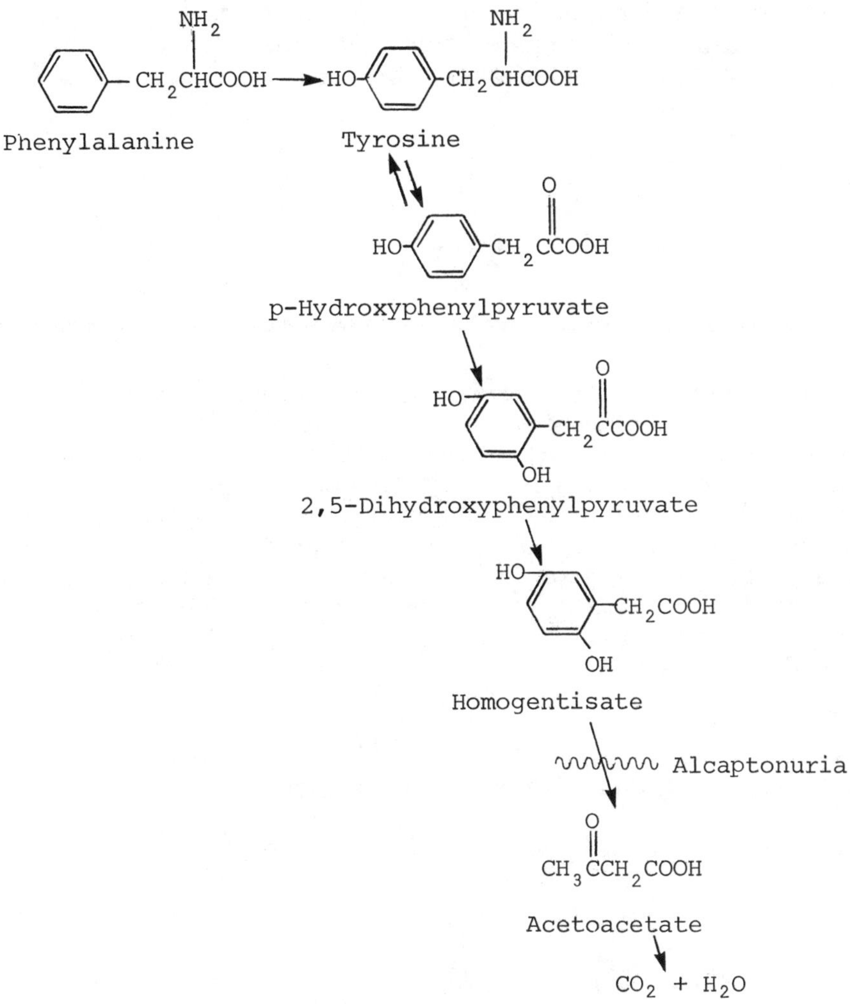

Fig. 1. THE CHEMICAL BLOCK IN ALCAPTONURIA

Solution: This condition is due to an inherited metabolic disorder called alcaptonuria. This disorder is another inborn error of metabolism; it is caused by an inherited defect in a single enzyme. The enzyme that is defective in alcaptonuria is homogentisate oxidase.

A person who is homozygous for the recessive allele

at the alcaponuria gene produces urine that turns black because he lacks the enzyme that converts homogentisate to acetoacetate in the phenylalanine and tyrosine catabolic pathway (see Figure 1). An affected individual excretes homogentisate into his urine. Homogentisate is oxidized and polymerized to a melanin-like compound when it remains exposed to air. This gives the urine its black color.

Alcaptonuria is relatively benign. It has no very harmful effects in young people. However, later in life it usually results in degenerative arthritis. This may be caused by the crystalization of homogentisate in the cartilages of the body.

● **PROBLEM** 11-6

A wild-type and four mutant strains of Neurospora are used in an experiment to study the biosynthesis of arginine. The mutants have specific mutations that affect their ability to synthesize arginine. The mutations affect the enzymes that convert one intermediate to the next along the arginine pathway. They can only grow on minimal media when it is supplemented with the intermediate that they cannot produce due to their defective enzyme. The growth results are as follows:

	Supplement			
Strain	none	Ornithine	Citrulline	Arginine
wild-type	+	+	+	+
1	-	-	-	+
2	-	-	+	+
3	-	+	+	+
4	-	+	+	+

A plus sign indicates growth and a minus sign indicates no growth. What is the sequence of these intermediates in the arginine pathway? Where are the mutations?

Solution: Neurospora is a bread mold which is haploid throughout most of its life cycle. It can normally grow on minimal medium which has only a single carbon and nitrogen source, inorganic salts and the vitamin biotin. Biochemical mutants need additional nutrients in their media in order to grow.

Biosynthetic pathways are series of chemical reactions that result in the formation of end products. Along the way from precursor to end product, stable intermediates are created. The intermediates are converted stepwise by specific enzymes until the end product is produced in sufficient quantity. Schematically, a pathway may be as follows:

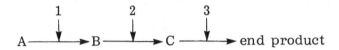

where A, B, and C are the precursor and intermediates, and 1, 2, and 3 are the enzymes. No end product will be made if there is a mutation in one enzyme of the pathway. For instance, if there is a mutation at 2 in the schematic pathway, no end product will be made. However, if the media is supplemented with C, the enzymatic block will be bypassed and an end product will be produced.

This problem involves two intermediates in the arginine pathway, citrulline and ornithine. From the information given, we can order the pathway. The wild-type strain can grow on all media, as expected. All strains can grow on arginine, which is expected if the mutations only affect the arginine pathway. Three of the four mutants can grow when supplemented with citrulline. This implies that citrulline is the intermediate directly before arginine. Similarly, two mutants grow when fed ornithine; ornithine is before citrulline in the pathway. The order of the intermediates is:

$$precursor \longrightarrow 0 \longrightarrow C \longrightarrow A$$

To find where the mutations lie, we must examine each strain individually to see where it can grow. Strain 1 can grow when supplemented with the end product, arginine. Its mutation, therefore, blocks the production of arginine. The rest of its pathway is fine. Strain 1's mutation is located in the enzyme that produces arginine:

$$precursor \longrightarrow 0 \longrightarrow C \xrightarrow{1} A$$

Strain 2 can grow when given citrulline and arginine. Since it requires citrulline, its faulty enzyme cannot convert ornithine to citrulline:

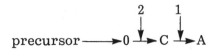

$$\text{precursor} \longrightarrow 0 \xrightarrow{2} C \xrightarrow{1} A$$

Strains 3 and 4 need ornithine, citrulline and arginine in their medium in order to grow. This places both mutations before the production of ornithine:

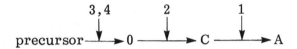

$$\text{precursor} \xrightarrow{3,4} 0 \xrightarrow{2} C \xrightarrow{1} A$$

The order of mutations 3 and 4 cannot be determined from this experiment. We would need to supplement the media of these strains with an additional intermediate that lies between the precursor and ornithine.

This experiment reveals only a part of the biosynthetic pathway of arginine. Further studies of this type are necessary to determine the complete pathway.

PROKARYOTIC REGULATION

● **PROBLEM** 11-7

What is the difference between negative and positive control of gene expression?

Solution: Compounds that bind to DNA can control the expression of the genes on that piece of DNA. This control can take two forms: positive and negative control.

Negative control is operative in some prokaryotic catabolic systems, see Figure 1. The lac operon of E.coli is under negative control. This form of control utilizes repressors and inducers to turn off a genetic system that would otherwise be turned on. The repressor molecule interacts with the DNA to inhibit the synthesis of the gene products. This inhibition is terminated when the inducer, the molecule that is to be catabolized, is present. Thus negative control involves substances that inhibit gene activity.

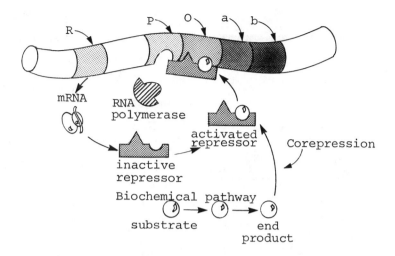

Fig. 1 Negative control in a repressible operon.

Positive control is found in biosynthetic as well as catabolic systems. The lac operon is under positive control as well as negative control. Positive control occurs when components enhance gene activity. Hormones, special proteins such as the catabolite activator protein (CAP), and cyclic AMP can act to enhance the transcription of genes, see Figure 2.

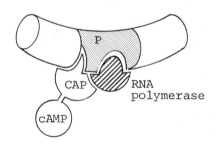

Fig. 2 Positive control by the cAMP-CAP complex.

Genes can be controlled by positive and/or negative control. Catabolic systems, such as the breakdown of lactose, utilize negative control since the genes need to be expressed only in the presence of the compound to be degraded. Biosynthetic systems, such as tryptophan biosynthesis, use positive control since they synthesize a product. There is still much to learn about the regulation of gene activity. But it seems that different forms of regulation are needed for different types of gene expression.

Given the lactose operon in the bacterium, Escherichia coli:

| i | | | | | | p | o | z | y | a |

where i = regulator gene

  p = promoter site

  o = operator site

  z = structural gene for β-galactosidase

  y = structural gene for β-galactoside permease

  a = structural gene for thiogalactoside transacetylase

Assuming that the inducer molecule, lactose, is present, what would be the result in terms of enzyme synthesis if the following mutational events took place:

a) mutation of i such that a defective repressor results that does not recognize o

b) mutation of i such that a "superrepressor" results which does not recognize lactose

c) mutation of o such that repressor will not recognize o

d) mutation of p.

Solution: Jacob and Monod first described the lac operon as a model to explain mutations such as these. Studies of mutations are an extremely important component of genetic analyses.

a) Since a defective repressor is produced, the normal repression of o will not occur; thus, there will be constitutive synthesis of the structural gene products regardless of the presence of an inducer molecule.

b) Since the product that results does not recognize the inducer molecule, the system will be permanently shut

444

off, and no structural enzymes will be produced.

    c) With the mutation of $\underline{o}$ resulting in nonrecognition by the repressor, no repression will occur regardless of the presence or absence of the inducer; thus, constitutive synthesis of all structural gene products will occur.

    d) With a mutation at $\underline{p}$, the most likely result is nonrecognition either by the mRNA polymerase, the CAP-cAMP (catabolite activator protein - cyclic AMP) or both; thus, no structural gene products will result.

● **PROBLEM** 11-9

Partial diploids can be produced in the bacterium, E.coli, for the lac operon. As a consequence, some mutations can be bypassed in terms of their disruption of the operon by production of the partial diploids with wild-type alleles at the sites of mutation. In each case the wild-type allele is dominant to its mutant homologue.

    Determine for each of the following partial diploids whether enzyme production will result constitutively or inducibly (normally) when the inducer molecule is introduced:

a) $\dfrac{\underline{i}^+ \quad \underline{o}^+ \quad \underline{z}^- \quad \underline{y}^- \quad \underline{a}^-}{\underline{i}^+ \quad \underline{o}^c \quad \underline{z}^+ \quad \underline{y}^+ \quad \underline{a}^+}$

b) $\dfrac{\underline{i}^- \quad \underline{o}^+ \quad \underline{z}^+ \quad \underline{y}^+ \quad \underline{a}^+}{\underline{i}^+ \quad \underline{o}^+ \quad \underline{z}^+ \quad \underline{y}^- \quad \underline{a}^-}$

c) $\dfrac{\underline{i}^+ \quad \underline{o}^c \quad \underline{z}^+ \quad \underline{y}^- \quad \underline{a}^-}{\underline{i}^- \quad \underline{o}^+ \quad \underline{z}^- \quad \underline{y}^- \quad \underline{a}^-}$

Solution: a) For this partial diploid, there will be only constitutive synthesis of the three normal enzymes, since the wild-type allele of the operator is in cis-configuration with mutant alleles of the structural genes. Since the

445

operator itself, and not a gene product, is the active component, it must work where it is. It cannot traverse to the other homologue to perform. Therefore the wild-type operator will not participate in any protein synthesis because the structural genes on that homologue are mutant. The wild-type structural genes have a mutant operator so the repressor won't bind to the operator; the genes' expression is constitutive.

b) All structural gene enzymes will be produced inducibly, because the normal repressor can be produced by the i^+ gene of one sequence, and the normal operator is in $\overline{cis}$-configuration with the wild-type structural genes. The $\underline{i}^+$ gene produces a protein product that is free to move. It can move to the other homologue to work in trans, away from its original site.

c) There will be no production of enzymes, since both chromosomes have mutant alleles for the structural genes.

VIRAL REGULATION

● **PROBLEM** 11-10

Explain how gene expression is regulated during phage λ infection.

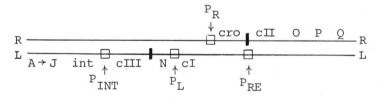

Fig. 1

Solution: The phage λ has a system of operons and regulatory proteins that regulate whether it will undergo lysis or lysogeny when it infects a host. Whether the virus undergoes lysis or lysogeny depends on environmental stimuli which affects gene expression. The genes that are involved in this regulation are ordered strategically on the λ chromosome. Contrary to most chromosomes, each strand of DNA is used as a sense strand - one is read towards the right and the other is transcribed towards the left. A linear representation of the λ chromosome is shown in Figure 1.

There are three phases that regulate λ's lytic cycle. They are the immediate-early, delayed early and late phases. The immediate-early phase begins immediately after the phage infects a cell. The host's polymerases bind to a promoter region (P_R) of the phage genome. P_R directs transcription on the R strand in the rightward direction. The second immediate-early transcript begins at the leftward promoter (P_L) which transcribes to the left. The transcription that begins at P_R leads to the production of Cro protein, and the transcription that begins at P_L leads to the production of N protein. N protein is an antiterminator. It enables the RNA polymerase to get over the chain terminating sequences that are denoted by black bars in Figure 1. N protein also stimulates the transcription of the delayed-early phase. The delayed early genes are cII and cIII, which are used only in lysogeny; genes O and P, which are needed for the replication of the phage chromosome; and gene Q which is needed for the stimulation of the next phase. When the Q gene has been transcribed, the Q protein, another antiterminator, stimulates the late phase genes. These genes, denoted A→J in Figure 1, encode the head and tail proteins of the phage. Once these proteins are made, the replicated phage chromosomes are packaged inside protein coats and the host cell is lysed. Figure 2 shows the three lytic phases. The genome is actually circular, so the third phase is not actually split as it appears in the diagram.

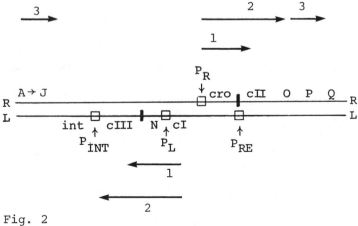

Fig. 2

Lysogeny requires two events: the repressor protein, cI, must be synthesized to turn off the lytic cycle by binding to operator regions near the promoters, P_R and P_L , and the Int protein must be synthesized to mediate λ's integration into the bacterial host's genome. In order for cI to be transcribed, a polymerase must bind to the P_{RE} promoter. P_{INT} must be recognized by a polymerase for the Int protein to be transcribed. Both promoters are recognized by RNA polymerase only in the presence of cII and cIII proteins. The cII protein acts as an activator protein; it stimulates polymerase to bind to promoters.

The race between lysis and lysogeny pivots on the levels of Cro protein and cI. Cro protein can act as a repressor by binding to the operators that cI can bind. It is not as stable as cI, nor does it bind as strongly. Thus, when it binds it slows down but does not stop, the expression of N, cIII, cro, cII, O, P and Q genes. When there is a lot of Cro protein, little cII and cIII is transcribed, and thus no cI made. When there is no cI, there is no strong repression of the lytic cycle phases, so the phage lyses the cell. When there is a small amount of Cro, the cII and cIII levels are high because Cro is not slowing their synthesis. These proteins are necessary for cI transcription, so cI is produced. The cI protein strongly inhibits the lytic cycle genes and the phage undergoes lysogeny.

The state of the phage is influenced by the levels of the proteins that are produced. Cro protein levels are affected by temperature, the metabolic state of the host, the genotype of the host and the genotype of the infecting phage. The lytic cycle will be followed when the conditions are optimal for the survival of the phage's progeny. Otherwise, the lysogenic cycle will be followed.

● **PROBLEM** 11-11

Some of the phage λ genome are shown in Figure 1.

Will the phage undergo lysis or lysogeny if the following genetic sequences are deleted:

(a) cI
(b) Q
(c) N
(d) cro

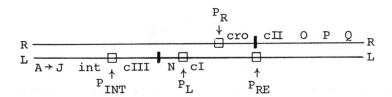

Fig. 1

Solution: Refer to the previous problem for a description of the gene expression of λ phage. The deletions of genes will affect this expression since the regulation depends on specific interactions of genes and gene products.

(a) If the cI gene is deleted, the phage will lyse the host cell. The cI protein is a repressor of the lytic cycle; without it the lytic cycle is free to be expressed.

(b) If the Q gene is deleted, the phage will undergo limited lysis. The Q protein is necessary for the full stimulation of the late genes of the lytic cycle. Without Q protein, the head and tail proteins (the late gene products) will be produced. The phage will undergo lysis, but only a few progeny will be released.

(c) A deletion of the N gene effectively blocks both lysis and lysogeny. The only proteins that would be produced are those whose genes lie before a terminator sequence.

(d) Lysogeny will occur if there is no cro gene. Cro protein at low levels enables the cI protein to block the lytic genes. Once blocked, the genes needed for lysogeny are read when RNA polymerase binds to the P_{RE} promoter.

(e) When P_{RE} is deleted, the lysogenic genes will not be read, so lysis will occur.

(f) The deletion of int gene makes it impossible for the phage to integrate into the host's genome. Whether the phage will be able to lyse the cell depends on the level of Cro and cI proteins.

(g) A deletion of the cII gene leads to lysis. The cII gene product is necessary for the production of cI. If there is no cII, there is no cI, so there is no repression of lysis.

EUKARYOTIC REGULATION

● **PROBLEM** 11-12

How can the expression of eukaryotic genes be regulated?

Solution: Eukaryotic organisms are decidedly more complex than prokaryotes. They have diploid rather than haploid genomes. They can surpass the one-celled state of most prokaryotes and grow into multicellular organisms whose numerous cells are highly specialized. This complexity complicates the study of eukaryotic regulation. But many forms of genetic regulation can be related to the processes of the expression of the genetic information. The genome can be regulated by DNA modification and through transcriptional, post-transcriptional and translational control.

DNA can be modified by the methylation of its cytosine residues. Specific methylation patterns exist, for example, the cytosine residues that are methylated are usually next to guanine residues. These patterns are not random; they are tissue specific and clonally inherited. Undermethylation of DNA is correlated with active gene expression. Conversely, methylation is correlated with nonexpression.

Control of transcription can account for the differential gene activity that occurs during development. Ovalbumin transcription can be initiated by the steroid hormone estrogen in immature chicken oviduct cells.

The separation of the genetic material in the nucleus from the translation apparatus in the cytoplasm introduces post-transcriptional control.

The RNA molecule that is produced in the nucleus is different from the one that is translated at the ribosomes. The nuclear RNA (hnRNA) contains sequences called introns or intervening sequences that are exised and never translated. The RNA that reaches the ribosomes (mRNA) is considerably shorter than the hnRNA. The hnRNA of different types of cells is similar even though their mRNAs are different. The processing of the hnRNA to create the specific mRNAs may be involved in the control of gene expression. The introns that are spliced out of the hnRNA may have a role in the regulation of some genes. This has been shown in the virus SV40 but not in prokaryotic or eukaryotic cells.

Other mechanisms of regulation of eukaryotic gene expression may occur during translation. Translation may be modulated by one or more factors that are involved in protein synthesis. For instance, in the unfertilized sea urchin egg, there is a lot of masked mRNA which may be inactive for months. Once the egg is fertilized, the masked mRNA is translated into protein. The gene products are produced when they are needed.

Eukaryotic gene regulation is not a well-defined area of genetics. Much of the information is speculative and has been derived from other experimental systems. Eventually these theories will be genetically analyzed in the eukaryotic system.

● PROBLEM 11-13

What is the heat shock response?

Solution: Heat shock is a response found in many eukaryotic cells. When the temperature is raised, the cells stop transcribing the genes that were previously active and instead transcribe a new set of genes called heat shock genes. Translation of the original genes also stops and the heat shock genes are preferentially translated. This event occurs in Drosophila, yeast, corn and in cultured mammalian cells. Drosophila's giant salivary gland chromosomes show nine new chromosomal puffs as a result of high temperatures.

How this regulation is achieved is not known. But four heat shock genes have been cloned and sequenced. They have promoter regions and areas of imperfect dyad symmetry upstream from the promoters. These areas are perfect places for regulatory proteins to bind, since many known controlling elements have such symmetry.

How can some hormones regulate gene action?

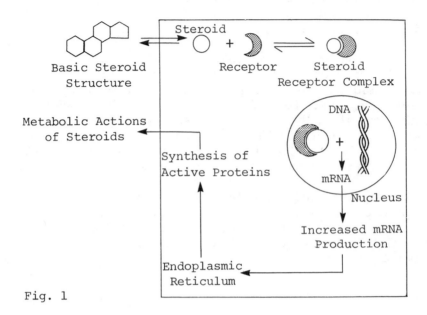

Steroid

Basic Steroid
Structure

Receptor   Steroid
          Receptor Complex

Metabolic Actions
of Steroids

DNA

Synthesis of
Active Proteins

mRNA

Nucleus

Increased mRNA
Production

Endoplasmic
Reticulum

Fig. 1

Solution: Hormones are control chemicals produced by cells in both plants and animals. They are produced in small amounts in specialized cells that are far removed from their sites of action. In higher plants, they are transported via the vascular system and in animals they are carried by the blood. They are effective in small concentrations, so they probably influence the synthesis or activity of enzymes. Some hormones that influence genetic activity are gibberellic acid, abscisic acid, ecdysone, and estrogen.

Gibberellic acid and abscisic acid are plant hormones that are involved in plant growth and development. Gibberellic acid has a role in controlling the early phases of growth. It activates stem lengthening, stimulates pollen germination, induces flower formation and stimulates seed germination. The stimulation of seed germination is a very important function. Just prior to germination, the seed embryo secretes gibberellins which induce the production of the enzyme α-amylase. This enzyme hydrolyzes stored starch and activates the other enzymes of the seed. An inhibitor of RNA synthesis, actinomycin D, effectively inhibits the synthesis of α-amylase. This suggests that gibberellic acid initiates the transcription of α-amylase.

Somehow it interacts with genetic material to induce its expression. Abscisic acid inhibits the production of α-amylase. It may bind to the DNA or interact with gibberellic acid in such a way that the transcription is turned off.

Ecdysone is one of the hormones involved in insect maturation. Ecdysone is a steroid hormone that acts as shown in Figure 1. When small amounts of ecdysone are injected into Drosophila, chromosome puffs are observed at certain sites. Chromosome puffs are visible in the salivary glands since they have very large (polytene) chromosomes. Chromosome puff formation is an indication of the activation of certain genes or sets of genes. Thus, ecdysone activates gene expression in Drosophila.

Estrogen is another steroid hormome. Estrogen is produced by the ovaries in mammals. It stimulates the development and maintenance of female reproductive structures and secondary sexual characteristics and it stimulates the growth of the uterine lining. Estrogen increases the transcription in uterine tissue.

These are only a few of the many hormones that exist. Many other hormones probably act in similar ways.

● **PROBLEM** 11-15

Do histones control gene activity?

Solution: Histones are the proteins that complex with eukaryotic DNA to form chromosomes. Histones are very similar from cell to cell and from organism to organism; therefore, they cannot be responsible for specific gene regulation. However, they do bind to the DNA so they can insulate it from transcription.

As shown in Figure 1, histones can repress the transcription of DNA. They can physically block the polymerases and other enzymes from interacting with the DNA. This repression may be overcome by the action of RNA. RNA may hybridize to the nontranscribing (antisense) strand of the DNA, thus freeing the sense strand for transcription. This occurs in a restricted area of the genome; only a few selected genes are open for transcription.

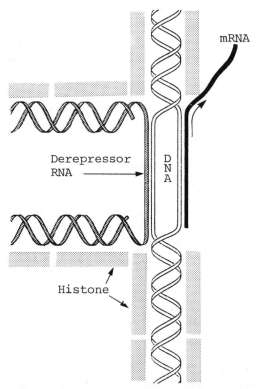

Fig. 1 MODEL FOR GENE REPRESSION
AND SELECTIVE DEREPRESSION BY
HISTONES

Thus, histones have a physical role in the regulation of gene expression. They protect the DNA from transcription enzymes until a signal arrives to initiate proper transcription. The specific regulation may be carried out by the other proteins found in chromosomes: the nonhistone proteins.

SHORT ANSWER QUESTIONS FOR REVIEW

Choose the correct answer

1. Melanin is formed from the product of the
    hydroxylation of (a) dopa. (b) 3,4 -
    dihydroxyphenylalanine. (c) tyrosinase. (d)
    all of the above (e) none of the above

    e

2. Which of the following substances do all albinos
    lack? (a) dopa (b) 3,4 dihydroxyphenylalanine
    (c) tyrosinase (d) all of the above (e) none
    of the above

    c

3. The production of melanin is determined by a
    gene which codes for the production of (a)
    dopa. (b) tyrosinase. (c) tyrosine. (d) all of
    the above

    b

4. Some albinos are found to have small amounts
    of melanin. This albinism is due to (a) a
    heterozygous recessive condition. (b) a homo-
    zygous recessive condition. (c) a mutant gene
    which codes for melanin production. (d) a
    mutant gene which codes for abnormal melanin
    cell absorption.

    d

5. The mutated gene in galactosemia codes for (a)
    an autosomal recessive allele. (b) a sex-linked
    dominant allele. (c) an autosomal dominant allele.
    (d) none of the above

    a

6. Galactosemia results from the failure of one
    gene to (a) produce an enzyme. (b) facilitate
    absorption. (c) activate a regulator gene. (d)
    none of the above

    a

7. The clinical symptoms in homozygous
    galactosemics are (a) lethal and cannot be
    treated. (b) in no need of treatment. (c)
    regressive if treated with galactose-free
    products. (d) all of the above

    c

8. The enzyme phenylalanine hydroxylase converts
    (a) tyrosine to galactose. (b) tyrosine to dopa.
    (c) phenylalanine to tyrosine. (d) phenylalanine
    to galactose.

    c

9. Alcaptonuria is a (an) (a) autosomal recessive
    disorder. (b) sex-linked recessive disorder. (c)

455

autosomal dominant disorder. (d) sex-linked
recessive disorder.

a

10. The enzyme homogentisic acid oxidase, which
is lacking in individuals affected with
alcaptonuria, converts homogentisic acid
(homogentisate) to (a) uridyl transferase.
(b) oxidase. (c) acetoacetate. (d) hydroxylase.

c

The table below shows the growth and non-growth
pattern of four mutant strains of Neurospora
cultured in growth factors A,B,C and D. Answer
questions 11-13 based on the information on this
table.

Strain	A	B	C	D
1	0	0	+	+
2	0	0	0	+
3	+	0	+	+
4	0	+	+	+

11. If A, B, C and D are part of a metabolic
pathway which is the order of synthesis? (a)
A → B→ C→ D (b) A → C → B → D (c)
C → A → B→ D (d) A⟩→C → D
      B

d

12. Where is the chain blocked in strain number
one? (a) between A and B (b) between C
and D (c) between B and D (d) between
AB and C

d

13. Where is the chain blocked in strain number
two? (a) between A and B (c) between B
and D (c) between C and D (d) between
AB and C

c

14. In essence, negative gene control is a
mechanism by which (a) inducer genes are
used to turn on a genetic system. (b)
inducer genes are used to turn off a mutated
genetic system. (c) inducer genes are used
to turn off a genetic system that would otherwise be turned on. (d) repressor genes are
used to turn off the action of an enzyme.

c

SHORT ANSWER QUESTIONS FOR REVIEW

15. Activity of identical genes vary from cell to cell during development. This phenomenon is due to control of DNA (a) transcription. (b) translation. (c) methylation. (d) cytoplasm.

a

16. Hormones which influence genetic activity are (a) gibberellic acid. (b) abscisic acid. (c) ecdysone. (d) all of the above

d

17. Histones directly influence genes by (a) physically blocking the polymerases from interacting with DNA. (b) transcribing antisense codons on the DNA strand. (c) transcribing sense codons on the DNA strand. (d) none of the above

a

Fill in the blanks.

18. Albinism results from a failure to form the pigment _____.

melanin

19. _____ is an inherited disorder in which normal metabolism of galactose is blocked.

Galactosemia

20. Individuals affected with galactosemia lack the enzyme_____.

galactose 1-
phosphate
uridyl trans-
ferase

21. Tay-Sachs disease is an _____ recessive disorder.

autosomal

22. _____ is a disease characterized by the absence of phenylalanine hydroxylase.

Phenyl-
ketonuria

23. Homozygous individuals affected with PKU accumulate _____ in all body fluids and excrete up to one gram a day.

phenyl
pyruvic
acid

24. A child heterozygous for PKU whose mother is homozygous for the disease is often born with severe _____.

mental
retardation

25. Alcaptonoria is an inborn error of metabolism due to a lack of the enzyme _____.

homogentisate
oxidase

26. When homogentisate is oxidized, it is converted to a _____ compound.

melanin-
like

457

27. A repressor molecule interacts with the _____
    molecule of a given gene to inhibit its enzyme
    synthesis.

    DNA

28. Negative gene control occurs in such _____
    organisms as E. coli.

    prokaryotic

29. The breakdown of lactose utilizes _____
    gene control.

    negative

30. In eukaryotic cells, DNA can be modified by
    the methylation of its _____ residues.

    cytosine

31. Methylation of DNA is correlated with _____
    of genes.

    non-
    expression

32. The set of genes which starts transcribing
    when temperature goes up is called _____
    genes.

    heat shock

Determine whether the following statements are
true or false.

33. Histones are lipids which form a complex with
    eukaryotic DNA to form chromosomes.

    False

34. Heat shock is a response found in eukaryotic
    cells, which results in a rise in temper-
    ature stimulating the cells to transcribe
    faster.

    False

35. The λ (lambda) phage has a system of
    regulatory lipids which determines whether
    the cell will undergo lysis of lysogeny.

    False

36. Positive gene control utilizes components
    such as hormones and special proteins to
    augment gene activity.

    True

37. Negative gene control involves the production
    of repressor molecules which interact with
    the enzyme produced by a given gene.

    False

38. The intermediates of a biosynthetic pathway
    are converted stepwise by specific enzymes
    until a final product is obtained.

    True

39. Alcaptonuria is a lethal disease in adults but
    it only produces mild arthritis in adolescents.

    False

40. Individuals affected with PKU produce urine which turns black when exposed to air.

False

41. Albinos have a subnormal number of melano-cytes on their skin.

False

42. The production of melanin is controlled by several gene loci.

False

43. Some albinos have a small amount of melanin thus, they are phenotypically normal.

False

44. Most galactosemics who have more than 50% of the required enzyme do not present overt symptoms.

True

45. Normally, individuals heterozygous for PKU are not affected with the disorder because one normal allele produces the necessary amount of enzyme.

True

46. Individuals who are heterozygous for Tay-Sachs disease have only 50% of the enzyme N-acetyl hexosaminidase.

True

CHAPTER 12

BEHAVIORAL GENETICS

BACTERIA

● **PROBLEM** 12-1

E.coli, a flagellated species of bacteria, is attracted to and repelled by various chemical substances. When capillary tubes with different substances are introduced to a culture of bacteria, the cells are attracted, repelled or unaffected. The results of a series of such experiments are shown in the graph in Figure 1.

What conclusions can be made about chemotaxis of E.coli from this experiment?

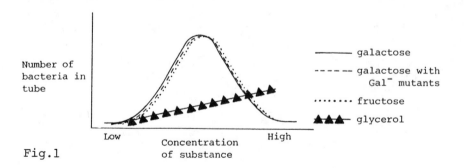

Fig.1

Solution: Chemotaxis is a behavior of E.coli that has been extensively studied. In 1973, J. Adler found that bacteria could be attracted or repelled by chemical substances in their environment. As the graph shows, this behavior is very specific.

The graph shows that E.coli is attracted to galactose and fructose when the concentration is not too high. Mutants that cannot metabolize galactose are also attracted by that sugar. Cells are indifferent to glycerol. Several important factors in chemotaxis are implicated in this study. First, this behavior is not necessarily correlated with metabolism. Mutant cells that cannot metabolize galactose are attracted to galactose-filled capillary tubes just as strongly as wild-type cells. Also, glycerol, a neutral fat that is used as an energy storage molecule and an energy source by many organisms, does not influence the bacteria's movement significantly. Fructose produces a strong effect even though it is not the sole carbon source. The second aspect of chemotaxis that this graph illustrates is that there is a concentration effect. The maximum number of bacteria are attracted to a test substance when it is present in an ideal concentration. When too much of the substance is present, little chemotaxis is observed.

These results can be explained by the presence of specific receptors on the cell surface. When a substance binds to its cellular receptor, it may trigger a response that induces the flagella to orient its movement towards (or away) from the areas of high concentration around the capillary tube source. As the concentration of the substance increases, it will diffuse throughout the cell solution so that the bacteria will no longer need to travel to the tube.

This behavior of E.coli has been found to have a genetic basis. There are protein products that act to initiate movement. These proteins interact to produce a flagellar response. Studies of various mutant E.coli strains has led to the conclusion that the mere movement of E.coli is controlled by a complex of genes. Each gene of the complex has a very specific function. Thus, behavior in even a "simple" organism is a result of coordinated interactions at the genetic and physiological levels.

● **PROBLEM** 12-2

Various substances in capillary tubes were introduced to bacterial suspensions with specific additives. The relative concentrations of the E.coli were measured.

Explain the results from these competitive chemotactic experiments.

Substances in capillary tube	% bacteria	Substance in bacterial suspension	% bacteria
galactose & fructose	0	galactose	100
galactose & fructose	0	fructose	100
glucose & galactose	0	glucose	100
glucose & galactose	40	galactose	60

Solution: In the previous problem, receptors on the bacterial surface were implicated in chemotactic response to chemicals. The results of this experiment reveal information about the binding capacity of the receptors.

The chemical that is in the bacterial suspension occupies the receptors that are able to bind to that substance. For instance, the first set of conditions in the chart of results includes galactose in the bacterial suspension. Thus, all of the receptors that can bind to galactose should be occupied as long as there is sufficient galactose. The substances that are in the capillary tubes are placed in after the cells have been in their suspension for a while.

The first part of this experiment shows that when galactose is in the bacterial suspension, neither galactose nor fructose can attract the bacteria - 0 percent are found in the capillary tube. Similarly, when fructose is in the bacterial suspension, none of the bacteria are attracted to galactose and fructose. This implies that the receptor protein for both galactose and fructose is the same.

When glucose and galactose are compared, the results are somewhat different. With glucose in the bacterial suspension, neither glucose nor galactose can attract the bacteria. However, when galactose is in the suspension, 40 percent of the bacteria are attracted to a capillary tube containing glucose and galactose. This implies that glucose can bind to receptors sensitive to glucose and galactose. But galactose cannot cover all of the receptors sensitive to glucose. So when these cells are given glucose, they have receptors free to bind and initiate chemotaxis towards the capillary tube.

INSECTS

The percentage of successful single pair matings observed for one hour in <u>Drosophila melanogaster</u> cultures showed the following:

Matings	Before crossing wild stock with <u>Yellow</u> stock for 7 generations	After crossing wild stock with <u>Yellow</u> stock for 7 generations
WT male x WT female	62	75
<u>Yellow</u> male x WT female	34	47
WT male x <u>Yellow</u> female	87	81
<u>Yellow</u> male x <u>Yellow</u> female	78	59

<u>Yellow</u> is a recessive mutant strain of flies that is phenotypically expressed as a yellow rather than gray body. Explain how this mutation affects the mating behavior of <u>D. melanogaster</u>.

Solution: Mating behavior in <u>Drosophila</u> involves a series of activities performed by the male and female flies. The courtship beings with "orientation" - the male follows the female. "Vibration", which involves wing movements and displays, and "licking" where the male's proboscis contacts the female's genitalia, are preludes to mounting. Wild-type flies show long bouts of licking and vibrating. <u>Yellow</u> mutants show shorter intervals for everything but orientation. The males with the <u>yellow</u> mutation are therefore less successful in mating with wild-type gray females than are wild-type males.

This experiment shows that the background genotype may be relevant to the effects of a mutation such as <u>yellow</u>. M. Bastock performed this experiment in 1956. She crossed wild-type flies with <u>yellow</u> flies for seven generations so that the wild-types were similar to the <u>yellow</u> at all loci except the <u>yellow</u> locus. A comparison of the percentages of successful matings before and after such a homogenizing process shows that the rest of the genotype does have an effect on behavior. After the seven generations were crossed, yellow x yellow matings were less frequent than wild-type x wild-type. The percentage of yellow male x wild-type female success is lower than that of wild-type males x yellow females. Bastock concluded that the males with the yellow mutation had a much lower success rate than crosses involving wild-type males regardless of the genotype of the female. However, before the strains were made homologous, there was a significant difference between females as well as between males. There is a big difference between the success of the crosses when there is either a yellow male or a yellow female as compared to their wild-type counterparts. This initial high receptivity in the females is partly dependent on the rest of the genotype. Perhaps there is selection for yellow females with a high receptivity when there is a low level of stimulus offered by the yellow males in the yellow x yellow crosses.

This experiment shows how important the entire genotype is in regard to behavioral traits. Single genes cannot be analyzed separately and then related to the organism as a whole unless all interactions are taken into account.

● **PROBLEM 12-4**

Geotaxis is gravity oriented locomotion. The genetics of this behavior has been well studied in Drosophila melanogaster with the use of plastic mazes with vertical units. The flies are attracted through the maze with food or light. Those flies that can orient themselves through the vertical units exhibit positive geotaxis; those that do not, show negative geotaxis. After selection based on their ability to travel through the maze, the following results were recorded:

Population	Chromosome		
	X	II	III
Selected for positive geotaxis	1.4	1.8	0.1
Unselected	1.0	1.7	-0.3
Selected for negative geotaxis	0.5	0.3	-1.1

Each unit represents one notch on the maze. Explain these results.

Solution: Drosophila melanogaster has a haploid chromosome complement of four. From the chart of data, three of these chromosomes, X, II and III, are involved in geotaxis. The ability to travel through the maze is reflected in the number of notches that the strain of fly is able to move through. These numbers appear in the chart and can be compared in order to assess the effects of selection on the chromosomes' ability to produce geotaxis.

Chromosomes X and II assert a positive effect on geotaxis while chromosome III asserts a negative effect. A comparison of each selected population with the unselected population will show the effects of each type of selection on the chromosomal effects. When positive geotaxis is selected for, little effect on chromosome II results. However, the ability of chromosome X to create a positive effect is increased and the ability of chromosome III to produce a negative effect is changed to slightly positive. Selection for negative geotaxis reduces the positive effects of chromosomes X and II and increases the negative effect of chromosome III.

This experiment confirms that there are three genetic loci distributed on three of Drosophila's chromosomes which affect the ability of the fly to use gravity-oriented locomotion. The exact functions of these genes is not presently known.

● **PROBLEM 12-5**

A cross between a hygienic nest cleaning queen bee, uurr, and a nonhygienic drone honeybee, UR, yields nonhygienic bees, UuRr. Would a backcross with a hygienic bee result in any hygienic bees in the F_2 generation?

Solution: American foulbrood is a disease of honeybee larvae caused by the pathogen Bacillus larvae. The immediate removal of the dead larvae from the hive is required for the maintenance of a safe, hygienic environment. If the diseased bees are not removed, they remain a source of continuous contamination. The honeybees have two independent genes which control their nest cleaning activities. One gene, U, controls the uncapping of cells and the other R, controls the removal of their contents. Bees of a hygienic colony have the genotype uurr.

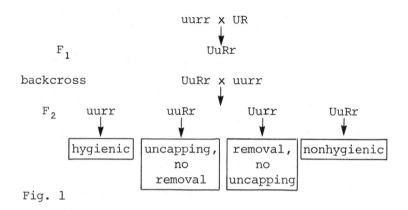

Fig. 1

The cross of a hygienic queen, uurr, and a nonhygienic drone, UR, and the backcross are outlined in the diagram shown in Figure 1.

From this cross, only one of the four offspring would have the genetic ability to both uncap the contaminated cell and remove the dead larvae.

● **PROBLEM 12-6**

How is the mating response in houseflies, <u>Musca domestica</u>, controlled?

<u>Solution</u>: Female houseflies produce (Z)-9-tricosene, a pheromone that attracts male flies. This pheromone has been named muscalure. The effects of the pheromone on the individual mating responses of different males was studied by using extracts containing the pheromone.

Pseudoflies were made from knotted black shoelaces

sprinkled with benzene extracts from female flies which contained the pheromone. Controls were made by sprinkling knotted shoelaces with only the solvent benzene. The quantity and quality of the pheromone, the female flies from which the chemical was extracted, and the light and the temperature were controlled in this study. A total of 347 males were individually observed in their responses.

The results of this experiment showed that two components of behavior are involved in the mating response. These are a pheromone-mediated attraction to the treated pseudoflies and the activity of the individual male flies. The pheromone-mediated attraction is under genetic control since a receptor protein is needed for chemical binding. The activity of the individual males is also under some sort of genetic control. Such characteristics as the number of mating strikes (number of times from flight to mount) are inheritable. Selective breeding from males with the most or fewest mating strikes was performed through the F_4 generation with virgin females. The responsiveness of each generation indicated the inheritance of genes from the parents.

● **PROBLEM 12-7**

Are there any mutations in mice that display behavioral as well as morphological, physiological or biochemical abnormalities?

Solution: To date, no genes have been found that affect behavior directly. The behavior changes that occur are the indirect result of genetic effects on hormones, enzymes, and cellular morphologies. In mice, there are many genes that create abnormal behaviors when mutated. Many of these mutations affect the nervous system during the development of the embryo. Others affect the morphology of the inner ear leading to disorder in the embryonic central nervous system.

These mutations have been given names that resemble those of the Seven Dwarfs: hairless, furless, short ear, pintail, looptail, waltzer, wobbler lethal, jerker, ducky, reeler, jumpy. All of these mutations affect the behavior of the carrier. However, the behavior is usually so abnormal that it is difficult to relate the mutant behavior to any normal behavior. Thus it is difficult to pinpoint genes which affect normal behaviors.

Some single gene mutations have been found that have an influence on behavior.

Gene	Phenotype	Behavior
Brown	Brown fur instead of black pigment	Increased grooming
Misty	Dilute fur color	Decreased nibbling
Pintail	Short tail	Fast avoidance instinct
Yellow	Yellow fur and black eyes	Failure of male to mate properly because of faulty courtship activities

These four mutations, along with ten others, were studied for their effect on behavior. Of the 14 genotypes tested, 71 percent showed an affect on behavior. This suggests that almost any mutation will be found to effect behavior as long as the analysis is comprehensive enough. In other words, it may be possible that every mutation affects behavior somewhat.

● **PROBLEM 12-8**

An abnormal behavior pattern called waltzing is seen in some mice. Waltzers twirl aimlessly and irregularly until they collapse exhausted. When waltzers and wild-type mice are crossed, the F_1 generation exhibits normal behavior but the F_2 generation produces normal and waltzer mice in a 3:1 ratio. Explain.

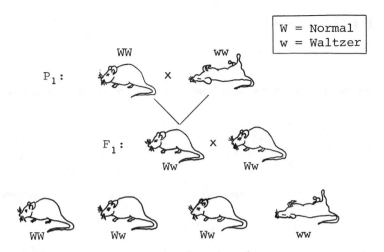

P₁: WW × ww

F₁: Ww × Ww

WW   Ww   Ww   ww

Fig. 1: Waltzing behavior in mice.

Solution: The waltzing behavior in mice has been associated with an abnormality in a single gene. This is an example of a behavioral trait that has direct genetic connections.

The 3:1 ratio indicates a Mendelian relationship. We can let WW represent the genotype of a mouse with normal behavior and let ww represent a mouse with waltzing behavior. We can see that a cross will yield the 3:1 ratio in the F_2 generation.

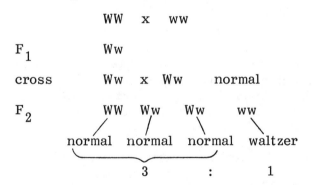

Thus, if the trait is inherited as an autosomal recessive, the 3:1 ratio will result. Since an abnormality in only one gene is sufficient to cause this behavior, a biochemical mechanism has been sought. A nervous disorder has been blamed. This disorder is associated with deafness and with abnormalities of the inner ear. In the homozygous recessive condition there is a lack of the correct information needed for the normal development of the inner ear. Thus, a physiological defect can lead to a behavioral abnormality.

VERTEBRATES

> Hybrids between two species of African parrots, Agapornis roseicollis and A. fischeri, have difficulty in preparing their nests. Why do these lovebirds have such difficulty?

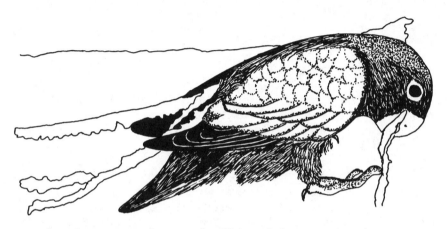

Fig. 1: Agapornis roseicollis with paper strips tucked between her feathers.

Solution: Each of these lovebird species has its own way of carrying nest-building material. Hybrids try to use both methods similtaneously and hence get confused. It takes the hybrids about three years before they can successfully build nests.

Agapornis roseicollis females carry strips of nesting material (bark, leaves or paper) tucked between their lower back feathers, Figure 1. They can carry several strips at one time. A. fischeri females carry the same types of nesting materials in addition to twigs individually in their beaks. Hybrids almost always try to carry the strips of material in their feathers; they are never successful. The hybrid bird awkwardly attempts to tuck the strips in its feathers. It uses the wrong movements and cannot carry any materials to its nest site. The hybrid female can only carry material in her beak, but it takes her three years to successfully learn this. Even then, she is not as adept at carrying strips as an A. fischeri female.

This behavior is controlled polygenically. But further studies of crosses need to be done for a more detailed analysis of the genes that control the nest-building activity of these birds.

● **PROBLEM 12-10**

What do you get when you cross a basenji, an African hunting dog, with a cocker spaniel?

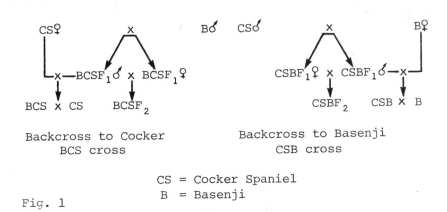

Backcross to Cocker
BCS cross

Backcross to Basenji
CSB cross

CS = Cocker Spaniel
B = Basenji

Fig. 1

Solution: This is a very complex question involving the genetics of behavior. In the 1960s, J.P. Scott and J.L. Fuller systematically varied the genetic constitution of dogs by performing crosses while keeping all other factors as constant as possible. Two of the breeds of dogs that they studied were basenji and cocker spaniel. These breeds are behaviorally very different. Cocker spaniels are nonaggressive and relate well to people. Basenjis are highly aggressive and fearful of humans when young. With handling and human contact, the basenjis tame rapidly.

The crosses that were carried out are shown in Figure 1.

The characteristics of each breed of dog shown in Table 1 were analyzed in the F_1, F_2 and backcrosses. Possible modes of inheritance were inferred from the data on the dog's behavior.

Table 1

Characteristic	Basenji	Cocker Spaniel	Mode of inheritance
1. Avoidance in reaction to handling	High	Low	One dominant gene for wildness
2. Struggle against restraint	High	Low	One gene with no dominance
3. Playful aggressiveness (13-15 weeks of age)	High	Low	Two genes with no dominance
4. Threshold of stimulation for barking	High	Low	Two dominant genes for low threshold
5. Tendency to bark a small number of times	High	Low	On gene with no dominance
6. Time of estrus	Annual	Semi-annual	Basenji type as a recessive gene

The modes of inheritance for these behaviors lie somewhere between a simple Mendelian inheritance pattern and polygenic inheritance. Complex traits such as behavior may be affected by very few genes, which is surprising since behavior seems so interrelated with environmental stimuli. Thus, to answer the original question, when we cross a basenji with a cocker spaniel we get a reliable way to study some behavioral genetics.

● **PROBLEM 12-11**

Do genetic factors influence human IQ performance?

Solution: Intelligence is defined as the ability to learn or understand. It is the requirement that is most important for achievement in the schools of the Western world. IQ (intelligence quotient) tests have been used as a basis to measure intelligence. Whether or not intelligence can be measured fairly, or even at all, in all populations by such a test is debatable. Attempts have been made to develop tests that measure intellectual ability cross-culturally, Figure 1. The analysis of various test scores of different groups of people and the comparison of the performances of siblings and twins have shown that the abilities measured by these tests has a hereditary basis. The environment that an individual is taught and raised in also has an effect on test scores. Because humans can never be totally separated from environmental influences by being placed in controlled experimental situations, the exact genetic basis of intelligence is extremely difficult to determine. However, several studies indicate that both the environment and genetics can influence IQ performance.

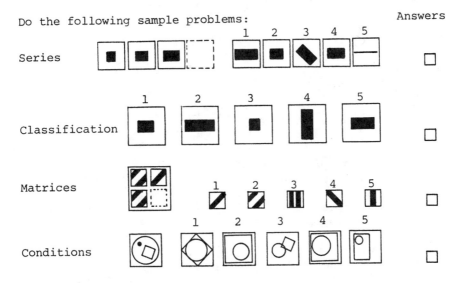

Fig. 1 A culturally fair test.

Twin studies have indicated that heritability is important in the acquisition of intelligence in a child. These studies have shown that the closer the degree of relationship, the higher the correlation coefficient (a high coefficient indicates heritability). A genetic component to intelligence has been implicated because twins (both mono- and dizygotic) that were reared apart (different environmental influences), and twins that were reared together (similar environmental influences), showed this high coefficient.

Studies of adopted children indicate that the environment has a large role in the development of the type of intelligence that is measured by intelligence tests, Figure 2. Adopted children's IQ scores show more correlation with those of their biological mother than with those of their adoptive mother. The prenatal environment also influences IQ scores. In 1956, R.F. Harrell, E.R. Woodyard and A.I. Gates published a study which showed that dietary supplementation during the last half of pregnancy had a positive effect on the IQ scores of their children later on. Children whose mothers had an enriched diet during pregnancy scored higher on intelligence tests than children whose mothers did not.

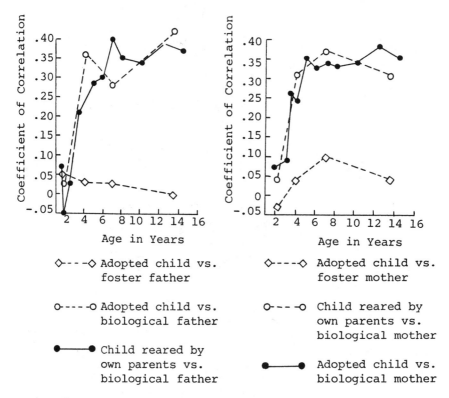

◇- - -◇ Adopted child vs. foster father

○- - - -○ Adopted child vs. biological father

●———● Child reared by own parents vs. biological father

◇- - - -◇ Adopted child vs. foster mother

○- - - ○ Child reared by own parents vs. biological mother

●———● Adopted child vs. biological mother

Fig. 2 Correlation of the IQ of children with the educational level of actual and foster parents.

In 1965, R.B. Cattell defined two components of general ability. These components encompass both hereditary and environmental influences. The first he called fluid intelligence, which is a function of brain development. This type of intelligence is completed by age 14 when the brain stops growing. It can theoretically be measured by tests that are free of cultural and environmental bias. The second component is crystallized intelligence. This component is a function of training and education. It, unlike fluid intelligence, can change after the completion of brain growth.

Problems are very easily encountered when data

concerning intelligence are analyzed. In 1969, Arthur Jensen concluded that white people do better than black people on IQ tests because of a hereditary difference. He argued that one half to three quarters of the difference between IQ scores was due to genetic factors. His theory cannot be proved or disproved because the experimental situation needed is unavailable and probably unobtainable. But since the publication of his paper, many reports have been published that dispute his claims. For instance, the difference in the IQ scores of northern groups is less than the difference between southern populations. Also, blacks and whites generally segregate into separate residential areas and hence schools. The schools that teach black students are less adequate than those that teach white students, since the blacks tend to live in economically deprived areas. Therefore, the same number of years in school does not amount to the same level of education. Studies have also shown that blacks score higher when tested by blacks than when tested by whites. These and many other variables, such as diet, cultural beliefs and societal attitudes, interplay to such an extent that Jensen's hypothesis has been almost completely discredited.

It has been noted that if a problem of this type were encountered in studies of laboratory animals, it would have been resolved long ago because their genotypes can be replicated and their environments controlled. Human populations have been morally barred from such studies, so the scientific proof necessary for judgement on the extent that genes play in the acquisition of intelligence is not available. Many more studies are needed before any definite conclusions can be reached. For the time being, however, it appears that environmental factors influence the extent to which the full genetic potential regarding intelligence is reached.

● **PROBLEM 12-12**

Can an extra Y chromosome (XYY) modify behavior?

Solution: In 1967, a study in a maximum security hospital in Scotland suggested that the antisocial behavior of some of the inmates was due to an XYY chromosome set. W. Price and P. Whatmore compared the crimes and sex-chromosomes of a group of men. They concluded from their examination of the men and their lives that the XYY males did not have a family background that was responsible for their wayward behavior. They blamed the men's behavior on their extra Y chromosome.

This conclusion is conveniently reached. D.L. Rimoin and R.N. Schimke indicate that XYY may occur in as many as 1 in 300 live births and that this is more frequent than the incidence of troublesome behavior. A survey in England has not revealed the significantly greater incidence of XYY men in institutions that would be expected in nonrandom distributions.

The extra Y chromosome may predispose a male to a more aggressive attitude. However, with the amount of environmental factors that influence behavior, a genetic basis for man's violent and antisocial behavior is extremely difficult to isolate and identify.

● **PROBLEM** 12-13

Is there a genetic basis for schizophrenia?

Solution: Schizophrenia affects people of all countries, races and socioeconomic groups. Estimates of its occurance range from 1 percent of the population to 2.9 percent. There are varying degrees of schizophrenia, but almost all schizophrenics tend to withdraw from reality so that they cannot distinguish between their own inner fantasies and the physical realities of the outside world.

There are two groups of theories of genetic influence on schizophrenia: monogenic and polygenic. Monogenic theories cite a single crucial genetic locus as the determinant of whether schizophrenia will manifest. A monogenic theory issued by I.L. Heston includes both cases of schizophrenia and schizoidia (a pre- or potentially schizophrenic state). When these cases are considered together, the number of observed cases approximates the proportions expected if the influence of a single dominant gene is assumed. Polygenic theories blame many gene loci for the manifestation of the disorder. Most of these theories concur with the diathesis-stress theory proposed by D. Rosenthal. This theory states that the schizophrenic does not inherit schizophrenia itself but is genetically predisposed to develop it. Environmental stress induces schizophrenia in predisposed individuals. The environmental stress could disturb a number of relatively minor genes which exhibit little or no dominance or recessiveness. The effect could then be additive; greater environmental stress causes higher degrees of schizophrenia. Theories of this sort do not exclude the possibility of the involvement of multiple alleles. Thus, different alleles could produce different degrees of effect.

A genetic basis for schizophrenia is implicated through twin studies and biochemical studies. In dizygotic twins the concordance rate is from 4 to 10 percent. Monozygotic twins show a concordance of from 25 to 40 percent. The higher concordance in monozygotic twins implies that the genotype of the individual has an influence on the occurance of schizophrenia. Biochemical analyses of schizophrenics have shown abnormal neurochemical activity. Monoamine oxidase, which inactivates some neurotransmitters, has been found in less than normal levels of activity in schizophrenics. Serotonin, a neurotransmitter present in platelets, of schizophrenics, is significantly different from normal platelet serotonin.

The genetics of a disorder such as schizophrenia are very complex because of the tremendous amount of influencing factors and the great deal of diversity that is observed in those with the abnormality.

● **PROBLEM** 12-14

About 0.5 percent of the American population have epilepsy, the falling sickness. Discuss the genetics of this disease.

Solution: Epilepsy is a nervous disorder which usually results from injuries to the cerebral cortex. Such damage can be from heredity, infection or trauma. Some doctors have singled out the hereditary basis of epilepsy as the most important.

Epileptic attacks occur when neurons are discharged in a spontaneous and uncontrolled fashion. When these discharges spread for short distances, the attacks are mild. However, when the discharges spread for long distances, severe seizures containing convulsions and unconsciousness result.

This disease is due to an autosomal recessive trait. One form of epilepsy follows Mendelian inheritance so it is passed from heterozygous parents to their children with a 1/4 ratio. Studies of twins show that the concordance in monozygotic twins is higher than the concordance in dizygotic twins. Thus the genotype plays a very important part in the acquisition of epilepsy.

● **PROBLEM** 12-15

Are there any differences in sensory, perceptual and motor processes among races?

Fig. 1

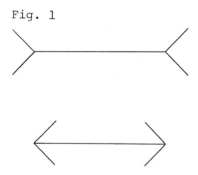

Solution: Not many studies have attempted to investigate genetic aspects of sensory and motor processes. The answer to this question is therefore very sketchy.

Late in the 1800s, American Indian subjects were found to have the lowest average latency for reaction time to visual, auditory and tactile stimuli. African-Caucasian hybrids followed and Caucasians were the slowest to react. In a later study, Torres Strait Islanders were found to have greater visual acuity than European groups. Weight discrimination, pain threshold and olfactory acuity were discussed by Spuhler and Lindzey in 1967. More recent studies have shown that certain illusions, such as the Muller-Lyer illusion shown in Figure

1, are more common among Americans than among African Bushmen.

At the present however, there is little compelling evidence, one way or the other, for racial difference or equality in sensory and motor processes.

SHORT ANSWER QUESTIONS FOR REVIEW

Choose the correct answer.

1. E. coli has genes which code for the production
   of _____ which are sensitive to a given chem-
   -ical concentration. (a) neurotransmitters (b)
   enzymes (c) receptor molecules (d) none of
   the above   c

2. The receptors in E. coli are the same for (a)
   galactose and glucose. (b) galactose and
   fructose. (c) fructose and glucose. (d) all of
   the above   b

3. E. coli has the advantage of having chemoreceptors which respond to changes in (a)
   temperature. (b) concentration. (c) surface
   tension. (d) density. (e) all of the above   b

4. It is highly beneficial for E. coli to have
   chemoreptors because the chemoreceptors can
   (a) signal for quick movement away from a
   toxic substance. (b) help maintain E. coli in
   a favorable surface tension. (c) detect
   concentrations of substances and help E. coli
   remain in a favorable concentration. (d) both
   b and c   c

5. The Bastock experiment with the yellow and
   wild type Drosophila flies demonstrated a
   difference in mating behavior. The results
   Bastock obtained indicate the the genes coding
   for (a) yellow color would disappear. (b) yellow
   color would increase in the population. (c) any
   trait cannot be analyzed individually; the whole
   genotype should be taken into account.   c

6. The nest cleaning behavior of bees is controlled
   by (a) one gene. (b) two genes. (c) three
   genes. (d) all the genotypes.   b

7. In the housefly Musca domestica, the female
   produces a pheromone which attracts males.
   In the male, the genes code for (a) a protein
   which acts as the receptor. (b) a specific
   neurological network. (c) the formation of a
   sex-specific brain area. (d) none of the above   a

8. Many of the studies on the inheritance of

480

vertebrate behavior are conducted on mice because mice, like pea plants, (a) have a prototypical genetic make up. (b) have simple behaviors. (c) are inexpensive to keep and produce a large progeny every few months. (d) are vertebrates. (e) both a and c

c

9. The behavioral changes that occur in mice can usually be traced to (a) a few mutated genes. (b) the effect of mutated genes on hormones and enzymes. (c) the effect of mutated genes on cellular morphology. (d) both a and c

d

10. In general, it is very difficult to isolate vertebrate genes which control certain behaviors because (a) there is no correlation between vertebrate behavior and genotype. (b) in vertebrates, every single gene may affect behavior somewhat. (c) in vertebrates, behavior is not genetically controlled.

b

11. The cross between two heterozygous waltzer mice (Ww) produced a ratio of 3 non-waltzers: 1 waltzer in the F_1 generation. What is the mode of inheritance of the waltzer trait? (a) sex-linked recessive (b) epistatic (c) autosomal recessive (d) sex-linked dominant.

c

12. The nest building behavior of love birds is controlled by (a) many genes. (b) one autosomal gene. (c) a holandric gene. (d) a gene on the X chromosome.

a

13. A hybrid resulting from a cross between an A. fischeri and an A. roseicollis takes ____ to efficiently learn nest building. (a) 5 years (b) 3 years (c) 2 years (d) 1 year

b

14. Estrus cycles are more or less stereotypic behaviors in the cocker spaniel and the basenji breed of dogs. The results of several crosses between these two breeds indicated that estrus timing is controlled by a (a) dominant gene in the basenji breed. (b) dominant gene in the cocker spaniel breed. (c) a recessive gene in the basenji breed. (d) none of the above

a

15. In 1969, Arthur Jensen argued that black people scored lower than whites in I.Q. tests because of a difference in heredity. This theory cannot be proved or disproved because (a) Jensen was not qualified to make such statements. (b) the genes for intelligence are the same for blacks and whites. (c) the experimental conditions were not controlled. (d) none of the above

c

16. W. Price and P. Whatman concluded from their study on the behavior of male criminals that aggressive behavior in man was due to (a) an extra Y chromosome (XYY). (b) an extra X chromosome (XXY). (c) 2 extra Y chromosomes (XYYY). (d) 2 extra X chromosomes (XXXY).

a

17. The diathesis-stress theory proposes that schizophrenia is (a) monogenically inherited. (b) polygenically inherited. (c) epistatic to a normal gene. (d) induced by environmental stress when the predisposing gene is present.

d

Fill in the blanks.

18. The movement by an organism toward or away from a chemical is called _____.

chemotaxis

19. The yellow Drosophila male courts the female for a shorter period of time than the _____ male.

wild type

20. _____ is movement oriented toward or away from gravity.

Geotaxis

21. Flies that cannot orient themselves over vertical planes exhibit _____ geotaxis.

negative

22. The specific cleaning behavior of bees involves the _____ of cells and the _____ of their contents.

uncapping
removal

23. The female housefly produces _____, a pheromone which attracts the male fly.

muscalure

24. The waltzing disorder of mice is associated with deafness and abnormal development of the _____.

inner ear

	Answer To be covered when testing yourself

25. The A. fischeri love birds carry nest materials on their back feathers and also carry twigs in their _____ . — beaks

26. The results of crosses between the cocker spaniel and the basenji dog breed showed that wildness is inherited through one _____ gene. — dominant

27. The _____ environment of an individual, as well as his outside environment, have a marked effect on the development of intelligence. — pre-natal

28. The genetic component of intelligence has been termed _____ intelligence. — fluid

29. Schizophrenia is believed to be _____ influenced. — mono-genically

30. Biochemical analysis of schizophrenics have shown that they have less than normal levels of the enzyme _____ . — monoamine-oxidase

31. Epilepsy has been found to be an _____ _____ trait. — autosomal recessive

Determine whether the following statements are true or false.

32. E. coli is attracted to galactose and fructose when the concentration is not too high. — True

33. In Drosophila, the yellow female is much more responsive to a shorter courting series than the wild type. — True

34. Flies that orient themselves on vertical planes exhibit positive geotaxis. — True

35. The dusting behavior in bees is controlled by a single gene. — False

36. Hygienic behavior in bees is controlled by two linked genes. — False

37. The mating behavior of the housefly, Musca domestica is controlled by the environment. — False

38. Studies show that only three specific genes control grooming behavior in mice.

False

39. The mating sequence of the male housefly is probably controlled by a single gene.

True

40. Many of the mutations that occur in mice, which produce abnormal behavior, also produce abnormal central nervous system morphology.

True

41. Agapornis roseicollis love birds build their nest by carrying strips of materials on their back feathers and on their beaks.

False

42. Regardless of one's culture, the I.Q. test is a reliable measure of intelligence.

False

43. Only 1/3 of the expression of intelligence is controlled by the environment.

False

44. The hereditary component of intelligence can be determined by comparing I.Q. scores of two separate populations.

False

45. The genetic basis of sensory and motor processes were clearly defined in the late 1800's.

False

CHAPTER 13

IMMUNOGENETICS

BASICS

● **PROBLEM** 13-1

What is the difference between T cells and B cells?

Solution: T cells and B cells are activated forms of lymphocytes that result in response to antigens. Morphologically, T and B cells are indistinguishable from each other. They arise from the same type of undifferentiated stem cell. Their difference lies in the location in which they differentiate and in their function.

Figure 1 shows how a stem cell originating from bone marrow can differentiate into two types of cell. T cells arise when the stem cells migrate to the thymus. B cells arise when the stem cells migrate to an intestinal gland, called the bursa, in chickens.

An animal whose thymus has been removed is unable to mount a cell-mediated attack on antigens. Likewise, an animal whose bursa has been removed cannot produce circulating antibodies. T cells, when activated by an antigen, can produce lymphokines that act in the cell-mediated immune response. When B cells are activated, they produce antibodies which react with freely circulating antigens in the humoral immune response.

Fig. 1

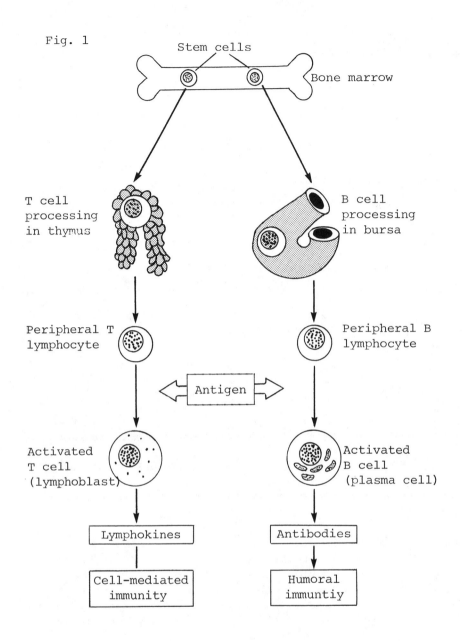

Stem cells

Bone marrow

T cell
processing
in thymus

B cell
processing
in bursa

Peripheral T
lymphocyte

Peripheral B
lymphocyte

Antigen

Activated
T cell
(lymphoblast)

Activated
B cell
(plasma cell)

Lymphokines

Antibodies

Cell-mediated
immunity

Humoral
immuntiy

● **PROBLEM 13-2**

Describe the structure of an antibody molecule.

Solution: Purified antibody molecules have been obtained from individuals with multiple myelomas. Multiple myelomas are cancerous antibody-producing tumors. Individuals with this form of cancer can make only one kind of antibody. The immunoglobulins can be collected from the blood or urine of affected individuals. These "purified" proteins have been analyzed extensively and their structure has been revealed in considerable detail.

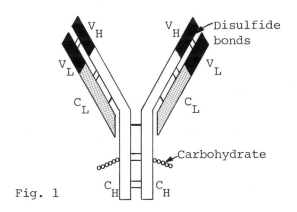

Fig. 1

Antibody molecules consist of four polypeptide chains. Two of the chains are long and are called the heavy (H) chains. These chains are identical to one another. The other two chains are shorter and are called the light (L) chains. The light chains are identical in an individual molecule. In human immunoglobulins, there are two types of light chains, kappa (κ) and lambda (λ). The light and heavy chains are held together by disulfide bonds. Each chain, whether light or heavy, has a constant portion and a variable portion. These regions line up to give the antibody molecule its unique Y shape. Most of the specificity of an antibody molecule is due to the variable portions of the four chains. These areas constitute the antigen binding sites of the molecule. The constant areas are relatively constant from one antibody molecule to another. They are responsible for somehow eliciting the immune responses of the organism.

There are five types of human immunoglobulins, (Ig). They are: IgG, IgM, IgA, IgD and IgE. Each of these have characteristic structures and functions. IgG molecules constitute about 80 percent of the antibodies in the blood serum. It is by far the best studied antibody class. These are the antibodies that are involved in the destruction of most invading antigens. IgM molecules are the first immunoglobulins to appear in response to an antigen. IgA molecules are found in saliva, tears and milk. The function of IgD is unknown, but it is also found in milk. IgE is involved in allergic reactions. There are four types of IgG heavy chains, γ_1, γ_{2a}, γ_{2b} and γ_3. There are similar notations used to describe the types of heavy chains of the other classes of immunoglobulins: IgM has μ types, IgA has α types, IgD has δ and IgE has ε. Thus, if 20 different human IgG molecules are examined, 11 might have the κ type of constant region on their light chains (C_κ) and the remaining 9 might have the λ variety. Of the 11 with κ types, 5 might have γ_1 heavy chains, 3 might have γ_{2a} and 3 might have γ_{2b} heavy chains. Thus even the constant regions of antibody molecules are varied. The variable regions are much more varied. This gives antibodies the tremendous amount of variety that they need for the recognition of many different antigens. The precise arrangement of genes in the chromosome enables such diversity in one type of protein molecule.

● **PROBLEM** 13-3

Any protein can elicit an antibody response. How can an organism make so many specific antibodies?

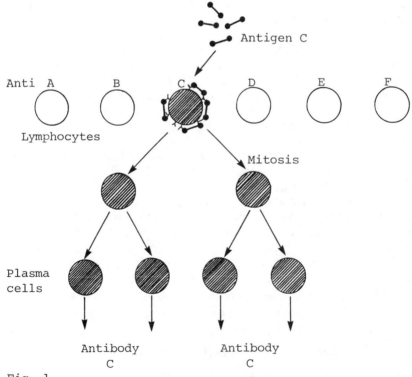

Fig. 1

Solution: The clonal selection theory was proposed in the 1950s by Sir Macfarlane Burnet to explain immunity. His theory states that millions of specific lymphocytes exist in the body. Each secretes an antibody that is specific for a single antigen. When the antigen is introduced to the body, its specific antibody becomes activated. It divides mitotically to form a clone of identical cells (see Figure 1). Each of these cells is specific for that antigen. When these lymphocytes are no longer needed, they circulate in a relatively unreactive state throughout the body.

The next time the same antigen is encountered, the cell's immune response is much quicker since the supply of the specific antibody producing lymphocytes has been greatly increased by the mitotic process. The persistence of these long-lived lymphocytes is the basis for immunological memory.

● **PROBLEM** 13-4

Supposing that the clonal selection theory is correct; how can an organism genetically make such diverse proteins?

Solution: There are three theories that account for this diversity. They are the germline hypothesis, the somatic mutation theory, and the rearrangement theory.

The germline hypothesis states that all of the possible sequences are carried in the DNA. This means that each mammalian genome would need to carry the information to make more than 10^8 antibodies.

The somatic mutation theory says that the actual number of antibody genes was initially small. The diversity arose through mutation. This implies that the immunoglobulin system is very random.

The rearrangement theory suggests that separated germline sequences come together in all possible combinations via recombination. The variable gene segments can come together in this way to create immense diversity.

To some extent, all of these theories are based on actual mechanisms. These mechanisms, among others, diversify the antibody sequences so that the millions of antigens can be recognized by a single class of protein.

Distinguish between the germline hypothesis, the somatic recombination hypothesis and the somatic hypermutation hypothesis.

Solution: These three very different theories attempt to explain the mechanism of how different variable-region sequences are generated. They try to answer the questions about when and how the diversity is generated.

The germline hypothesis starts with the assumption that the diversity is already present in the genome. This implies that a very large number (greater than 10^4) of genes exist in the genome. Thus, the diversity of the variable regions arose in the course of evolution by mutation and selection.

The somatic recombination hypothesis assumes a much smaller number of genes (about 100) for the variable regions of antibodies. Throughout the lifetime of an individual, these similar genes undergo recombination in the antibody-producing cell. Recombination among 100 genes could lead to millions of combinations and, hence, enormous variability is possible. This type of mechanism is not evolutionary; it occurs somatically, throughout the life of an individual.

The somatic hypermutation hypothesis disregards polygenic variability. It assumes that there is only one gene for the variable region of a particular subclass. Point mutations in this region can then create the diversity that is found in antibody molecules. An extremely high mutation rate would then be needed to produce the amount of diversity that is required for a lifetime of immunity. This may be achieved by a DNA repair mechanism designed especially to make mistakes in the antibody-producing cell. This theory is, again, somatic rather than evolutionary.

All of these mechanisms are probably used by the immune system in order to create the diversity of antibodies needed to fight antigens. For instance, somatic mutation may be responsible for the variation in the V_λ genes, of which there are only two in mice. In contrast, there are at least 4500 kinds of V_K genes that are formed by the recombinations of V and J regions. Thus, the somatic recombination hypothesis has applications. The germline mechanism is evident in the existence of 4500 light chain genes. Thus the three mechanisms, although very different, are probably used to create enormous diversity among antibody molecules.

GENES

● **PROBLEM** 13-6

Explain the following experimental results:

Labelled myeloma mRNA from a mouse hybridizes to DNA that has been cut in half by the restriction enzyme EcoRI, Figure 1.

When the same experiment is performed with mouse embryonic cells, the hybridization pattern is as shown in Figure 2.

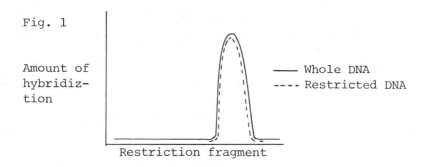

Fig. 1

Amount of hybridiz-tion

——— Whole DNA
---- Restricted DNA

Restriction fragment

Solution: This experiment was done in the mid 1970s by Hoziumi and Tonegawa. The results of this experiment revealed information about the construction of immunoglobulin genes.

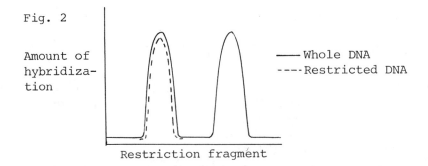

Fig. 2

Amount of hybridiza-tion

——Whole DNA
----Restricted DNA

Restriction fragment

In general, hybridization techniques are used to find if a particular sequence is on a piece of DNA. Specific pieces of mRNA will hybridize to homologous areas of DNA under certain conditions. By radioactively labelling the mRNA, the amount of hybridization, and hence homology, can be determined by autoradiography. In this experiment, myelomas were used as a source of mRNA. Since myelomas produce only one type of immunoglobulin, samples of mRNA that are greater than 50% pure can be obtained. This mRNA can be used to probe for antibody genes on DNA. The DNA was cut by the restriction enzyme EcoRI. This enzyme recognizes a specific palindrome in the DNA, where it makes its cut. EcoRI cuts the particular DNA molecule, where the antibody-specifying sequences reside, in half. This enables investigators to locate a homologous region of the DNA more precisely.

The first graph of the experimental results shows that both the whole DNA and the restricted DNA can hybridize to the mRNA. In other words, the mRNA that was transcribed from the antibody-specifying gene can bind to an area of the DNA that was not disrupted by the action of EcoRI. The sequence for antibody production lies on one restriction fragment and is therefore one gene. A sequence that contains more than one gene would be disrupted by the restriction enzyme. The second graph shows a difference between embryonic and differentiated DNA. There are now two areas on the uncut DNA to which the mRNA can bind. Only one of these regions appears when EcoRI is used. This implies that the second region is cut by the enzyme. This indicates that embryonic DNA has two antibody-specifying genes.

As a whole, these sub-experiments have shown that two embryonic genes join to form the single segment found in differentiated cells. Further experimentation has shown that in the embryo one of these genes encodes the variable portion of an immunoglobulin molecule and the other encodes the constant portion.

Describe how the variable region of embryonic light chains are genetically processed to yield antibody diversity in the differentiated organism.

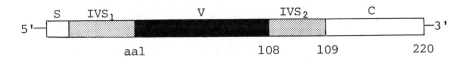

aal   108   109   220

S = signal sequence
IVS = intervening sequence
V = varible
C = constant

Fig. 1: Numbers refer to position of amino acid in completed antibody molecule.

Solution: The previous problem described how it was found that mouse embryonic genomes contain two antibody genes. More detailed analyses have revealed further differences between the embryonic and differentiated (or adult) genome. A major difference has been found that helps to diversify the variable regions of the light chain.

An adult DNA sequence resembles the diagram shown in Figure 1.

This differs drastically from the same area of the embryonic genome shown in Figure 2.

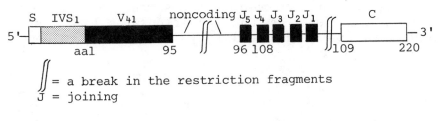

aal   95   96 108   109   220

$\int\!\!\int$ = a break in the restriction fragments
J = joining

Fig. 2

To make the adult V region, one of the J regions joins with V_{41}. The noncoding regions are spliced out and the remaining J sequences become IVS_2. How this splicing is regulated is unknown. The IVS_2 of the adult DNA is also removed by splicing of the RNA. This brings the V and C regions together to enable translation to occur.

There are up to 200 different regions in a cell. If this number is multiplied by the number of functional J regions, which is 4 since J_3 is nonfunctional, there is a total of 800 possible light chains. Even further variability is introduced at amino acid 96 due to the recombination process. Amino acid 96 lies near the antigen binding site so its change can confer changes in the specificity of the binding site.

● **PROBLEM** 13-8

How are the variable portions of heavy chains combined to create diversity in the antibody sequences?

Solution: The variable portions of heavy chains are organized like the variable portions of light chains. The major difference between them is that three separate DNA regions must be combined in heavy chains. These regions are called V, D (for diversity) and J_H. In heavy chains two joining events, V-D and VD-J, must occur.

DNA hybridization studies have detected 10 D regions. The current estimates for V and J_H regions are 200 and 4 respectively. The possible V-D-J_H joining reactions can make 200 x 10 x 4 = 8000 different variable genes for heavy chains.

Since the sequences for the heavy chains and light chains are on separate chromosomes, recombination between them is rare. This almost ensures that a light chain's variable sequence does not combine with a heavy chain's J sequence.

● **PROBLEM** 13-9

How can the genes for an IgM molecule encode for an IgG molecule with the same specificity later in the immune response?

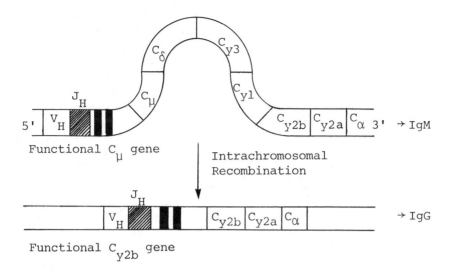

Fig. 1

Solution: The five immunoglobulin classes, IgM, IgG, IgD, IgA, and IgE, differ only in the constant regions of their heavy chains. These constant regions are encoded by a cluster of genes on the same chromosome. Class switching is the term used to describe the change from one immunoglobulin class to another.

There are two recombination events that are needed in order for IgG to be produced, see Figure 1. The first event attaches a V_H gene to a C_μ gene at one of the J segments. This sequence is used to synthesize IgM. The second recombination event attaches $V_H J_H$ to a C_γ gene. The IgG molecule which is synthesized from this sequence has the same variable sequences as the previous immunoglobulin and, hence, the same specificity.

● **PROBLEM** 13-10

How can crosses involving strains of highly inbred mice be used to determine a genetic basis for transplant incompatibility?

Solution: Mouse strains that are homozygous at nearly all loci can be obtained by mating brothers and sisters for many generations. Different inbred strains will have different alleles that are homozygous. We can test two such inbred strains for histocompatibility.

| | RECIPIENT | | |
DONOR	MALE PARENT STRAIN	FEMALE PARENT STRAIN	PROGENY
Male parent strain	+(1)	−(2)	+(3)
Female parent strain	−(2)	+(1)	+(3)
Progeny	−(4)	−(4)	+(3)

(1) grafts within a strain
(2) grafts between strains
(3) grafts from parents or siblings
(4) grafts from progeny

Table 1

Any skin transplant made within a strain is readily and permanently accepted. A transplant between two individuals of different strains does not take. When these strains are crossed and the F_1 generation is tested for hybrid graft rejection, the results are as in Table 1. These results show that a graft from either parent or from the hybrid will be accepted when the recipient is a hybrid. The results also show that a graft from the F_1 hybrid will not take on either of the parents, but it will on siblings.

This experiment suggests that transplant rejection (or acceptance) has a genetic basis. It also suggests that codominant alleles are involved because the progeny exhibit antigenic properties of both of the parents.

TRANSPLANT REJECTION

● PROBLEM 13-11

The rejection of foreign skin grafts in mice depends on a group of antigenic proteins on the cell surfaces that the immune system recognizes as foreign. Describe the genes that code for these proteins.

Solution: The histocompatibility complex is the system that differentiates "self" from "nonself". The system probably evolved to protect the body from its own cells when they are infected with viruses or become cancerous. However, medical practices have shown the importance of this recognition system in regard to transplants from one individual to another. The lymphocytes of the immune system that are involved in this response are called T cells since they are secreted by the thymus. T cells can migrate to various lymphoid tissues around the body to elicit cell-mediated immunity. This immunity is possible because the histocompatibility complex codes for cell surface antigens that differ from individual to individual.

So far, all of the organisms that have been studied have one major histocompatibility complex (MHC). In humans, this complex (HLA) is on chromosome 6 and in mice, the complex (H-2) is on chromosome 17. In addition to the major locus, there are many minor loci. These genetic loci code for the cell-surface antigens. The major locus gives rise to antigens that evoke a more vigorous response than the antigens specified by the minor loci.

In humans and mice, three polymorphic genes are responsible for producing the proteins involved in cell-mediated immunity. In mice the genes code for three very different classes of protein that are the histocompatibility complex antigens on cell surfaces. Class I proteins are found on almost all cell surfaces. They are the antigens that are recognized as foreign in transplants. They elicit the cytotoxic activity of killer T cells in the host. Class II proteins are suppressor and helper proteins. Found only on lymphocytes, these molecules control the extent of certain immunological responses. Class III proteins are several components of the complement system. The complement system contains proteins in the blood serum that destroy antigenic cells once they have been bound by antibodies. Complement provides binding sites of its own to aid in the removal of the antigenic cells. Complement proteins can also make holes in the plasma membrane of foreign cells. The class III proteins are a link between an immune response and the destruction of an unwanted foreign cell.

The three genes are inherited as a closely linked group. This gives great specificity to an individual's histocompatibility complex. A daughter cell will receive a block of these genes from the mother and another from the father. Since the genes are highly polymorphic and the alleles of both gametes are expressed, there are many possible allelic combinations; except in identical twins, exact matches are rare. This leads to many kinds of cell surface antigens giving individuality to an organism's cells. An organism will have cells that contain antigens that are different from those of virtually all other cells. The basis for skin graft rejection lies in this difference.

● **PROBLEM** 13-12

Differentiate between killer T cells (cytotoxic T-lymphocytes), helper T cells and suppressor T cells. What are the functions of each?

Solution: T cells are secreted by the thymus. They are the lymphocytes utilized in the cell-mediated immune response. They are part of the histocompatibility complex.

Cytotoxic T-lymphocytes, or killer T cells, are responsible for skin graft rejection, killing tumor cells and killing virus infected cells. These T cells recognize foreign cells and abnormal cells in ways that the humoral system cannot. The humoral system works through the blood and responds to free antigens. The cell-mediated immune system responds to antigens bound to cell surfaces.

Helper T cells interact with B-lymphocytes of the humoral immune system to enable them to produce antibody molecules. Macrophages are also involved in this reaction:

Helper T cell+macrophage+B-lymphocyte→antibody

Suppressor T cells suppress, and hence, mediate the activities of killer and helper T cells.

The T-lymphocytes work to rid the body of unwanted foreign cells. They interact in ways that are not fully understood. Someday we may understand their interaction and be able to use the knowledge to our medical advantage.

498

A mouse of strain A was infected with viral strain 1, creating A_1 cells. The spleen was removed after one week. The T cells were extracted from the spleen and tested against various cells: noninfected A cells (A); noninfected cells of mouse strain B (B); A cells infected with viral strain 2 (A_2); A cells infected with viral strain 1 (A_1); and B cells infected with viral strain 1 (B_1). The following results were observed:

A	no killing
B	no killing
A_2	no killing
A_1	killing
B_1	no killing

Explain these results in terms of cell-mediated immunity.

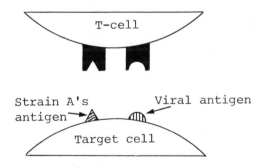

Solution: This experiment was performed by Peter Dougherty and Rolf Zinkernagel of the Australian National University. The results led them to propose a theory about the cell-mediated immune response.

The cell-mediated immune response was elicited when the mouse of strain A was infected with virus 1. The immune response was given one week to produce lymphocytes specific for the viral antigen. The T cells that were removed from the spleen were specific for its own cells that had been infected by virus 1, (A_1 cells). The results show that the T-lymphocytes can kill only those cells. The T cells could not kill A cells alone. This was an expected result because otherwise normal cells of the mouse would have been killed - an autoimmune response. A different virus was not recognized even when it was in the proper cell type, A_2. The T cells could not recognize B cells or B_1 cells. This indicates that the virus alone could not be recognized even when it was in a cell foreign to the system. The virus was only recognized by these specific T cells when it was in the A type cell. Therefore, two receptors on the T cell must match perfectly with the infected cell to elicit an immune response, see diagram. The T cell has a receptor that recognizes the cell type and a receptor that recognizes the viral type. This is called the dual receptor theory.

● **PROBLEM** 13-14

How can mutation and recombination contribute to the process of tissue graft rejection?

Solution: In a solution to a previous problem, it was mentioned that there are two groups of histocompatibility loci - the major locus and the minor loci. This creates different groups of antigens on the surfaces of cells:

H = antigens of an individual's own major histocompatibility complex

X = antigens of the individual's own minor histocompatibility complex

H' = antigens of a foreign major histocompatibility complex

X' = antigens of a foreign minor histocompatibility complex

A T cell must recognize one of its own sequences to elicit an immune response. Thus, T cells can recognize HX' or H'X cells. They do not respond to HX or to H'X' cells. This can be explained by mutation and recombination that occurs during T cell maturation in the thymus.

The thymus is composed of two zones - the outer cortex and the medulla. The outer cortex contains large lymphocytes that are undergoing rapid division in spite of an absence of foreign antigen. The medulla contains smaller inactive lymphocytes that are not dividing. Experiments using labelled stem cells show that they enter the cortex, divide and then go to the medulla or the bloodstream. Many cells die of exhaustion in the cortex. They are T cells that have the makeup HX. They respond to their own antigen, divide rapidly and then die. The only cells that escape death are those that, through mutation or recombination, have become H'X' or HX'. These leave the thymus and become killer T cells. H'X' cells involve a double mutational or recombination event which is highly unlikely. Therefore, H'X' do not survive to become killer T cells.

● **PROBLEM** 13-15

What do the diseases myasthenia gravis, rheumatoid arthritis and multiple sclerosis have in common?

Solution: These disorders are autoimmune diseases. They are characterized by immune responses against cells of the individual's own body; "self" cells are recognized as "nonself". The exact causes of autoimmune diseases are speculative. Mutations in a protein may cause the protein to be so changed that it elicits an antibody response. Mutations could also affect the cells of the immune system so that they recognize "self" cells as foreign invaders and destroy them. A virus that has been repressed may be derepressed and it may synthesize an antigen that triggers antibody production. The exact etiology of these diseases is not known. However, their symptoms indicate that the immune system is attacking its own cells. "Self" cells are recognized as "non-self" and destroyed.

Myasthenia gravis, in Latin, describes a grave problem which causes muscles to have no strength. After the muscle of an affected individual has been used a few times, it loses its power to contract. With sufficient rest it will contract again, so it is not a form of paralysis. Somehow, antibodies are made against the individual's own acetylcholine receptors. This leads to defective neuromuscular transmission. Since the removal of the thymus drastically improves a patient's condition, the immune system, specifically the T-lymphocytes, is involved in this autoimmune response.

Rheumatoid arthritis is a chronic inflammatory condition that affects the small joints of the hands and feet. The factor that causes this condition is found in the blood of affected individuals. The rheumatoid factor is a macroglobulin antibody or antigen-antibody complex which originates in the lymphocytes and plasma cells. The disease is characterized by a superabundance of these cells. They attack many joints in the body and lead to the destruction of the articular cartilage.

Multiple sclerosis is a disease of the nervous system that shows its symptoms in individuals around 30 years old. It is chracterized by the presence of demyelination associated with the hardening (sclerosis) of scattered areas of gray and white matter of the brain stem and spinal cord. The nerve fibers degenerate and are replaced by scar tissue. Most patients have antibodies to measles virus present. Another possible viral origin is the virus that causes canine distemper. Patients usually belong to two HLA groups, so the disease may be an inherited abnormality of the major histocompatibility complex.

SHORT ANSWER QUESTIONS FOR REVIEW

Choose the correct answer.

1. B cells are (a) produced in the bursa and
    produce lymphokines. (b) produced in the
    bursa and are responsible for cell-mediated
    immunity. (c) functionally the same as T-cells.
    (d) responsible for humoral immunity.   d

2. Antibodies are characteristically shaped like
    the letter (a) X. (b) Y.(c) K. (d) M.   b

3. The clonal selection theory states that (a)
    millions of specific lymphocytes exist in the
    body. (b) upon activation, specific antibodies
    begin to reproduce mitotically. (c) both a and
    b (d) neither a nor b   c

4. The different human immunoglobulins differ
    only in the (a) variable region of the light
    chain. (b) variable region of the heavy chain.
    (c) constant region of the light chain. (d)
    constant region of the heavy chain.   d

5. _____ recombination events are needed in
    order for immunoglobulin G to be produced.
    (a) 2 (b) 4 (c) 6 (d) 8   a

6. The histocompatibility complex (a) differentiates
    between self and non-self. (b) cannot function
    genetically in certain organisms. (c) plays a
    role in transplant rejection. (d) a and c   d

7. The human histocompatibility complex is located
    on (a) chromosome 4. (b) chromosome 6. (c)
    chromosome 17. (d) chromosome 21.   b

8. Cytotoxic T-lymphocytes are responsible for
    (a) mediating the responses of the other T-cells.
    (b) binding with B-lymphocytes and macro-
    phages to form antibodies. (c) skin graft
    rejection. (d) a, b and c   c

9. Autoimmune diseases are characterized by (a)
    response of the body to foreign antigens. (b)
    rejection of transplanted organs. (c) only cell
    mediated responses to foreign antigens. (d)
    immune responses against cells in the individual's
    own body.   d

SHORT ANSWER QUESTIONS FOR REVIEW

10. An example of an autoimmune disease is (a) myocardial infarction. (b) rheumatoid arthritis. (c) tetralogy of fallot. (d) patent ductus arteriosus.

b

In questions 11-13 match the immunoglobulin with the phrase that best fits the description.

11. IgA   (a) involved in allergic reactions

b

12. IgM   (b) found in saliva and tears

c

                 (c) the first immunoglobulin to appear in response to an antigen

13. IgE

a

In questions 14 through 16 match the theory to the choice that best describes it.

14. Germline hypothesis   (a) separate sequences come together in all possible combinations via recombination

c

15. Somatic mutation theory

a

16. Rearrangement theory   (b) actual number of initial antibodies is small

b

                         (c) all possible sequences are carried on the DNA.

Fill in the blanks.

17. Both T cells and B cells arise from the same type of undifferentiated _____.

stem
cells

18. Antibody molecules consist of _____ polypeptide chains.

four

19. The _____ portions of antibodies constitute the antigen binding sites.

variable

20. In the variable portions of heavy chains _____ separate DNA regions must be combined.

three

21. The constant regions on human heavy chains are encoded by a cluster of genes on _____.

the same
chromo-
some

22. In mice, the mating of brothers and sisters for many generations will produce strains that are _____ at nearly all loci.

homo-
zygous

23. A transplant between two separate strains of
an organism will usually be _____ .

rejected

24. T cells are secreted by the _____ .

thymus

25. The human histocompatibility complex is
known as _____ .

HLA

26. Mice show _____ different classes of proteins
on skin surfaces responsible for cell surface
antibodies.

three

27. _____ always show an identical match
between histocompatibility complexes and cell
surface antibodies.

Identical
twins

28. There are _____ different types of T cells.

three

29. In myesthenia gravis, an autoimmune disease,
antibodies are made against the individual's
own _____ receptors.

acetyl-
choline

30. Multiple sclerosis, another autoimmune disease,
may be an _____ abnormality of the major
histocompatibility complex.

inherited

Decide whether the following statements are true
or false.

31. T and B cells are morphologically alike.

True

32. Patients with multiple myelomas produce
multiple types of antibodies.

False

33. Each chain of an antibody, whether light or
heavy, has either a constant portion or a
variable portion.

False

34. There are five types of human immunglobulins.

True

35. In mouse embryos, it was shown that one
gene codes for the constant portion of an
antibody chain, while another gene codes for
the variable portion of the chain.

True

36. Recombination between heavy and light chains
of an antibody is common.

False

37. In a specific strain of mouse that is homozygous for almost all traits, any skin
transplant between mice is readily accepted.

True

38. It has been suggested, and experimentally
proven, that transplant rejection or
acceptance has a genetic basis.

True

39. In human cells, surface antigens are alike in
all people.

False

40. The only histocompatibility locus is the major
locus.

False

41. A mouse and a human can be histocompatible
for a certain trait.

True

CHAPTER 14

GENETIC ENGINEERING

METHODS

● PROBLEM 14-1

What are restriction enzymes? Why was their discovery an important step in genetic engineering? What is a restriction map?

Solution: Restriction enzymes are nucleases that recognize very specific sequences of DNA. They can cut a double-stranded molecule of DNA at these recognition sites. Their discovery has enabled the detailed analysis and manipulation of DNA.

A series of experiments in the 1960s led to the discovery of the first restriction nuclease in 1970. In the 1960s, methylated DNA from E.coli was found that did not degrade when introduced into another strain of E.coli. Normally, DNA that is introduced from one strain to another is broken apart. Chemical analysis revealed the presence of two types of bacterial enzymes: one that methylated nonmethylated DNA and another that cut nonmethylated DNA. In 1970, Hamilton Smith of Johns Hopkins University discovered a restriction enzyme in Haemophilus influenzae that could break down E.coli DNA but not Haemophilus DNA. This enzyme, Hin dII, very specifically binds to the following sequence and cuts at the arrows:

```
5'  G T Py  ↓  Pu A C  3'

3'  C A PU  ↑  Py T G  5'
```

Pu represents any purine residue and Py represents any pyrimidine residue.

Since 1970, restriction enzymes have been isolated from about 230 bacterial strains, and over 91 different specific cleavage sites have been found. Table 1 shows a very limited list.

Table 1.

Microorganism	Abbreviation	Sequence $\begin{smallmatrix}5'\to3'\\3'\leftarrow5'\end{smallmatrix}$
Bacillus amyloliquefaciens H	BamH1	G↓GATCC CCTAG↑G
Escherichia coli RY13	EcoR1	G↓AATTC CTTAA↑G
Haemophilus aegyptius	Hae III	GG↓CC CC↑GG
Haemophilus parainfluenzae	Hpa I	GTT↓AAC CAA↑TTG
Haemophilus parainfluenzae	Hpa II	C↓CGG GGC↑C

Most restriction enzymes recognize sequences of four or six base pairs. Those that recognize four nucleotides usually cut more often in a given DNA than those that recognize six nucleotides. Sometimes, a restriction enzyme that recognizes a hexanucleotide sequence will not be able to cut a molecule of DNA at all. For instance, EcoRI cannot cut phage T7 DNA. The necessary GAATTC CTTAAG sequence is not present in the 40,000 nucleotide long phage DNA.

Another property of restriction enzymes is their ability to recognize palindromes - sequences that read the same backwards and forwards. These palindromic sequences may figure in the recognition mechanism. Once the proper sequence is recognized, one of two types of nicks can be made. Either a staggered cut, like that made by Bam H1, or a blunt end cut, like that made by Hae III, is produced. Staggered cuts produce "sticky" ends that can be exploited in cloning techniques.

The fragments that are generated when the DNA is cut by restriction enzymes can be separated by gel electrophoresis. Small fragments move faster than large fragments, so relative sizes can be determined. The molecular weights of fragments can be estimated by comparisons to the travelling ability of fragments with known molecular weights. Restriction maps can be made using these techniques. The order of the fragments can be determined by overlapping intermediate-sized fragments. In 1971 Daniel Nathans of Johns Hopkins University completed a restriction map of the virus SV40. This map locates the relative sites on the DNA that are attacked by specific restriction enzymes. This map and technique enabled scientists to study the initiation sites of SV40 replication. The specific base sequence of the DNA could only be determined indirectly by the RNA-sequencing procedure developed by Fred Sanger in the mid 1960s. This was done by using RNA polymerase to synthesize the DNA's complementary RNA strands and then using stepwise degradation processes to determine the sequence. Since then, less time-consuming methods have been developed that allow the direct sequencing of DNA. Restriction enzymes have contributed greatly by opening the door to a whole realm of genetic analyses.

● **PROBLEM** 14-2

Three fragments are produced when a piece of RNA is treated with pancreatic RNase. According to the amount of phosphate, these fragments are highly acidic (much phosphate), moderately acidic, and slightly acidic (little phosphate). Each of these fragments is further hydrolyzed with NaOH. The resulting nucelotides are:

1. highly acidic fragment: Gp, pAp, Cp

2. moderately acidic fragment: Gp, Up

3. slightly acidic fragment: G, Gp.

What is the sequence of this piece of RNA?

Solution: This problem illustrates how RNA molecules can be sequenced. This technique utilizes nucleases that cut RNA molecules after specific bases. The fragments that are produced by such action are separated chemically and then treated further with alkali. An alkaline compound breaks the oligonucleotide fragments into single nucleotides. This breakage occurs so that the 3' phosphate group remains bonded to the nucleotide.

Pancreatic RNase was used to cut the RNA into managable fragments. This nuclease specifically cuts RNA after a pyrimidine. Thus, each of the three fragments must end with either uracil or cytosine, the two pyrimidines of RNA. NaOH was the basic chemical used to cut the fragments into single nucleotides. It left the nucleotides with their 3' phosphate group (if they had one), and their 5' hydroxyl group.

We now have enough information to piece together this stretch of RNA. Starting with the most acidic fragment, notice that the adenine residue has both a 5' and a 3' phosphate. Since RNA nucleotides have a phosphate group only on their 3' side when treated with alkali, the adenine must not have had any base preceding it that could take the extra phosphate group. Adenine must be the first base of the entire RNA piece. Since each fragment must end with a pyrimidine because of the action of pancreatic RNase, cytosine must be the last base of this fragment. That leaves guanine in the middle. The sequence of the highly acidic fragment is: pApGpCp.

The moderately acidic fragment can be ordered similarly. The last nucleotide of the fragment must be uracil, since it is the only pyrimidine. Only one other nucleotide is in this fragment, so the order is: GpUp.

The least acidic fragment has one nucleotide without a phosphate group. This must be the base at the 3' end of the RNA molecule, where there is a free hydroxyl group. Again, with only two nucleotides in the fragment, ordering is simple: GpG.

Piecing together the fragments so that there is a phosphate group between each nucleotide, with a phosphate group at the 5' end and a hydroxyl at the 3' end, we arrive at the final sequence:

$$5' \; pApGpCpGpUpGpG_{OH} \quad 3'.$$

If we had more fragments and a lot more time, we would be able to sequence stretches of RNA hundreds of nucleotides long.

What is the sequence of the DNA that has been analyzed to produce the electrophoretic gel (Figure 1) whose bands are shown by autoradiography? How was the information on this gel obtained?

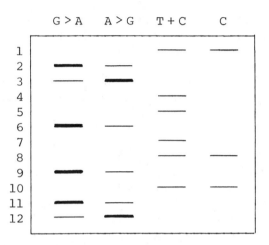

Solution: Gels of this sort are used to sequence DNA molecules. The procedure was developed by Allan Maxam and Walter Gilbert of Harvard University in 1977. It utilizes several laboratory techniques: radioactive labelling, denaturation, gel electrophoresis, molecular modification and degradation, and autoradiography.

1. The pure DNA (a restriction fragment eluted from a gel, for example) is enzymatically labelled with ^{32}P at the 5' ends of both strands.

2. The duplex DNA fragments are dissociated by treatment with heat or alkali which weakens the hydrogen bonds. These are separated into two single-stranded fragments by gel electrophoresis. One of these fragments travels farther in the gel because it contains more purines than the other; this is the heavy strand.

3. One of these fractions, either heavy or light, is subjected to further tests. It is divided into four portions. One portion is tested to indicate the positions of every G; one indicates the positions of all A residues;

one indicates the positions of all Ts; and one indicates every C. Each sample is analyzed by applying specific chemicals and conditions. They are then analyzed together on a gel like the one shown in the problem.

To find every G, the sample is treated with dimethyl sulfate under conditions that allow the methylation of one purine per strand on the average. Guanine residues are methylated preferentially over adenine. The presence of warm alkali· causes the strand to break at the site of methylation. When these pieces are run on a gel they separate. The lengths (and therefore the ability to move through the gel) depend on the distance of the base that was destroyed to create the break from the labelled end of the molecule. Only those fragments that contain the ^{32}P label will appear with autoradiography. Strong bands indicate the position of G and weak bands show the position of A.

To find the A residues, the purines are methylated in the same way but the sample is exposed to cold dilute acid. This causes the strand to preferentially break at A positions. The dark bands of this sample are at the A positions and the weak bands are at G positions.

To find Ts, the sample is treated with hydrazine under conditions that favor the hydrazinolysis of one pyrimidine per strand. T and C are equally sensitive. Piperdine is used to make the strands sensitive to breakage at the modified T and C positions. The pattern on the gel shows both C and T positions.

To differentiate the Cs, hydrazine and piperdine are used in the presence of high salt which suppresses the hydrazinolysis of T. The bands on the gel show the positions of the Cs.

Thus, the gel given in the problem can be read to determine the DNA sequence. The shorter pieces move fastest and farthest through the gel since they are not hindered by bulkiness. The bands at the bottom of the gel result from nucleotides that were closer to the 5' labelled phosphate than those at the top of the gel. By reading the darker bands to find A and G residues and by differentiating the T and C residues by noticing which of the T+C bands are T alone, we obtain the following sequence:

5' AGCGCTGTTAGC 3'

What is a plasmid vector?

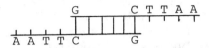

Fig. 1: Sticky ends of a piece of DNA cut with
the restriction enxyme, E co Rl.

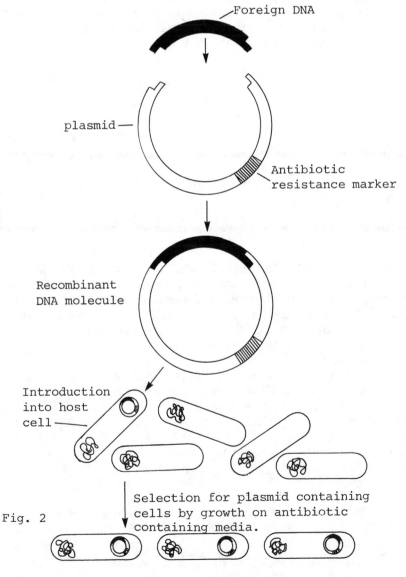

Fig. 2

513

Solution: Plasmids are extrachromosomal, circular pieces of bacterial DNA. They are self-replicating accessory chromosomes. They carry genes for antibiotic resistance, metabolism of natural products, and production of toxins. Plasmids have become important components in the manipulation of genes in cloning experiments.

When the restriction enzyme EcoR1 is used to cut a piece of DNA, it leaves "sticky" ends, Figure 1. Such a fragment can be inserted into a circular plasmid DNA that has been similarly treated. As shown in Figure 2, these hybrid plasmids can be used to infect bacteria.

A plasmid can be used as a means of introducing a foreign piece of DNA into a bacterial cell. Since the plasmid is self-replicating, the foreign DNA will remain a part of the plasmid and a part of the bacterial strain as long as the plasmid stays in a cell. Thus, clones of cells containing a piece of foreign DNA can be produced. This is the basis of the recombinant DNA industry.

● **PROBLEM** 14-5

How has the action of reverse transcriptase been exploited by biologists?

Solution: In 1970, Howard Temin and David Baltimore independently discovered reverse transcriptase. Since its discovery, this viral enzyme has been used in many ways by research biologists. Its unique ability to catalyze the synthesis of DNA from RNA has established it as an important tool in genetic research.

Reverse transcriptase is coded for by the nucleic acid of retroviruses. When retroviruses infect a bacterial host, their RNA genomes are transcribed into DNA by reverse transcriptase which is present in small amounts in the viral protein coat. Once in the DNA form, the viral genome integrates into the host chromosome as a provirus. The provirus is then replicated as a part of the bacterial genome.

The mechanism of this enzyme is similar to that of other DNA polymerases. The DNA is synthesized in the 5' to 3' direction. It needs a primer to begin this synthesis. The primer is a noncovalently bound tRNA that was picked up from the host during the previous round of replication. The DNA chain can be added to the 3' end of this tRNA molecule. Somehow, double-stranded circular DNA molecules are made from this single-stranded DNA copy. These circular proviruses are now ready for insertion into the host genome.

This enzyme has proven to be a useful tool to the molecular biologist. It can be used to make DNA copies of any RNA that can be purified. This function can be useful in many types of experiments. Purified mRNA can be obtained from cells that are specialized to make specific proteins (e.g. hemoglobin from red blood cells and insulin from mammalian pancreas cells). The DNA copy of mRNAs from these cells can be used to find the sequence in the cells' own DNA. Thus, a specific area of the mass of DNA can be focused on. In similar ways, split genes and differences between hnRNA and mRNA can be studied. But perhaps most importantly, reverse transcriptase is a necessary reagent for genetic engineering with recombinant DNA. The complementary DNA (cDNA) that is transcribed from an mRNA is what is inserted into plasmids to create recombinant DNA molecules. Thus, this enzyme is a very significant part of the blossoming genetic technology.

● **PROBLEM 14-6**

You receive an anonymous gift box which contains:

pBR322 (plasmid)	$CaCl_2$
human DNA gene library	oligo-dT
Hind III (restriction enzyme)	terminal transgerase
reverse transcriptase	replica plating equipment
ligase	Petri dishes
ampicillin	growth media
tetracycline	S1 nuclease (single-strand specific nuclease)
radioactively labeled human hemoglobin	Hind III linkers

mRNA	DNA polymerase
E.coli	NaOH

What would you do with the contents of this box?

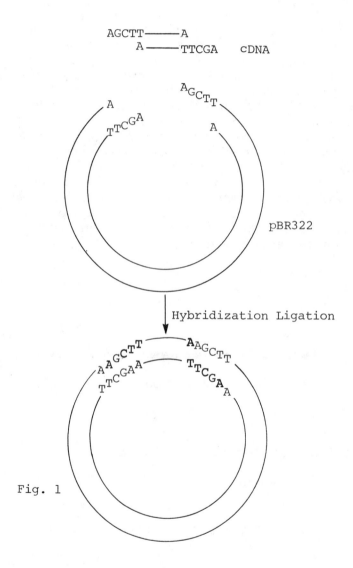

Fig. 1

Solution: You know immediately, from the contents of this box, who the anonymous donor was - your friend, Dr. Gamma, who has been doing genetic experiments in his basement laboratory for years. Since you also have some genetic knowledge, you know that the contents of this box are the ingredients necessary to produce recombinant DNA-carrying bacteria. You carry the box down to your own basement laboratory and start to work.

The radioactively labeled hemoglobin mRNA can be used to probe for its complementary sequence in the gene library. A gene library is from a whole DNA complement of an organism that has been cut into fragments with a restriction enzyme. The fragments are joined to plasmid vectors and the plasmids are introduced into a population of bacteria. The result is a culture of bacteria containing the entire genome. Each recombinant bacteria has a piece of the genome. If one wants to find a particular gene, one is faced with the problem of trying to find a needle in the haystack. However, this difficult procedure does not have to be done. Instead, one can mix the short chains of oligo-dT with the mRNA provided by Dr. Gamma. These chains will hybridize to the poly-A tails that are present on almost every eukaryotic mRNA molecule. This will act as a primer for the action of reverse transcriptase. This enzyme catalyzes the synthesis of DNA from the mRNA. A hairpin loop forms when the enzyme turns around and starts to copy itself. This loop can serve as the primer that is needed for DNA polymerase to finish synthesizing the DNA. The hairpin loop can be removed with S1 nuclease and the mRNA can be degraded with NaOH. Since by this time the sun is beginning to rise, you decide to postpone further experiments until the next evening.

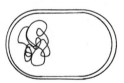
No plasmid →
    no resistance

Fig. 2

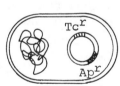
Plasmid →
    resistant to
    ampicilin and
    tetracyclin

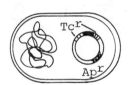
Recombinant
plasmid →
    resistant to
    ampicillin;
    sensitive to
    tetracyclin

The following evening, you take your sample of double-stranded cDNA and prepare it for insertion into the plasmid. You attach the Hind III linkers, 8 to 10 base pair oligonucleotides that contain Hind III recognition sites, with the catalytic activity of ligase. You treat the DNA fragment with Hind III so that staggered cuts are made. You also treat the plasmid, pBR322, with Hind III. As shown in Figure 1, the "sticky ends" may join to form a recombinant plasmid. The pieces are sealed with DNA ligase. The final step for the day is to treat the E.coli cells with CaCl$_2$ to make them better able to pick up

DNA. The cells and plasmids are mixed under conditions that facilitate this uptake. The cells are then plated on ampicillin containing media and then incubated. They are grown on media containing ampicillin to select for those cells with the plasmid. The plasmid, pBR322 has some important characteristics: it contains a gene for ampicillin resistance (Ap^r) and a gene for tetracyclin resistance (Tc^r). Ap^r has a recognition sequence for the restriction enzyme Pst1 and Tc^r does not; Tc^r has a Hind III site and Ap^r does not. These are very useful characteristics which enable a researcher to determine exactly which cell colonies contain the recombinant plasmid: those cells with no antibiotic resistance have no plasmid; those with resistance to both ampicillin and tetracyclin have the plasmid but no foreign DNA; and those with resistance to ampicillin but not to tetracyclin have the plasmid with a piece of foreign DNA interrupting its tetracyclin resistance gene (Figure 2).

When colonies appear on the Petri plates, you know that some of the E.coli has picked up the plasmid. But only those that are resistant to ampicillin and sensitive to tetracyclin have the human hemoglobin gene. Using the replica plating equipment that Dr. Gamma was so thoughtful to provide, you plate the colonies onto media which contains tetracyclin. Those colonies that can survive when ampicillin is added but not when tetracyclin is added are the recombinant clones. You have succeeded in creating a bacterial cell that contains a human gene. You rush to tell Dr. Gamma the good news.

● **PROBLEM** 14-7

How can transposons be used to genetically engineer Drosophila?

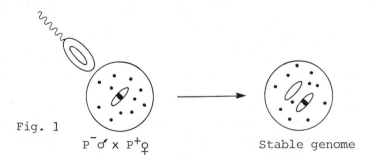

Fig. 1

$P^- ♂ \times P^+ ♀$

Stable genome

<u>Solution</u>: Transposons are genetic elements that can integrate into a chromosome or plasmid and, later, excise themselves or replicate themselves for insertion into another piece of DNA. Transposons have no origin of replication, so they must be integrated into a chromosome or plasmid in order for them to be replicated. Transposons have been found in bacteria, <u>Drosophila</u> and maize. Bacterial transposons carry genes for antibiotic resistance. A typical <u>Drosophila</u> genome has many copies of a transposon known as copia element. Another transposable element in <u>Drosophila</u> is called the P element. Although these transposable elements are present in most <u>Drosophila</u> genomes, they appear at different chromosomal locations. In maize, transposable elements can cause mutations during transposition.

The P element can be used as a vector to mediate gene transfer in <u>Drosophila</u>. Flies that have the P element are P$^+$ and those that lack the element are P$^-$. P element insertions into P$^-$ gametes may cause mutations that render the adult fly sterile. This is probably due to the presence of a repressor molecule in the cytoplasm of P$^+$ gametes. This repressor may inhibit the transposition of the element, thus stabilizing the genome. When P$^-$ males are mated to P$^+$ females, the progeny are normally fertile, Figure 1.

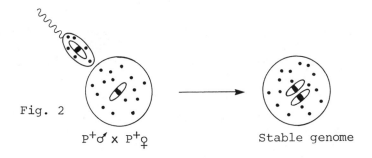

Fig. 2

P$^+$♂ x P$^+$♀   Stable genome

When both gametes contain the P element, fertile progeny are produced as shown in Figure 2.

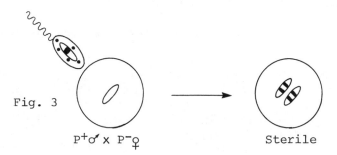

Fig. 3

P$^+$♂ x P$^-$♀   Sterile

However, when P$^+$ males are mated with P$^-$ females, the resulting progeny have unstable genomes; they are sterile. This occurs because the male gamete only donates its DNA to the female; no cytoplasmic contents are exchanged. The zygote contains no repressor so the P element is free to insert into many areas of the germ cells' genomes. The resulting flies are sterile, Figure 3. This process is called hybrid dysgenesis. The fact that the P element is mobile in embryos arising from P$^-$ eggs has been used to genetically engineer Drosophila embryos.

A cloned copy of the rosy gene, which codes for xanthine dehydrogenase, an eye color marker, can be inserted into a cloned copy of a P element. This insertion disrupts the transposase gene that is necessary for the P elements' ability to move. Without this gene, the P-rosy hybrids are not mobile. The recombinant P element can then be inserted into the plasmid pBR322 and propogated in E.coli. The P-rosy hybrids can then be microinjected into a P$^-$rosy$^-$ Drosophila embryo. But these hybrids are not mobile unless wild-type P elements are also injected. The wild-type P elements code for the enzyme necessary for transposition, so the hybrid P element will be able to insert into the genome and function normally. Successful gene transfer is indicated by flies with altered eye color due to the rosy gene.

This type of gene transfer has several advantages. The transfers occur at high frequencies and do not result in a detectable rearrangement of the integrated DNA. Also, relatively large DNA segments can be transferred.

● **PROBLEM 14-8**

Why is yeast an important organism in genetic engineering? How have studies of the genetics of yeast contributed to the study of genetics in general?

Solution: Baker's yeast, Saccharomyces cerevisiae, is a very useful eukaryote. It has certain properties that make it ideal for genetic manipulation. Some important aspects of eukaryotic genetics have been elucidated by the manipulation of this unicellular organism.

Yeast is a relatively simple eukaryote. It has a small genome (only four times that of E.coli). It has a generation time of only a few hours, so effects of genetic changes can be seen quickly. Yeast can be maintained in either the haploid or diploid state. The haploid state makes it easy to follow recessive markers. Complementation can be studied in the diploids that result from the mating of pairs of haploids containing appropriate mutations. These properties make baker's yeast very useful in the study of the regulation of gene expression in eukaryotic genomes.

Many studies can be done using yeast to learn about eukaryotic genetics. Yeast can take up external DNA very easily once its cellulose wall has been enzymatically removed. Yeast can take in recombinant bacterial plasmids. External DNA can even integrate into the yeast genome if the homologous sequences necessary for the integration via crossing over are present in the foreign DNA. Cloned genes can be mutagenized and reintroduced into their proper places in the genome to study the effects of mutations on the function of genes. This is known as "reverse genetics".

The analysis of the genetics of yeast has shown the presence of positive and negative regulatory functions that control the gene expression in eukaryotes. Cell mechanics and physiology (such as chromosomal origins of replication) sequences of the centromere that attach to the mitotic spindle and functional chromosome ends (telomeres), have been studied through yeast genetics. The role of chromatin proteins in the regulation of gene expression has similarly been studied. These investigations are in their infancy. Much has been learned already, but there is such complexity in eukaryotes not present in prokaryotes that we know more about prokaryotic genetic mechanisms than their eukaryotic counterparts. Further analyses will increase our knowledge of eukaryotic genetics. Yeast will surely help in those studies.

● PROBLEM 14-9

What is a shuttle vector?

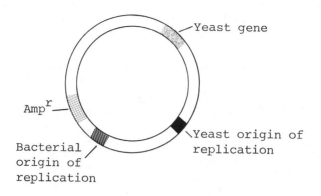

Yeast gene

Amp^r

Bacterial
origin of
replication

Yeast origin of
replication

Solution: Shuttle vectors contain sequences that signal
DNA replication in E.coli and sequences that signal
replication in yeast. Thus, the plasmid can be shuttled
back and forth between yeast and E.coli and be replicated
in both organisms. Shuttle vectors can be used to clone
many genes. Total genomic yeast DNA is cut with a
restriction enzyme. The fragments are inserted into
shuttle vectors using recombinant DNA techniques. These
plasmids are propogated in E.coli. This mixed population
of plasmids is introduced into mutant yeast spheroplasts.
Any recombinant that complements the mutation in yeast
can be identified and reintroduced into E.coli. Once in
E.coli, it can be grown in large amounts and studied
further. Theoretically, any gene for which a mutation can
be identified can be cloned this way.

● **PROBLEM 14-10**

How can foreign genes be introduced into the genomes
of dicotyledonous plants?

Solution: The subclass Dicotyledoneae includes oaks,
willows, beans, roses, clover and tomatoes. Increased
disease resistance, weather resistance and crop yield for
many of the dicots would benefit both agriculture and
livestock farming. Traditionally, genes have been
introduced from one plant variety to another by sexual
crosses. This process spans several years and is
restricted to sexually compatible species. Recent
discoveries have enabled the use of genetic engineering
techniques in dicots. The major discovery is a plasmid
found in a tumor-inducing bacteria that transforms only

dicotyledonous cells. Through manipulation of this plasmid, foreign genes can be introduced into plants quickly and cross sexual boundaries.

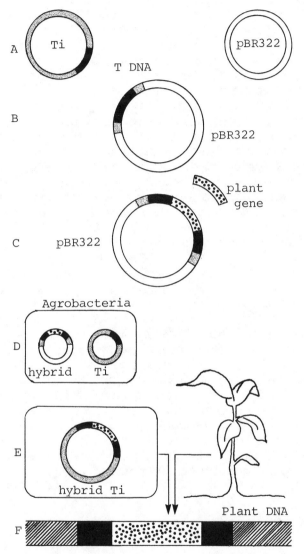

Fig. 1: How to introduce a foreign gene into a plant. A: Ti plasmid and pBR322 cut with a restriction enzyme and the T DNA is incubated with pBR322 to form hybrid pBR322, B; plant gene inserted into non-essential region of T DNA to form hybrid C; hybrid C used to infect Agrobacteria containing normal Ti plasmid D; recombination between homologous regions of plasmids forms hybrid Ti plasmid E; hybrid Ti plasmid used to infect plant which incorporates foreign plant DNA into its chromosome F.

Several species of Agrobacterium can infect plants and cause a crown gall tumor to form. A crown gall tumor is a mass of tumor tissue that grows in an undifferentiated way at the site of infection. A particularly strong species, Agrobacterium tumefaciens, contains a tumor inducing (Ti) plasmid. Ti plasmids, like other bacterial plasmids, are self-replicating circular DNA molecules. Studies have shown that one section of the plasmid, called T DNA, is integrated into the host's chromosome upon infection. Once inserted, T DNA behaves like a normal Mendelian plant gene. This T DNA-containing Ti plasmid can be used as a vector to transfer DNA to plants.

Foreign genes can be introduced into plants by the method shown in Figure 1. Shortcuts have recently been found to simplify this process considerably. Only an intact T DNA region and another area of the Ti plasmid called "vir" are needed for Agrobacterium to infect and transform cells. These two regions need not even be on the same plasmid. This eliminates the step where the hybrid plasmid and the native Ti plasmid undergo recombination to produce a hybrid Ti plasmid.

The long term goals of plant genetic engineering are manifold. Basically, the goals are to find ways to introduce foreign genes into plants and to study the development of plants. But, as far as plant breeding, the engineering techniques have serious limitations. So far, transformation of monocotyledons, such as corn and wheat, with Ti plasmids has proven to be impossible. Also, there is great difficulty in identifying specific genes responsible for such broad traits as increased yield. Once these genes have been identified, they still need to be cloned and properly inserted into the T DNA. When ways have been found to circumvent and solve these problems, genetic engineering of plants can become as important as the genetic engineering of bacteria.

● **PROBLEM** 14-11

How can genes be transferred into mammalian cells?

Solution: Since geneticists are humans and humans are mammals, geneticists are extremely interested in mammalian genetics. Recently, techniques to genetically engineer mammalian cells have been developed. Cloned genes can be routinely introduced into the genomes of many mammalian cells.

Several special techniques have been devised to enable genes to be incorporated into mammalian genomes. The first of these techniques utilizes calcium. Vertebrate cells are stimulated to take up DNA when Ca^{++} is added. The reasons for this are largely unknown. The next technique enables the small fraction of cells that incorporate the foreign DNA into their genomes to be selected for and easily identified. The most ideal "marker" is thymidine kinase (tk). TK is the enzyme used in the salvage pathway of pyrimidine biosynthesis. Its presence is not essential for cells to survive. Tk⁻ mutants can be used to take up DNA. These mutants can be isolated by giving the cells a nucleoside analog that is lethal only when it is phosphorylated. In the presence of this analog, bromodeoxyuridine (BrUdr), only tk⁻ cells can survive. The tk gene could be used as a selective marker for the integration of other genes linked to it. Thus, it can be used as a vector to transfer genes into eukaryotic cells. This technique is problematic because it is very time consuming to make eukaryotic cells th⁻ since both of the tk alleles of the diploid cells must be inactivated.

Further genetic research to the rescue! Two new vectors have been successfully used. Both vectors contain bacterial genes connected to genes of the SV40 virus. These vectors, called SVgpt and SVneo, utilize biochemical reactions that are similar in the bacterial gene and the mammalian host cell. For instance, SVneo contains the bacterial gene that confers resistance to neomycin, an antibiotic that is toxic to ribosomes. This gene is ligated into a region of the SV40 genome. Eukaryotic cells are sensitive to a neomycin-like molecule, G418, which is also inactivated by the enzyme produced by the Neo^R gene. This vector can then be used to transform mammalian cells that are resistant to G418.

There are other ways that genes can be introduced into mammalian cells. A process called cotransformation involves the ligation of a cloned gene to a cloned selectable marker. Prior ligation outside of the cells is not necessary in this procedure. Any gene can be introduced into a mammalian cell in this way. Another method involves the microinjection of DNA into the nuclei of tissue culture cells with a glass micropipette. This technique needs sophistocated equipment to draw out the pipette to a diameter of only 0.1 to 0.5 microns. A great deal of practice is needed to perfect this tedious technique. However, up to 50 percent of the injected cells (of a practiced scientist) will stably integrate and express the added genes. This technique has two distinct advantages: any piece of DNA can, in principle, be introduced into any cell and, no selective pressure is needed to maintain the foreign gene. Disadvantages are the expense, practice and the relatively small number of cells that can be treated (500-1000 cells/hour).

Genetic engineering of mammalian cells has added much to the understanding of genetics. The DNA sequences are responsible for controlling the expression of some eukaryotic genes. Human cancer genes can be cloned and identified in this way, also.

● **PROBLEM** 14-12

What are the possible hazards of molecular cloning?

Solution: As with all new technologies, cloning has possible hazards. Virulent strains of the ubiquitous E.coli could spread disease throughout human populations if experiments introducing viral genes into the bacterial genome were performed carelessly. Most scientists in the early days of cloning, the 1970s, were concerned about the potential military applications of virulent bacteria as part of biological warfare. Another potential hazard surfaced in 1972. The fear was about the finding that the DNA of mice, and possibly all higher cells, harbored latent RNA tumor virus genes. There was then the possibility of introducing cancer causing genes into human cells in the search for antibody genes.

In 1975 in California, the Asilomar Conference proposed guidelines for recombinant DNA research. Among the guidelines were rules for the safe handling of recombinants. The development of "safe" bacterial hosts and vectors was demanded. The first "safe" bacteria was the E.coli strain K12 named χ1776. This strain cannot live without diaminopimelic acid in its environment. This compound is not present in human intestines, so the bacteria would be unable to survive in human hosts. This bacteria also has a fragile cell wall that lyses in low salt concentrations or in traces of detergent. However, the introduction of recombinant DNA molecules was difficult in this strain. Other "safe" bacteria have since been developed that greatly lessen the risk of an accidental spread of disease.

APPLICATIONS

> Insulin, interferon and growth hormone have been successfully manufactured in large quantities by the pharmaceutics industries. Explain the importance of genetic engineering in this process.

Solution: These proteins are manufactured through the use of the recombinant DNA techniques that have been described throughout this chapter. Since many commercially valuable proteins are present in very small amounts in animal cells and tissues, and since the expression of the cloned gene is essential for the organism, most of the commercial research has focused on the cDNA cloning of the cells' mRNA. However, human insulin was obtained by the actual chemical synthesis of a gene.

Insulin is necessary for the treatment of diabetes mellitus. Previously, it was obtained from animals such as pigs and cows. Unfortunately, many people developed side effects and severe allergic reactions, probably due to impurities. Through the production of insulin by recombinant bacteria, a protein product identical to human insulin has been made.

Interferons are proteins that can inhibit virus replication. Interferons are made by the body in extremely small amounts, so the production of a recombinant bacteria with the gene for human interferon was a perfect candidate for the pharmaceutics industry. Since the gene is generally translated in such small amounts, mechanisms had to be found to enable the host vector systems to produce commercially valuable amounts. One step towards this goal was achieved by precisely positioning the interferon sequence adjacent to bacterial promoter regions. Now, these vector systems are producing much more interferon than before so the protein can be tested for its therapeutic values.

Growth hormone controls the growth of our bodies; dwarfs have a deficiency of the protein. Previously, it was obtained from the pituitary glands of corpses. Thus it was difficult to obtain amounts sufficient for clinical use. The growth hormone gene has been cloned and the gene has been inserted into bacterial vectors. However, the bacteria are unable to remove the initial methionine residue of the polypeptide. The necessary enzyme probably cannot get to the required position due to the folding of the polypeptide. This is not critical and we can settle for a very good second best.

The production of these proteins by bacteria has lowered their prices since they are not as difficult to obtain as they were previously. Recombinant DNA production of medically significant molecules is a very promising aspect of genetic engineering.

● **PROBLEM** 14-14

Can vaccines be made by genetic engineering techniques?

<u>Solution</u>: Vaccines against viruses consist of either inactivated virulent viral particles or weakened live particles that immunize against the virulent strains. However, vaccinations can cause a few cases of disease if one or more viral particles have survived the inactivation. Also, since the viruses of both types of vaccines are grown in animal cells, the vaccines are sometimes contaminated with cellular material that can cause adverse reactions. Since the surface proteins of the viruses are what induce immunity, the proteins themselves can be used as vaccines. These proteins can be synthesized by recombinant vectors and thus vaccines can be made which are less risky than whole viral vaccines.

Foot-and-mouth disease virus (FMDV) infects cattle. The major antigenic viral protein (VPI) has been cloned and synthesized. However, this isolated protein was not as antigenic as the macromolecular assemblies of the same protein. Two laboratories have produced peptides between 8 and 41 amino acids in length corresponding to antigenic segments of VPI. These synthetic peptides were linked to protein carriers to increase their immunogenicity. Studies on cattle, guinea pigs and rabbits have shown that some of the synthetic peptides induced an antibody specific to FMDV. These results are encouraging, but the synthetic vaccine must be able to compete with existing vaccines in terms of purity, safety and efficiency in order to be a commercial success.

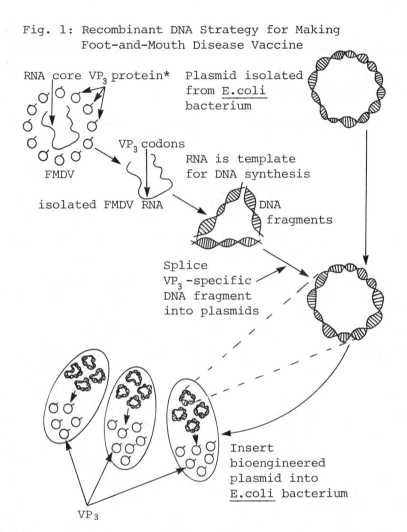

Fig. 1: Recombinant DNA Strategy for Making
Foot-and-Mouth Disease Vaccine

RNA core VP$_3$ protein*   Plasmid isolated
                            from E.coli
                            bacterium

FMDV

VP$_3$ codons

RNA is template
for DNA synthesis

isolated FMDV RNA

DNA
fragments

Splice
VP$_3$-specific
DNA fragment
into plasmids

Insert
bioengineered
plasmid into
E.coli bacterium

VP$_3$

*VP$_3$ is the protein from the shell of the virus,
which can act as a vaccine for immunizing livestock
against foot-and-mouth disease.

The hepatitis B antigen has been cloned and its gene
has been inserted into bacterial vectors. This protein is
being studied and used to diagnose the existence of
antibodies in the blood of infected people. Until this clone
was developed, the hepatitis B virus was very difficult to
study since it cannot be grown in cultured cells. As of
yet no vaccine has ever been made against this virus.
Eventually the hope is that one will be made by using
yeast as a vector to synthesize antigenic protein.

Vaccines are being developed for these and other
diseases. The use of recombinant vectors to produce
synthetic peptides that can be used as vaccines is
another high technology possibility in the medical field.

How can genetic engineering be used to improve agricultural crops?

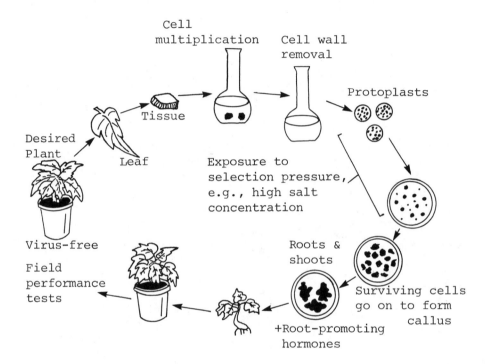

Cell multiplication

Cell wall removal

Protoplasts

Tissue

Desired Plant

Leaf

Exposure to selection pressure, e.g., high salt concentration

Virus-free

Field performance tests

Roots & shoots

Surviving cells go on to form callus

+Root-promoting hormones

Fig. 1: The process of plant propagation form single cells in culture can produce plants with selected characteristics. These selections must be tested in the field to evaluate their performance.

Solution: Agriculture has been using the principles of Mendelian genetics for thousands of years. The yields of wheat and corn have steadily increased over the past 50 years by the use of close inbreeding and rigorous artificial selection. This produces distinct and genetically uniform varieties with both desired and undesired traits. These varieties have improved crop yields and introduced hybrid vigor. For instance, genes were introduced, by sexual crosses, from a semi-dwarf variety of Japanese wheat to a Mexican wheat strain. The hybrid had greater wind resistance and needed less growth before flowering because the straw was shorter and stiffer; this meant greater adaptability to the region and greater disease and insect resistance.

The recent discovery of the crown gall plasmid system has created the possibility for recombinant DNA techniques to be applied to plants. This would be much faster than conventional breeding and would enable the introduction of genes from one sexually incompatible species to another. However, the isolation of specific genes that affect crop yield is extremely difficult.

Thus, plant breeders have been using genetics for a long time. The techniques of recombinant DNA may eventually be used to improve agricultural crops with greater specificity and speed than is available in the traditional methods.

SHORT ANSWER QUESTIONS FOR REVIEW

Choose the correct answer.

1. Restriction enzymes can usually recognize a sequence of _____ base pairs. (a) 1 to 3 (b) 2 to 4 (c) 3 to 5 (d) 4 to 6

   d

2. _____ help to plot the locations attacked by specific restriction enzymes on DNA molecules. (a) Gene maps (b) Restriction maps (c) Chromosomal attack maps (d) Point maps

   b

3. Gel electrophoresis, autoradiography and molecular modification allow for (a) DNA sequencing. (b) RNA sequencing. (c) enzymatic enucleation. (d) enzymatic restriction.

   a

4. Plasmids are found _____ (a) on selected chromosomes. (b) on every chromosome. (c) extrachromosomally. (d) in plant cells only.

   c

5. Reverse transcriptase is an enzyme that catalyzes the synthesis of _____ (a) RNA from DNA. (b) DNA from RNA. (c) mRNA from rRNA. (d) mRNA from tRNA.

   b

6. Hybrid dysgenesis is the process by which _____ (a) the P element is introduced into Drosophila embryos for the purpose of genetic engineering. (b) all mutations occur in Drosophila. (c) DNA is uncoiled to allow specific point mutations to occur. (d) mutations are corrected in Drosophila embryos.

   a

7. Reverse genetics involves the (a) hybridization of mutated clones. (b) mutation and then replacement of cloned genes. (c) mutation of non-cloned hybrids. (d) mutation of all wild type organisms and subsequent study of the offspring.

   b

8. DNA fragments are inserted into shuttle vectors using _____ (a) recombinant techniques. (b) hybridization over many generations. (c) restriction enzymes. (d) micropipettes.

   a

9. Some vertebrate cells will only take up DNA in the presence of _____. (a) K^+ (b) Cl^- (c) Na^+ (d) Ca^{++}

   d

To be covered
when testing
yourself

10. Two vectors which have recently been
discovered for use with eukaryotic cells are
_____ (a) SVgpt and SVopt. (b) SVgpt
and SVneo. (c) SVgk and SVopt. (d) SVgk
and SVneo.

b

11. Any gene can be introduced into a mammalian
cell by _____ (a) transformation. (b) any
vector method. (c) Ca^{++} uptake. (d) cotransformation.

d

12. One possible hazard of molecular cloning is
(a) formation of a new dominant species. (b)
widespred disease due to human infection. (c)
a and b (d) none of the above

b

13. Which one of the following substances has not
been recently manufactured in large quantities by the pharmaceutical industry (due
to the use of genetic engineering)? (a)
cerebrospinal fluid (b) insulin (c) interferon (d) growth hormone

a

14. A property of all restrictive enzymes is their
ability to recognize _____. (a) purine
residues. (b) pyrimidine residues. (c)
palindrome sequences. (d) a,b and c

c

15. The first "safe" bacteria was the (a) E. coli
strain named K12. (b) Proteus vulgaris. (c)
P. aeriginosa. (d) none of the above

a

In questions 16 through 19 match the bases on the
left with the correct gel electrophoretic ident-
ification tests on the right.

16. guanine   (a) treatment with hydra-   d
                        zine, piperidine and a
17. cytosine   high salt concentration   a
                    (b) treatment with hydrazine
18. thymine   (c) addition of dimenthyl   b
                        sulfate and exposure to
19. adenine   cold, weak acid   c
                    (d) addition of dimenthyl
                        sulfate and exposure to
                        an alkali

SHORT ANSWER QUESTIONS FOR REVIEW

	Answer
	To be covered when testing yourself

Fill in the blanks.

20. Restriction enzymes are _____ that recognize specific DNA sequences.

> nucleases

21. A(n) _____ compound breaks oligonucleotides into single strands.

> alkaline

22. Reverse transcriptase is coded for by nucleotides present in _____.

> retroviruses

23. Two examples of transposable elements in Drosophila are P element and _____.

> copia element

24. It is easier to follow recessive markers in baker's yeast than it is in the _____ state.

> haploid

25. Removal of the _____ in baker's yeast cells readily permits the taking up of external DNA.

> cellulose wall

26. _____ proteins also play a role in gene expression.

> Chromatin

27. Shuttle vectors can signal DNA replication both in baker's yeast and in _____.

> E. coli

28. Agrobacterium tomefaciers is a specific bacteria which contains a plasmid which can be used as a _____ to transfer DNA to plants.

> vector

29. The most ideal marker for cells which incorporates foreign DNA into their genomes is _____.

> thymidine kinase

30. _____ involves the ligation of a closed gene to a closed selectable marker.

> Cotransformation

31. Recombinant vectors produce _____ that can be used as vaccines.

> synthetic peptides

Decide whether the following statements are true or false.

32. Restriction enzymes have allowed for detailed studies of DNA because they can permit manipulation of the DNA molecule without cutting it.

> False

SHORT ANSWER QUESTIONS FOR REVIEW

33. By knowing the relative ptt's of several RNA fragments, and the enzyme that caused the fragmentation, the original RNA sequence can be determined.

True

34. Plasmids cannot self-replicate.

False

35. Plasmids allow for foreign DNA to be produced in a cell by cloning.

True

36. Transposons cannot self replicate.

True

37. Although baker's yeast has a large genome, it is still very useful for genetic studies.

False

38. Baker's yeast can be maintained in either the haploid or the diploid state.

True

39. There is more information available about prokaryotic genetic mechanism than about eukaryotic genetic mechanisms.

True

40. In the study of mammalian genetics, cloned genes are routinely introduced into the genome of many mammalian cells.

True

41. Insulin is a large molecule that has never been produced synthetically.

False

42. Genetic engineering allows for the production of vaccines that cause less harm than whole viral vaccinations.

True

43. With the advent of genetic engineering techniques, sexual reproduction in plants has become obsolete.

False

44. Restriction enzymes that recognize four nucleotides work more often than those that recognize six nucleotides.

True

CHAPTER 15

PROBABILITY AND STATISTICS

MEASURES OF CENTRAL TENDENCY AND DISPERSION

● **PROBLEM** 15-1

From a patch of garden peas, a random sampling of 13 plants is made. Their height in centimeters is as follows:

161 183 177 157 181 176 180
162 163 174 179 169 187

Calculate:

(a) the mean;
(b) the median;
(c) the mode;
(d) the variance;
(e) the standard deviation.

Solution: (a) The mean of a sample ($\bar{x}$) is the sum of all the quantities in the sample (Σx) divided by the number sampled (n).

$$\bar{x} = \frac{\Sigma x}{n}$$

$$\bar{x} = \frac{2249}{13} = 173 \text{ cm}$$

(b) The median is the middle value in a group of numbers arranged in order of size.

157 161 162 163 169 174 (176)
177 179 180 181 183 187

The median value is 176 cm.

If our sample had contained 12 plants instead of 13 we would not have been able to find a median data point because there is no middle value. It would lie instead between points 6 and 7. In this case we would take the mean ($\overline{x}$) between these 2 values as the median, i.e.

157 161 162 163 169 (174 176)
177 179 180 181 183

$$\overline{x} = \frac{350}{2} = 175 \text{ cm}$$

(c) The mode is the observation or observations that occur with the greatest frequency. In our sample of the garden pea all the heights occur with the same frequency. No single number is observed more than once. In a case such as this, it is necessary to arrange our data in classes, and to find the modal class.

Class	Individuals in each class	Frequency
156 - 160	157	1
161 - 165	161, 162, 163	3
166 - 170	169	1
171 - 175	174	1
176 - 180	176, 177, 179, 180	4
181 - 185	181, 183	2
186 - 190	187	1

In our sample of the garden pea, the modal class is 176-180.

(d) Variance (s^2) describes the variation or dispersion in a sample. In other words, how different each plant is from the others in the sample. The formula for sample variance is:

$$s^2 = \frac{\Sigma(x_i - \overline{x})^2}{n - 1}$$

In this case, x_i is the height of an individual plant. We already know $\overline{x}$ is 173 cm and, as before, n is the number sampled. To aid calculations it is advisable to arrange any data in tabular form as shown next.

x_i	$x_i - \bar{x}$	$(x_i - \bar{x})^2$
157	-16	256
161	-12	144
162	-11	121
163	-10	100
169	-4	16
174	1	1
176	3	9
177	4	16
179	6	36
180	7	49
181	8	64
183	10	100
187	14	196

$$s^2 = \frac{1108}{12} = 92.33 \text{ cm}^2$$

(e) Standard deviation is simply the square root of the variance.

$$s = \sqrt{s^2} = \sqrt{\frac{\Sigma (x_i - \bar{x})^2}{n - 1}} = \sqrt{92.33 \text{ cm}^2} = 9.61 \text{ cm}$$

Standard deviation is slightly more preferable than variance because it is expressed in more meaningful units - centimeters as opposed to (centimeters)^2.

● **PROBLEM** 15-2

A sample of 25 female <u>Drosophila</u> were measured for number of eggs laid in a 24-hour period, and the following counts were recorded:

97	79	88	91	88
86	104	89	91	92
103	96	101	94	91
92	94	95	88	89
90	93	84	87	93

Calculate for this sample:

a) mean number of eggs laid;

b) variance and standard deviation;

c) standard error of the mean.

Solution: a) The sample mean can be calculated using:

$$\overline{X} = \frac{\Sigma X}{N}$$

where $\overline{X}$ = mean,

ΣX = sum of the individual observations and

N = total number of observations

Thus: $\overline{X} = \frac{2,295}{25} = 91.8$ eggs/female.

b) The sample variance can be calculated using the formula: $s^2 = \frac{\Sigma (X - \overline{X})^2}{N}$, which represents the average squared deviation from the mean. However, computationally, the formula can be more conveniently presented as:

$$s^2 = \frac{X^2 - \frac{(\Sigma X)^2}{N}}{N-1}$$

Thus,

$$s^2 = \frac{211,453 - \frac{(2,295)^2}{25}}{24} = \frac{772}{24} = 31.17$$

The standard deviation can be determined by:

$$s.d. = \sqrt{s^2} = \sqrt{31.1667} = 5.58$$

c) The standard error of the mean can be determined by the formula, $S.E. = \frac{s.d.}{\sqrt{N}}$; thus, $S.E. = 1.11$.

The radii of five different brands of softballs (in inches) are 2.03, 1.98, 2.24, 2.17, 2.08. Find the range, variance, standard deviation, mean deviation about the median, and coefficient of variation.

Solution: The range gives a measure of how dispersed our sample may be. It is defined as the difference between the smallest and largest observations. In this case the range equals 2.24 in. - 1.98 in. = 0.26 in.

To compute the variance, $s^2 = \frac{1}{n} \Sigma(X-\overline{X})^2$, we first need the mean, $\overline{X}$.

$$\overline{X} = \frac{\Sigma X}{n} = \frac{2.03 + 1.98 + 2.24 + 2.17 + 2.08}{5} = 2.10.$$

Variance $= \frac{1}{n} \Sigma(X-\overline{X})^2$. The computations involved are represented in tabular form.

X	X - $\overline{X}$	$(X - \overline{X})^2$
2.03	2.03 - 2.10 = - .07	$(- .07)^2 = .0049$
1.98	1.98 - 2.10 = - .12	$(- .12)^2 = .0144$
2.24	2.24 - 2.10 = .14	$(.14)^2 = .0196$
2.17	2.17 - 2.10 = .07	$(.07)^2 = .0049$
2.08	2.08 - 2.10 = - .02	$(- .02)^2 = .0004$
		$\Sigma(X - \overline{X})^2 = .0442$

$$\frac{1}{n} \Sigma(X - \overline{X})^2 = \frac{.0442}{5} = .00884.$$

The standard deviation is the square root of the variance $s = \sqrt{.00884} = .094$.

Since we have 5 observations, the third from the lowest, 2.08, is the median. We will compute the mean deviation about the median with the aid of a table:

X	X - n	|X - n|
2.03	2.03 - 2.08 = - .05	|- .05| = .05
1.98	1.98 - 2.08 = - .10	|- .10| = .10
2.24	2.24 - 2.08 = .16	|.16| = .16
2.17	2.17 - 2.08 = .09	|.09| = .09
2.08	2.08 - 2.08 = 0	|0| = 0

Mean deviation about median $= \dfrac{\Sigma |X - n|}{n}$

$$= \frac{.05 + .10 + .16 + .09 + 0}{5} = \frac{.4}{5} = .08.$$

The Coefficient of Variation is defined as

$$V = \frac{s}{\overline{X}} .$$

Sometimes we want to compare sets of data which are measured differently. Suppose we have a sample of executives with a mean age of 51 and a standard deviation of 11.74 years. Suppose also we know their average IQ is 125 with a standard deviation of 20 points. How can we compare deviations? We use the coefficient of variation:

$$V_{age} = \frac{s}{\overline{X}} = \frac{11.74}{51} - .23; \quad V_{IQ} = \frac{s}{\overline{X}} = \frac{20}{125} = .16.$$

We now know that there is more variation with respect to age.

In our example, $V = \dfrac{s}{\overline{X}} = \dfrac{0.094}{2.10} = .045.$

CALCULATING HERITABILITY

● **PROBLEM** 15-4

Measurements are made in mm of the length of the trumpet in two varieites of daffodil (A and B). Variety A is crossed with variety B and the same measurements are made on the F_1 and F_2 progeny.

The data is compiled in the following table:

Length in mm	Variety A (P_A)	Variety B (P_B)	F_1	F_2
20	1			
21	12			
22	50			
23	77			
24	48			
25	10			1
26	2			1
27				2
28				2
29				2
30			2	6
31			9	18
32			18	57
33			53	115
34			85	145
35			57	108
36			20	55
37			7	13
38			1	6
39				3
40				3
41				2
42				1
43		2		1
44		14		1
45		45		
46		81		
47		47		
48		10		
49		1		

(a) Calculate the mean, standard deviation, and standard error of the mean for each.

(b) Determine whether the difference in the P_1 and P_2 varieties is statistically significant.

(c) Determine if the difference between the F_1 and F_2 is statistically significant.

(d) Assuming that each parental variety was homozygous and that the genes involved are additive in their effect, estimate how many gene pairs are segregating and assorting in the F_2 generation.

Solution: (a) Applying the formula for the mean

$$\bar{x} = \frac{\Sigma fx}{n}$$

where f equals the observed frequency of each height, gives us the following means:

$P_A: \bar{x} = \frac{4597}{200} = 23$ mm $\qquad P_B: \bar{x} = \frac{9191}{200} = 46$ mm

$F_1: \bar{x} = \frac{8566}{252} = 34$ mm $\qquad F_2: \bar{x} = \frac{18379}{542} = 34$ mm

Now, to calculate the standard deviation we use

$$s = \sqrt{\frac{\Sigma f(x-\bar{x})^2}{n-1}} \; .$$

Compiling the following tables:

for P_A:

x	f	$x-\bar{x}$	$f(x-\bar{x})^2$
20	1	-3	9
21	12	-2	48
22	50	-1	50
23	77	0	0
24	48	1	48
25	10	2	40
26	2	3	18

$$P_A: \; s = \sqrt{\frac{\Sigma f(x-\bar{x})^2}{n-1}} = \sqrt{\frac{213}{199}} = 1.03$$

For P_B:

x	f	$x-\bar{x}$	$f(x-\bar{x})^2$
43	2	-3	18
44	14	-2	56
45	45	-1	45
46	81	0	0
47	47	1	47
48	10	2	40
49	1	3	9

$$P_B: \; s = \sqrt{\frac{\Sigma f(x-\bar{x})^2}{n-1}} = \sqrt{\frac{215}{199}} = 1.04$$

543

For F$_1$:

x	f	x − x̄	f(x−x̄)^2
30	2	−4	32
31	9	−3	81
32	18	−2	72
33	53	−1	53
34	85	0	0
35	57	1	57
36	20	2	80
37	7	3	63
38	1	4	16

$$F_1: \quad s = \sqrt{\frac{\Sigma f(x-\bar{x})^2}{n-1}} = \sqrt{\frac{454}{251}} = 1.34$$

For F$_2$:

x	f	x − x̄	f(x−x̄)^2
25	1	−9	81
26	1	−8	64
27	2	−7	98
28	2	−6	72
29	2	−5	50
30	6	−4	96
31	18	−3	162
32	57	−2	228
33	115	−1	115
34	145	0	0
35	108	1	108
36	55	2	220
37	13	3	117
38	6	4	96
39	3	5	75
40	3	6	108
41	2	7	98
42	1	8	64
43	1	9	81
44	1	10	100

$$F_2: \quad s = \sqrt{\frac{\Sigma f(x-\bar{x})^2}{n-1}} = \sqrt{\frac{2033}{541}} = 1.94$$

To find the standard error of the mean we use the following formula:

$$\delta_{\bar{X}} = \frac{s}{\sqrt{n}}$$

For P$_A$: $\quad \delta_{\bar{X}} = \frac{1.03}{\sqrt{200}} = 0.07$

For P_B: $\delta_{\overline{X}} = \dfrac{1.04}{\sqrt{200}} = 0.07$

For F_1: $\delta_{\overline{X}} = \dfrac{1.34}{\sqrt{252}} = 0.08$

For F_2: $\delta_{\overline{X}} = \dfrac{1.94}{\sqrt{542}} = 0.08$

(b) To determine whether the difference between P_A and P_B is statistically significant we must find the standard error of the difference in the means (δ_D) using the formula:

$$\delta_D = \sqrt{(\delta_{\overline{X}_A})^2 + (\delta_{\overline{X}_B})^2}.$$

This gives us $\delta_D = \sqrt{(0.07)^2 + (0.07)^2} = 0.10$

The actual difference between the means of the two samples is ± 23. This 230 times the standard error of the difference in the means. We can thus say that the difference between P_A and P_B is very significant.

(c) Using the same formula as above we get:

$$\delta_D = \sqrt{(0.08)^2 + (0.08)^2} = 0.11$$

The actual difference between the means of F_1 and F_2 is 0 and therefore $0/.11 = 0$. Obviously, there is no significant difference between F_1 and F_2.

(d) In this case the extremes of homozygosity present in F_2 occur 2 in 542 or 1 in 271. Therefore, we can say that there are probably 4 pairs of genes present, since in such a case either homozygote would be expected to occur 1 in 4^4 or 1 in 256 times (which is close to our observation).

The following table contains data on the variances of two phenotypic traits in sparrows (wing span and beak length):

	Wing Span		Beak Length
V_P	271.4	V_P	627.8
V_E	71.2	V_E	107.3
V_A	102.0	V_A	342.9
V_{GE}	98.9	V_{GE}	177.6

a) Calculate the heritability for each trait.

b) Tell which one of these two traits is more susceptible to selection pressure.

Solution: Upon examining any population for a particular trait, the observed variation among individuals of that population may be the result of genetic differences, environmental differences or any combined interaction of these two factors. Stated in a more mathematical sense, the total phenotypic variance (V_P) observed in a population is the sum of three factors: the environmental variance (V_E), the genetic variance (V_G) and the variance due to genetic and environmental interaction (V_{GE}). This can be expressed in the formula:

$$V_P = V_G + V_E + V_{GE}$$

The V_E component is the expression of all differences which are not genetically based. The V_G component represents all differences which are genetic. The V_{GE} component is a representation of how the genotypic expression varies in regard to the type of environment in which it is placed. Of these three components V_{GE} is the most difficult to measure quantitatively. Because of this, V_{GE} is' often disregarded and the following formula is used:

$$H = \frac{V_G}{V_P}$$

What this formula says is that heritability (H) is a measure of the degree to which a phenotype is genetically determined and the degree to which it is influenced by natural selection. It does not end there, however, as the component V_G can be further divided into three subcomponents. As we know, some genes are additive in their effect, some dominant, and some epistatic. These are represented by V_A, V_D and V_I respectively.

Therefore:

$$V_G = V_A + V_D + V_I$$

The most significant of these components is V_A, and it is usually the only value considered, hence:

$$H = \frac{V_A}{V_P}$$

A value of H = 1 would indicate a trait not influenced by the environment. A trait with H = 0 has no genetic basis.

So, from what we are given the heritability of wing span is:

$$H = \frac{V_A}{V_P} = \frac{102.0}{271.4} = 0.376$$

For beak length

$$H = \frac{V_A}{V_P} = \frac{342.9}{627.8} = 0.546$$

Since the heritability value of wing span is a smaller number than the heritability value of beak length, $0.376 < 0.546$, it is therefore farther away from one (no environmental influence involved) and closer to zero (no genetic basis). We can conclude that wing span is more susceptible to selection pressure (environment) than beak length.

It is important to keep in mind that heritability is only an approximation and, as mentioned earlier, many of the components are difficult to quantify.

According to early studies (performed by Wright) on guinea pig coat color, the total variance in a randomly mating strain was 0.573. The variance in an inbred strain was 0.340. From correlations between relatives in the randomly mating population the heritability (gene effect) was determined to be 38% of the total variance. Find the following: (a) variance due to the gene effect; (b) variance due to epistasis and dominance.

Solution: The variance of a population of animals or plants can be represented by the following formula:

$$V_t = V_g + V_d + V_i + V_e$$

where

V_t = total phenotypic variance

V_g = variance due to gene effect

V_d = variance due to epistasis

V_i = variance due to dominance

V_e = environmental variance

a) Since the gene effect is given to be 38% of the total variance, we can compute the following:

0.38 x 0.573 = 0.218 = variance due to gene effect

b) Since we are given 0.340 as the variance in the inbred strain (this can be considered to be the environmental variance) we can write the following:

$$0.573 = 0.218 + V_d + V_i + 0.340$$

$$0.015 = V_d + V_i$$

GENERAL PROBABILITY AND APPLICATIONS

A deck of playing cards is thoroughly shuffled and a card is drawn from the deck. What is the probability that the card drawn is the ace of diamonds?

Solution: The probability of an event occurring is

$$\frac{\text{the number of ways the event can occur}}{\text{the number of possible outcomes}}$$

In our case there is one way the event can occur, for there is only one ace of diamonds and there are fifty-two possible outcomes (for there are 52 cards in the deck). Hence the probability that the card drawn is the ace of diamonds is 1/52.

What is the probability of getting a 5 on each of two successive rolls of a balanced die?

Solution: We are dealing with separate rolls of a balanced die. The 2 rolls are independent; therefore, we invoke the following multiplication rule: The probability of getting any particular combination in two or more independent trials will be the product of their individual probabilities. The probability of getting a 5 on any single toss is $\frac{1}{6}$ and by the multiplication rule

$$P \ (5 \text{ and }) = \frac{1}{6} \cdot \frac{1}{6} = \frac{1}{36} \ .$$

Note also the problem could have been stated as follows: What is the probability of rolling 2 balanced dice simultaneously and getting a 5 on each?

If a pair of dice is tossed twice, find the probability of obtaining 5 on both tosses.

Solution: We obtain 5 in one toss of the two dice if they fall with either 3 and 2 or 4 and 1 uppermost, and each of these combinations can appear in two ways. The ways to obtain 5 in one toss of the two dice are:

$$(1,4),(4,1),(3,2), \text{ and } (2,3).$$

Hence, we can throw 5 in one toss in four ways. Each die has six faces and there are six ways for a die to fall. Then the pair of dice can fall in 6·6 = 36 ways. The probability of throwing 5 in one toss is:

$$\frac{\text{the number of ways to throw a 5 in one toss}}{\text{the number of ways that a pair of dice can fall}} = \frac{4}{36} = \frac{1}{9}.$$

Now the probability of throwing a 5 on both tosses is:

P(throwing five on first toss and throwing five on second toss).

"And" implies multiplication if events are independent, thus p(throwing 5 on first toss and throwing 5 on second toss)

= p(throwing 5 on first toss) x p(throwing 5 on second toss)

Since the results of the two tosses are independent. Consequently, the probability of obtaining 5 on both tosses is

$$\left(\frac{1}{9}\right)\left(\frac{1}{9}\right) = \frac{1}{81}.$$

The trait represented in the pedigree below is inherited through a single dominant gene. Calculate the probability of the trait appearing in the offspring if the following cousins should marry.

(a) $F_{2,2}$ x $F_{2,4}$;   (b) $F_{2,1}$ x $F_{2,3}$.

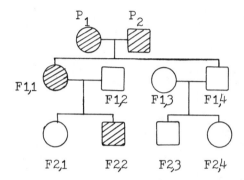

Solution: Let R represent the dominant allele for the trait, and r the recessive allele. First, we can determine the possible genotypes of the individuals involved. We know that $F_{1,2}$, $F_{1,3}$, $F_{1,4}$, $F_{2,1}$, $F_{2,3}$, and $F_{2,4}$ are homozygous recessive (rr), since they do not express the trait. P_1 and P_2 must be heterozygous dominant (Rr) since they produced a child ($F_{1,4}$) who is homozygous recessive. F_1, could be either RR or Rr. However, F_2 is homozygous recessive. Therefore, $F_{1,1}$ must carry the recessive allele and be Rr.

$F_{2,2}$ is also a heterozygote. We know this because one of his parents ($F_{1,2}$) is a homozygous recessive, and the cross (Rr x rr) is incapable of producing a homozygous dominant.

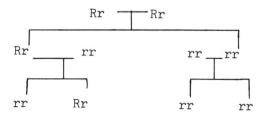

We can now do the crosses in question.

a)   P   Rr   x   rr

Gametes   R;r   r

F_1 1 Rr : 1 rr

In this cross, half the offspring are heterozygous dominant and half are monozygous recessive. Thus, we can say that there is a .5 probability that any offspring of the mating will express the dominant trait.

b)   P   rr   x   rr

gametes   r   r

F_1 rr

Since neither parent carries the dominant allele it should be obvious even without doing the cross that no offspring expressing the dominant trait will be produced.

Thus, we can say that there is 0 probability that any offspring will express the trait.

● **PROBLEM** 15-11

Polydactyly is a dominant genetic trait in which more than the normal five digits are present on hands or feet. If a man heterozygous for polydactyly marries a normal woman, (A) what is the probability that their first child will have polydactyly?, (B) what is the probability that their second child will have polydactyly?

Solution: Man heterozygous   Normal
                 for polydactyly   woman
                          Pp   X   pp

     Types of gamete   P p   p p

	P	p	Expected results in progeny
p	Pp	pp	1/2 Pp polydactyly
p	Pp	pp	1/2 pp normal

(A) The probability of a child (the first) having polydactyly is 1/2.

(B) Since each child is an independent event, the probability would be the same (1/2) in the second child.

Consider that in humans red-green colorblindness is controlled by a recessive X-linked gene, c. Assume that a normal-visioned woman, whose father was colorblind, marries a normal-visioned man.

What is the probability that their first child will be colorblind?

Solution: Since this trait is sex-linked, we first must consider whether sex of the child is important, and determine the genotypes of the parents. The woman has to be heterozygous, Cc, since her father was colorblind, and the man must be C/ since he was normal-visioned. As a consequence, the only children that can exhibit the trait will be sons. Therefore, the probability of the first child being colorblind means that the child must also be a male.

Thus, P = P(male) · P(colorblind) = 1/2 · 1/2 = 1/4.

● PROBLEM 15-13

Consider the following three traits in the fruit fly, Drosophila melanogaster, each controlled by a single pair of contrasting genes exhibiting complete dominance:

wing length	body color	eye color
Long wings = L	gray body = B	dull red eyes = R
short wings = l	black body = b	brown eyes = r

Assume that each pair of genes is located in a different pair of chromosomes (i.e., independent gene pairs). In a cross between two flies heterozygous for each pair of genes, what is the probability that the first adult fly emerging is short-winged, gray-bodied and red-eyed?

Solution: Since the three traits are controlled by independent gene pairs, we can use the Probability Law for Independent Events which states the probability of simultaneous occurrence of independent events is equal to the product of their separate probabilities.

The probability of getting short wings from this cross is 1/4, the probability of getting gray body is 3/4, and the probability of getting red eyes is 3/4. Thus, P = P(short)·P(gray)·P(red) = (1/4)(3/4)(3/4) = 9/64.

● **PROBLEM 15-14**

Given the following human pedigree:

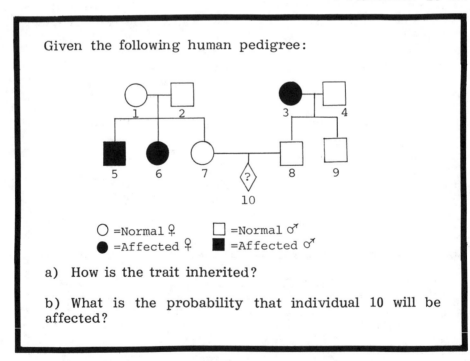

O =Normal ♀   □ =Normal ♂
● =Affected ♀   ■ =Affected ♂

a) How is the trait inherited?

b) What is the probability that individual 10 will be affected?

Solution: a) Since individual 3 is affected and none of her children are, and since individuals 5 and 6 are affected but neither of their parents are, the trait most likely is inherited as a recessive. There is also no apparent association with sex, so the trait most likely is autosomal as well.

b) Since individual 8 is known to be heterozygous, the probability that he will transmit the gene is 1/2. Since both parents of individual 7 are heterozygous, the probability that she also is heterozygous is 2/3, and if heterozygous, the probability that she **will** transmit the gene is 1/2. Thus, the probability that individual 10 will receive a defective gene from both parents is:

$$P = (1/2) \cdot [(1/2)(2/3)] = 1/6.$$

CONDITIONAL PROBABILITY

● **PROBLEM** 15-15

Find the probability that a face card is drawn on the first draw and an ace on the second in two consecutive draws, without replacement, from a standard deck of cards.

Solution: This problem illustrates the notion of conditional probability. The conditional probability of an event - event B - given the occurrence of a previous event - event A - is written $P(B/A)$. This is the conditional probability of B given A.

$P(B/A)$ is defined to be $\dfrac{P(AB)}{P(A)}$, where $P(AB) =$

Probability of the joint occurrence of events A and B.

Let A = event that a face card is drawn on the
first draw

B = event that an ace is drawn on the
second draw

We wish to find the probability of the joint occurrence of these events, $P(AB)$.

We know that $P(AB) = P(A) \cdot P(B/A)$.

P(A) = probability that a face card is drawn on the

$$\text{first draw} = \frac{12}{52} = \frac{3}{13}.$$

P(B/A) = probability that an ace is drawn on the
second draw given that a face card is drawn
on the first

= number of ways an ace can be drawn on the second
draw given a face card is drawn on the first divided by
the total number of possible outcomes of the second draw.

$= \frac{4}{51}$; remember there will be only 51 cards left in the

deck after the face card is drawn.

$$\text{Thus } P(AB) = \frac{3}{13} \cdot \frac{4}{51} = \frac{4}{13 \times 17} = \frac{4}{221}.$$

● **PROBLEM** 15-16

You are in your laboratory late one night, working
with eight separate containers holding the flour
beetle, Tribolium castaneum. Three of the containers
hold beetles homozygous for ebony bodies. The
remaining five containers hold beetles homozygous for
red bodies. Suddenly, the lights in your lab go out.
You decide to remove your beetles to another lab so
you can continue your work. If you can carry only
one container at a time, what is the probability that
the first container you select in the darkness contains
homozygous ebony beetles and the second container
contains homozygous red?

Solution: The probability that the first container you
select will contain ebony beetles will be denoted $P(e_1)$. It
is assumed that your selection is made at random. We can
apply the classical probability model to this problem:

$$P(e_1) = \frac{\text{number of containers with ebony beetles}}{\text{total number of containers}} = \frac{3}{8}$$

We now wish to calculate the conditional probability that a
container holding red beetles will be selected on the
second selection, given an ebony beetle container was

556

drawn on the first. This can be denoted by $P(R_2/e_1)$. Thus,

$$P(R_2/e_1) \;=\; \frac{\text{number of containers with red beetles}}{\text{total of containers after removal of 1 ebony}}$$

$$=\; \frac{5}{8-1} \;=\; \frac{5}{7}$$

The probability we wish to find is $P(R_2$ and $e_1)$. By the multiplication rule,

$$P(R_2 \text{ and } e_1) = P(e_1)P(R_2/e_1)$$

$$= \left(\frac{3}{8}\right)\left(\frac{5}{7}\right) = \frac{15}{56}$$

Thus, the probability of you selecting first a box with ebony beetles and then a box with red beetles is $15/56 = 0.268$.

● **PROBLEM** 15-17

Find the probability of throwing at least one of the following totals on a single throw of a pair of dice: a total of 5, a total of 6, a total of 7.

Define the events A, B, and C as follows:

    Event A: a total of 5 is thrown,

    Event B: a total of 6 is thrown,

    Event C: a total of 7 is thrown.

Solution: Only one of these three events can occur at one time. The occurrence of any one excludes the occurrence of any of the others. Such events are called mutually exclusive.

Let $A \cup B \cup C$ = the event that at least a 5, 6 or 7 is thrown. $P(A \cup B \cup C) = P(A) + P(B) + P(C)$ because the events are mutually exclusive.

Referring to a previous table we see that

557

$$P(A) = \frac{4}{36}, \quad P(B) = \frac{5}{36}, \quad \text{and} \quad P(C) = \frac{6}{36}. \quad \text{Therefore,}$$

$$P(A \cup B \cup C) = \frac{4}{36} + \frac{5}{36} + \frac{6}{36} = \frac{15}{36} = \frac{5}{12}.$$

HARDY-WEINBERG PROBABILITIES

● **PROBLEM** 15-18

Derive the Hardy-Weinberg probabilities in a population with random mating.

<u>Solution</u>: Assume that a sexually reproducing population contains N males and K females. The total population, T, is equal to N + K. Each individual carries two genes and each gene is represented by one of two alleles, A or a. The two genes together constitute that individual's genotype - AA, Aa, or aa.

In the process of mating, each partner contributes one gene to the offspring. For example, if a male of genotype Aa mates with a female of genotype AA, the following diagram illustrates the possible genotypes of the offspring:

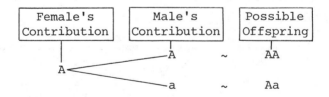

First, consider all of the male genes. Since there are N males, there are 2N total male genes. A certain number of these, r, are of the type A. The proportion of the frequency of gene A in the males can be represented by $p = \frac{r}{2N}$. The proportion of the remaining genes, type a, can be represented by $q = 1 - p$, or $q = 1 - \frac{r}{2N}$. For example, if there were 100 males, there would be 200 total genes (A + a). If r = 50, then $p = \frac{50}{200} = \frac{1}{4}$, and $q = \frac{3}{4}$. Similarly, realizing that the total number of female genes is 2K, we can define p' as the gene frequency of A, and q' as the frequency of a, in females.

Note that it is possible to have the same gene frequencies even though the genotype proportions might differ. Consider the following example: In a group of 100 organisms, we might have 50 AA, 0 Aa, and 50 aa, in which case p = 0.5. Another possibility is that there might be 25 AA, 50 Aa, and 25 aa, in which case p is also 0.5.

We now turn to the subject of random mating. We are said to have a random mating population if the determination of the genotype of an offspring obeys the following three rules: (1) A gene is selected simply at random from all the male genes in the population. (2) A gene is selected simply at random from all the female genes in the population. (3) The two experiments are independent.

In the first experiment there are 2N male genes in the sample space. Since the selection is random, each gene has the probability, $\frac{1}{2N}$, of contributing to the offspring, if there are r genes of type A. The probability, p, of choosing one is $\frac{r}{2N}$.

Analogous reasoning holds for the second experiment: the selection of a gene from a female. There are 2K simple events in the sample space. The probability of the event "the gene chosen is A" is p'; and that of "the gene chosen is a" is q'. Since the two experiments are independent, the following tree diagram can be constructed:

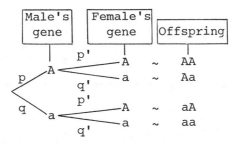

Recall that genotype Aa is the same as aA. From the diagram the probabilities of offspring genotypes are:

$P(AA) = pp'$; $P(Aa) = pq' + qp'$; $P(aa) = qq'$.

Usually we assume that the gene frequencies are the same in both males and females (i.e. $p = p'$ and $q = q'$). Then the probabilities become:

$P(AA) = p^2$; $P(Aa) = 2pq$; $P(aa) = q^2$.

These probabilities have been brought together in one formula, called the Hardy-Weinberg equation:

$$p^2 + 2pq + q^2 = 1.$$

This equation can be used to calculate the frequencies of two alleles of a gene in a sample population.

● PROBLEM 15-19

Referring to the independent random mating scheme of the previous problem, find the offspring genotype probabilities of the following two populations:

a)

	AA	Aa	aa
Males	600	0	400
Females	400	400	200

b)

	AA	Aa	aa
Males	400	400	200
Females	200	800	0

Solution: Each individual has 2 alleles. The homozygotes can be either AA or aa and the heterozygotes are Aa at this particular gene locus.

a) We must find the population gene frequencies.

Males: 600 AA ⟶ 600   x   2 A's ⟶ 1200 A

400 aa ⟶ 400   x   2 a's ⟶   800 a

Total =   2000 alleles

$$P(A) = p = \frac{\# A}{Total} = \frac{1200}{2000} = \frac{3}{5}$$

$$P(a) = q = 1 - p = \frac{2}{5} \; .$$

Females: 400 AA ⟶ 400   x   2 A's ⟶ 800 A

200 aa ⟶ 200   x   2 a's ⟶ 400 a

400 Aa ⟶ 400   x   1 A   ⟶ 400 A

400   x   a   ⟶ 400 a

Totals: 1200 A; 800 a; 2000 alleles

$$p' = \frac{\# A}{Total} = \frac{1200}{2000} = \frac{3}{5} \; ; \quad q' = 1 - p' = \frac{2}{5} \; .$$

From the Hardy-Weinberg probabilities:

$$P(AA) = pp' = \left(\frac{3}{5}\right)\left(\frac{3}{5}\right) = \frac{9}{25}$$

$$P(Aa) = pq' + p'q = \left(\frac{3}{5}\right)\left(\frac{2}{5}\right) + \left(\frac{3}{5}\right)\left(\frac{2}{5}\right) = \frac{12}{25}$$

$$P(aa) = qq' = \left(\frac{2}{5}\right)\left(\frac{2}{5}\right) = \frac{4}{25} \; .$$

b) The same technique can be used for the second population. We first find the population gene frequencies.

Males: 400 AA ⟶ 400   x   2 A's ⟶ 800 A

200 aa ⟶ 200   x   2 a's ⟶ 400 a

400 Aa ⟶ 400   x   1 A   ⟶ 400 A

400   x   1 a   ⟶ 400 a

Totals: 1200 A; 800 a; 2000 overall

$$p = \frac{\# A}{Total} = \frac{1200}{2000} = \frac{3}{5} \; ; \quad q = 1 - p = \frac{2}{5}$$

Females: 200 AA $\longrightarrow$ 200   x   2 A's $\longrightarrow$ 400 A

800 Aa $\longrightarrow$ 800   x   1 A $\longrightarrow$ 800 A

800   x   1 a $\longrightarrow$ 800 a

Totals: 1200 A; 800 a; 2000 overall

$$p' = \frac{\# A}{\text{Total}} = \frac{1200}{2000} = \frac{3}{5} \; ; \quad q' = 1 - p' = \frac{2}{5} \; .$$

We have the same p, p', q , q' as in part a. Therefore, the offspring genotype probabilities will be the same.

$$P(AA) = \frac{9}{25} \quad P(Aa) = \frac{12}{25} \quad P(aa) = \frac{4}{25} \; .$$

BINOMIAL DISTRIBUTION

● **PROBLEM** 15-20

What is the probability of getting exactly three heads in five flips of a balanced coin?

Solution: In this problem we can introduce the use of the binomial distribution. The binomial distribution is a method for determining the probability of occurrence of any of all the possible results for certain types of problems. In order for the binomial distribution to be applicable, the following three conditions must be met by the problem:

1) the same experiment is repeated several times;

2) there are only two possible outcomes each time the experiment is repeated;

3) events are independent (the probability of success or failure must remain the same on each trial).

When these three conditions are met, we can use the binomial distribution, which is stated as follows:

$$P(X) = \frac{N!}{X!(N-X)!} \; p^X \cdot q^{N-X}$$

where:

    N = the total number of times the experiment is repeated

    X = the number of occurrences or successes of an event in N trials

  N-X = the number of failures or occurrences in N trials

    p = the probability of occurrence or success on a single trial. (p must remain the same on all trials.)

    q = the probability of failure, or nonoccurrence, on a single trial. (q must remain the same on all trials.)
    Note:
    p + q must always equal one.

In this particular problem, the same experiment is repeated five times: N = 5.

There are only two possible outcomes on each trial of the experiment: heads or tails. In our case we wish to record a head as a success and a tail as a failure. The probability of getting heads or tails remains the same with each flip (independent events). Hence, p = 1/2, q = 1/2. Since we want to find the probability of getting exactly 3 heads, X = 3. So, plugging into the equation we get:

$$P(3) = \frac{5!}{3!(5-3)!} \; (\tfrac{1}{2})^3 (\tfrac{1}{2})^{5-3}$$

$$= \frac{5!}{3! \, 2!} \; (\tfrac{1}{2})^3 (\tfrac{1}{2})^2$$

$$= \frac{(5)(4)(3)(2)(1)}{(3)(2)(1)(2)(1)} \; (\tfrac{1}{2})^5$$

$$= \frac{(5)(\overset{2}{\cancel{4}})(3)(2)(1)}{(3)(2)(1)(2)(1)} \; (\tfrac{1}{2})(\tfrac{1}{2})(\tfrac{1}{2})(\tfrac{1}{2})(\tfrac{1}{2})$$

$$= 10(1/32)$$

$$= \frac{10}{32}$$

$$= 31.25\%$$

Therefore, the probability of getting exactly three heads in five flips of the coin is 0.3125 or 31.25%.

● **PROBLEM** 15-21

Suppose you are a geneticist confronted by two anxious parents, both of whom are known to be carriers for albinism. They want to know what the chance is for the following combinations if they choose to have four children:

(a)   all four are normal;
(b)   three normal and one albino;
(c)   two normal and 2 albino;
(d)   one normal and three albino.

Solution: Albinism is transmitted as an autosomal recessive. If both partners are carriers they will be normally pigmented and their genotypes will be Cc. Each child will have the following genotypic probabilities:

$$Cc \times Cc = \begin{array}{l} 1/4 \text{ CC} \\ 1/4 \text{ cc} \\ 1/2 \text{ Cc} \end{array}$$

The phenotypic results will be:

3/4 normal pigmentation
1/4 Albino

These probabilities predict the frequency of different phenotypes or genotypes arising from a particular cross. In situations where large populations are often obtained these probabilities are sufficient. However, when we have only a few fertilizations we wish to be able to predict the chance that a particular combination of phenotypes will occur in a specified number of fertilizations. This is most often the case in human genetics. The probability for any specific combination of genotypes or phenotypes can be calculated using the formula:

$$P = \frac{n!}{x!\,(n-x)!} \cdot (a)^x (b)^{n-x}$$

n = the number of events (children) specified (4)
x = the number of normal children specified
a = individual probability of a normal child (3/4)
b = individual probability of an albino child (1/4)

The symbol ! means factorial - the product of all the integers from 1 to the term specified. Thus, in this example,

n! = 4! = 1 x 2 x 3 x 4 = 24.

We are now ready to solve (a).

$$P = \frac{4!}{4!\,(4-4)!} \cdot (3/4)^4 (1/4)^{4-4}$$

$$P = \frac{81}{256} = 0.316$$

The probability of having 4 normal children is 0.316.

(b) $$P = \frac{4!}{3!\,(4-3)!} \cdot (3/4)^3 (1/4)^{4-3}$$

$$P = \frac{648}{1536} = 0.422$$

The probability of having 3 normal children and 1 albino is 0.422.

(c) $$P = \frac{4!}{2!\,(4-2)!} \cdot (3/4)^2 (1/4)^{4-2}$$

$$P = \frac{216}{1024} = 0.211$$

The probability of having 2 normal and 2 albino children is 0.211.

(d) $$P = \frac{4!}{1!\,(4-1)!} \cdot (3/4)^1 (1/4)^{4-1}$$

$$P = \frac{72}{1536} = 0.047$$

The probability of having 1 normal and 3 albino children is 0.047.

From our results we can see that having 3 normal children and 1 albino is the most probable combination for a couple having 4 children.

Assuming that a 1:1 sex ratio exists for humans, what is the probability that a newly married couple, who plan to have a family of four children, will have three daughters and one son?

Solution: We use the following formula to solve this problem:

$$P = \frac{n!}{x!\,(n-x)!} \; p^x q^{n-x}$$

where

n   = total number of children

x   = number of daughters

n-x = number of sons

p   = probability of a daughter

q   = probability of a son

Thus,

$$P = \frac{4 \cdot 3 \cdot 2 \cdot 1}{(3 \cdot 2 \cdot 1)(1)} \; (1/2)^3 (1/2) = 1/4.$$

NORMAL DISTRIBUTION

Distinguish between a discrete variable and a continuous variable and give examples of each.

Solution: A discrete random variable is a variable which can take on only isolated values.

Some examples of discrete variables are:

1) the number of offspring in a mouse litter;

2) the number of girls in families with 4 children;
3) the number of apples in a bushel;
4) the number of sparrows per acre of land.

All of these examples are counts. Many situations do not involve counting, but rather, measurement. In this case we could say that a boy is 65 inches tall or if measured more accurately 65.3 inches, or even more accurately 65.32 inches. In other words, a person's height may be a range of values, and not just isolated values such as 64, 65, 66 inches.

Some examples of continuous variables are:

1) the time it takes for an electric component to fail;
2) the cruising speeds of various airplanes;
3) the heights of a hybrid strain of plants;
4) the length of people's toes.

● **PROBLEM 15-24**

If a random variable X is normally distributed with a mean of 118 and a standard deviation of 11, what Z-scores correspond to raw scores of 115, 134 and 99?

Solution: To convert a raw score to a Z-score we subtract the mean and divide by the standard deviation. Thus

$$Z\text{-score} = \frac{\text{Raw score} - \text{mean}}{\text{standard deviation}}.$$

Thus,

$$\frac{115 - 118}{11} = \frac{-3}{11} = -.27:$$

a Z-score of -.27 corresponds to a raw score of 115.

$$Z = \frac{134 - 118}{11} = \frac{16}{11} = 1.45 \text{ or}$$

a Z-score of 1.45 corresponds to a raw score of 134. And

$$Z = \frac{99 - 118}{11} = -1.73,$$

or a Z-score of -1.73 corresponds to a raw score of 99.

● **PROBLEM** 15-25

Given that x has a normal distribution with mean 10 and standard deviation 4, find P(x < 15).

Solution: x is a normal random variable with a mean or location parameter of 10 and a standard deviation or scale parameter of 4. A graph of its density function might look like this:

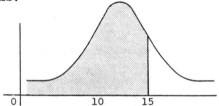

We wish to find the Pr(x < 15) or the area of the shaded area. It would be possible to construct tables which would supply such probabilities for many different values of the mean and standard deviation. Luckily this is not necessary. We may shift and contort our density function in such a way so that only one table is needed. How is such a change accomplished?

First the mean is subtracted from x giving a new random variable, x - 10. This new random variable is normally distributed but E(x - 10), the mean of x - 10, is E(x) - 10 = 0. We have shifted our distribution so that it is centered at 0.

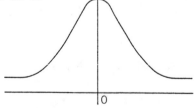

We can contort our new random variable by dividing by the standard deviation creating a new random variable $Z = \frac{x - 10}{4}$; the variance of Z is

$$\text{Var}\left(\frac{x - 10}{4}\right) = \frac{\text{Var } x}{16} = \frac{(\text{standard deviation of } x)^2}{16} = 1.$$

Fortunately, after all this twisting and shifting, our new random variable Z is still normally distributed and has mean 0 and variance 1. This new random variable is referred to as a Z-score or standard random variable and tables for its probabilities are widespread.

To solve our problem we first convert an x-score to a Z-score and then consult the following table:

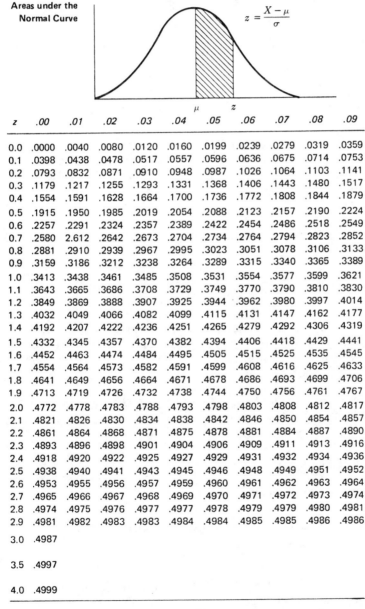

Areas under the Normal Curve

$z = \dfrac{X - \mu}{\sigma}$

z	.00	.01	.02	.03	.04	.05	.06	.07	.08	.09
0.0	.0000	.0040	.0080	.0120	.0160	.0199	.0239	.0279	.0319	.0359
0.1	.0398	.0438	.0478	.0517	.0557	.0596	.0636	.0675	.0714	.0753
0.2	.0793	.0832	.0871	.0910	.0948	.0987	.1026	.1064	.1103	.1141
0.3	.1179	.1217	.1255	.1293	.1331	.1368	.1406	.1443	.1480	.1517
0.4	.1554	.1591	.1628	.1664	.1700	.1736	.1772	.1808	.1844	.1879
0.5	.1915	.1950	.1985	.2019	.2054	.2088	.2123	.2157	.2190	.2224
0.6	.2257	.2291	.2324	.2357	.2389	.2422	.2454	.2486	.2518	.2549
0.7	.2580	2.612	.2642	.2673	.2704	.2734	.2764	.2794	.2823	.2852
0.8	.2881	.2910	.2939	.2967	.2995	.3023	.3051	.3078	.3106	.3133
0.9	.3159	.3186	.3212	.3238	.3264	.3289	.3315	.3340	.3365	.3389
1.0	.3413	.3438	.3461	.3485	.3508	.3531	.3554	.3577	.3599	.3621
1.1	.3643	.3665	.3686	.3708	.3729	.3749	.3770	.3790	.3810	.3830
1.2	.3849	.3869	.3888	.3907	.3925	.3944	.3962	.3980	.3997	.4014
1.3	.4032	.4049	.4066	.4082	.4099	.4115	.4131	.4147	.4162	.4177
1.4	.4192	.4207	.4222	.4236	.4251	.4265	.4279	.4292	.4306	.4319
1.5	.4332	.4345	.4357	.4370	.4382	.4394	.4406	.4418	.4429	.4441
1.6	.4452	.4463	.4474	.4484	.4495	.4505	.4515	.4525	.4535	.4545
1.7	.4554	.4564	.4573	.4582	.4591	.4599	.4608	.4616	.4625	.4633
1.8	.4641	.4649	.4656	.4664	.4671	.4678	.4686	.4693	.4699	.4706
1.9	.4713	.4719	.4726	.4732	.4738	.4744	.4750	.4756	.4761	.4767
2.0	.4772	.4778	.4783	.4788	.4793	.4798	.4803	.4808	.4812	.4817
2.1	.4821	.4826	.4830	.4834	.4838	.4842	.4846	.4850	.4854	.4857
2.2	.4861	.4864	.4868	.4871	.4875	.4878	.4881	.4884	.4887	.4890
2.3	.4893	.4896	.4898	.4901	.4904	.4906	.4909	.4911	.4913	.4916
2.4	.4918	.4920	.4922	.4925	.4927	.4929	.4931	.4932	.4934	.4936
2.5	.4938	.4940	.4941	.4943	.4945	.4946	.4948	.4949	.4951	.4952
2.6	.4953	.4955	.4956	.4957	.4959	.4960	.4961	.4962	.4963	.4964
2.7	.4965	.4966	.4967	.4968	.4969	.4970	.4971	.4972	.4973	.4974
2.8	.4974	.4975	.4976	.4977	.4977	.4978	.4979	.4979	.4980	.4981
2.9	.4981	.4982	.4983	.4983	.4984	.4984	.4985	.4985	.4986	.4986
3.0	.4987									
3.5	.4997									
4.0	.4999									

$$\Pr(x < 15) = \Pr\left(\frac{x - 10}{4} < \frac{15 - 10}{4}\right)$$

If Z is a standard normal variable, use the table of standard normal probabilities to find:

(a) Pr(Z < 0)
(b) Pr(-1 < Z < 1)
(c) Pr(Z > 2.54).

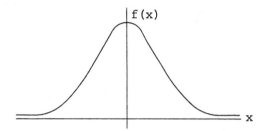

Solution: The normal distribution is the familiar "bell-shaped" curve. It is a continuous probability distribution that is widely used to describe the distribution of heights, weights, and other characteristics.

The density function of the standard normal distribution is

$$f(x) = \frac{1}{\sqrt{2\pi}} \exp\left(\frac{-x^2}{2}\right) \qquad -\infty < x < \infty.$$

See Figure 1. The probability of a standard normal variable being found in a particular interval can be found with the help of tables found in the backs of most statistics text books.

(a) To find the probability Pr(Z < 0) we can take advantage of the fact that the normal distribution is symmetric about its mean of zero. Thus,

Pr(Z > 0) = Pr(Z < 0). We know that

Pr(Z > 0) + Pr(Z < 0) = 1

because Z > 0 and Z < 0 are exhaustive events. Thus,

2Pr(Z < 0) = 1   or   Pr(Z < 0) = ½.

(b) To find the Pr(-1 < Z < 1) we use the tables of the standard normal distribution found in 15-25:

Pr(-1 < Z < 1) = Pr(Z < 1) - Pr(Z < -1).

Reading across the row headed by 1 and down the column labeled .00 we see that $Pr(Z < 1.0) = .8413$.

$Pr(Z < -1) = Pr(Z > 1)$ by the symmetry of the normal distribution. We also know that

$$Pr(Z > 1) = 1 - Pr(Z < 1).$$

Substituting we see,

$$Pr(-1 < Z < 1) = Pr(Z < 1) - [1 - Pr(Z < 1)]$$

$$= 2Pr(Z < 1) - 1 = 2(.8413) - 1 = .6826.$$

(c) $Pr(Z > 2.54) = 1 - Pr(Z < 2.54)$ and reading across the row labeled 2.5 and down the column labeled .04 we see that $Pr(Z < 2.54) = .9945$.

Substituting,

$$Pr(Z > 2.54) = 1 - .9945 = .0055.$$

● **PROBLEM** 15-27

Find $Pr(-.47 < z < .94)$.

Solution:

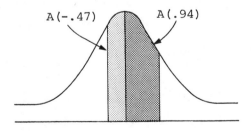

$Pr(-.47 \leq z \leq .94)$ is equal to the shaded area above. To find the value of the shaded area we add the areas labeled $A(-.47)$ and $A(.94)$.

$$Pr(-.47 \leq z \leq .94) = A(-.47) + A(.94).$$

By the symmetry of the normal distribution, $A(-.47)$ $= A(.47) = .18082$ from the table in 15-25.

Also   A(.94) = .32639 so

Pr(-.47<Z<.94) = .18082 + .32639 = .50721.

If X has a normal distribution with mean 9 and standard deviation 3, find P(5<X<11).

Solution: First, we convert our X-scores to Z-scores by subtracting the mean and dividing by the standard deviation. Next, we consult tables for the standard normal distribution found in problem 15-25.

Thus, $P(5<X<1) = P\left[\dfrac{5-9}{3}<\dfrac{X-9}{3}<\dfrac{11-9}{3}\right]$

$$= P\left[\dfrac{-4}{3}<Z<\dfrac{2}{3}\right] = \Phi(.66) - \Phi(-.133)$$

$$= .74537 - .09176 = .65361.$$

Given a mean of 50 and a standard deviation of 10 for a set of measurements that is normally distributed, find the probability that a randomly selected observation is between 50 and 55.

Solution: We wish to find $Pr(50 \le X \le 55)$, where X is normally distributed with mean 50 and standard deviation 10. We standardize X to convert our distribution of X scores to a distribution of Z-scores. Let $Z = \dfrac{X-\mu}{\sigma}$, where μ is the mean of X scores and s is the standard deviation of the X-scores. Then

$$Pr(50 \leq X \leq 55) = Pr\left[\frac{50 - \mu}{\sigma} \leq \frac{X - \mu}{\sigma} \leq \frac{55 - \mu}{\sigma}\right]$$

$$= Pr\left[\frac{50 - 50}{10} \leq Z \leq \frac{55 - 50}{10}\right] = Pr(0 < Z \leq .5).$$

$$Pr(Z \leq .5) - Pr(Z \leq 0) = Pr(0 \leq Z \leq .5).$$

From the table of standard normal, found in problem 15-25

$$Pr(Z \leq 0) = .5 \quad \text{and} \quad Pr(Z \leq .5) = .691.$$

Substituting we see that

$$Pr(50 \leq X \leq 55) = Pr(0 \leq Z \leq .5)$$

$$= Pr(Z \leq .5) - Pr(Z \leq 0) = .691 - .500$$

$$= .191.$$

● **PROBLEM 15-30**

Three hundred college freshmen are observed to have grade point averages that are approximately normally distributed with mean 2.1 and a standard deviation of 1.2. How many of these freshmen would you expect to have grade point averages between 2.5 and 3.5 if the averages are recorded to the nearest tenth?

Solution: To find the number of students with averages between 2.5 and 3.5 we first find the percentage of students with averages between 2.5 and 3.5. The averages are continuous random variables that are rounded to become discrete random variables. For example, any average from 2.45 to 2.55 would be recorded as 2.5. An average of 3.45 to 3.55 would be recorded as 3.5.

Thus, in computing the probability of an average lying between 2.5 and 3.5, we must account for this rounding procedure. Hence,

$$Pr(2.5 < X < 3.5) = Pr(2.45 < X < 3.55).$$

We now find this probability by standardizing the X-scores and converting them to Z-scores. Thus,

$$Pr(2.45 < X < 3.55) = Pr\left[\frac{2.45 - \mu}{\sigma} < \frac{X - \mu}{\sigma} < \frac{3.55 - \mu}{\sigma}\right]$$

$$= Pr\left[\frac{2.45 - 2.1}{1.2} < Z < \frac{3.55 - 2.1}{1.2}\right]$$

$$= Pr(.292 < Z < 1.21) = Pr(Z < 1.21) - Pr(Z < .292)$$

referring to the table in 15-25

$$= .8869 - .6141 = .2728,$$

or 27.28% of the freshmen have grades between 2.5 and 3.5. So, 27.28% of 300 is 81.84 or approximately 82 students have grade point averages between 2.5 and 3.5.

● **PROBLEM** 15-31

Miniature poodles are thought to have a mean height of 12 inches and a standard deviation of 1.8 inches. If height is measured to the nearest inch, find the percentage of poodles having a height exceeding 14 inches.

Solution: Let X be the height of a randomly selected poodle. X has mean 12 and standard deviation 1.8. Because the heights are measured to the nearest inch, any height that is greater than 13.5 or less than 14.5 is recorded as 14.

To find the percentage of poodles such that height, X, is greater than 14, we must find the percentage of poodles whose heights are greater than 13.5.

$Pr(X > 13.5)$ can be found by converting X to a random variable Z, that is normally distributed with mean 0 and variance 1.

$$Pr(X \geq 13.5) = Pr\left[\frac{X - \mu}{\sigma} \geq \frac{13.5 - \mu}{\sigma}\right]$$

$$= \Pr\left[Z \geq \frac{13.5 - 12}{1.8}\right] = \Pr(Z \geq .83).$$

From the table in problem 15-25 this is found to be

$$= .2033.$$

Thus, about 20% of these miniature poodles have heights that are greater than 14 inches.

● **PROBLEM** 15-32

The mean spread of a large group of guayule plants is 12 inches. The standard deviation is 2 inches. If the heights are normally distributed, find the probability that a plant picked at random from the group will have a spread: (a) between 10 and 14 inches; (b) greater than 16 inches; (c) of 12 inches. (Assume that heights are recorded to the nearest inch.)

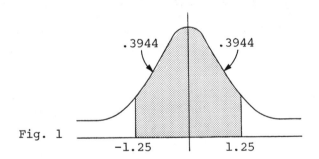

Fig. 1

.3944   .3944

-1.25   1.25

Solution: Any plant whose spread falls between 9.5 and 14.5 inches would be recorded as having a spread between 10 and 14 inches (since in recording spreads we round off to the nearest inch). Therefore, to find the probability that a plant picked at random will have a spread between 10 and 14 inches, we must find P(9.5 in< X<14.5 in). This is indicated by the shaded area on the normal curve (Figure 1).

The X value of 9.5 corresponds to a z value of -1.25 calculated by $z = \frac{x - \bar{x}}{s} = \frac{9.5 - 12}{2} = -1.25$. The X value of 14.5 corresponds to a z value of 1.25 calculated by z =

$$\frac{x - \bar{x}}{s} = \frac{14.5 - 12}{2} = 1.25.$$ Looking up the z values of -1.25 and 1.25 we get 0.3944 for both. The total area from 9.5 to 14.5 is 0.3944 + 0.3944 = 0.7888. Thus, the probability that a plant picked at random from our group will have a spread between 9.5 and 14.5 inches is 78.88%.

b) A plant with a spread of more than 16 inches must have a spread of at least 16.5 inches. Thus, we must find P(X>16.5 inches). This is shown by the shaded area under the following standard normal curve.

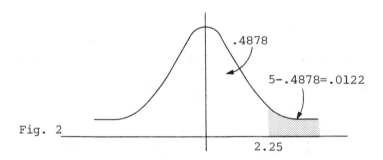

.4878

5-.4878=.0122

Fig. 2

2.25

The X value of 16.5 corresponds to a z value of $\frac{16.5 - 12}{2}$ = 2.25. Looking up 2.25 on our table of areas we find that the area under the curve is 0.4878. So to pick a plant greater than 16.5 inches we would subtract 0.4878 from 0.5 to find the area to the right of z = 2.25. In other words, there is a 1.22% chance of selecting a guayule plant from our group with a spread of greater than 16 inches.

c) The probability that a plant picked at random will have a spread of 12 inches means that P(11.5<X<12.5). This area is shaded in the following curve.

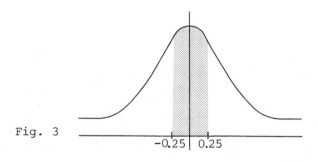

Fig. 3

-0.25   0.25

The X value of 11.5 corresponds to a z value of $\frac{11.5 - 12}{2}$ = -0.25 and the X value of 12.5 corresponds to a z value of $\frac{12.5 - 12}{2}$ = 0.25. Referring to the table of areas gives us values of 0.0987 and 0.0987. Thus, finding the total shaded area 0.1974 we can say that there is a 19.74% chance of picking a guayule plant with a spread of 12 inches.

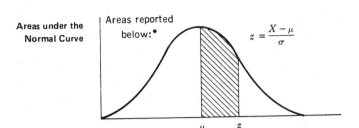

z	.00	.01	.02	.03	.04	.05	.06	.07	.08	.09
0.0	.0000	.0040	.0080	.0120	.0160	.0199	.0239	.0279	.0319	.0359
0.1	.0398	.0438	.0478	.0517	.0557	.0596	.0636	.0675	.0714	.0753
0.2	.0793	.0832	.0871	.0910	.0948	.0987	.1026	.1064	.1103	.1141
0.3	.1179	.1217	.1255	.1293	.1331	.1368	.1406	.1443	.1480	.1517
0.4	.1554	.1591	.1628	.1664	.1700	.1736	.1772	.1808	.1844	.1879
0.5	.1915	.1950	.1985	.2019	.2054	.2088	.2123	.2157	.2190	.2224
0.6	.2257	.2291	.2324	.2357	.2389	.2422	.2454	.2486	.2518	.2549
0.7	.2580	2.612	.2642	.2673	.2704	.2734	.2764	.2794	.2823	.2852
0.8	.2881	.2910	.2939	.2967	.2995	.3023	.3051	.3078	.3106	.3133
0.9	.3159	.3186	.3212	.3238	.3264	.3289	.3315	.3340	.3365	.3389
1.0	.3413	.3438	.3461	.3485	.3508	.3531	.3554	.3577	.3599	.3621
1.1	.3643	.3665	.3686	.3708	.3729	.3749	.3770	.3790	.3810	.3830
1.2	.3849	.3869	.3888	.3907	.3925	.3944	.3962	.3980	.3997	.4014
1.3	.4032	.4049	.4066	.4082	.4099	.4115	.4131	.4147	.4162	.4177
1.4	.4192	.4207	.4222	.4236	.4251	.4265	.4279	.4292	.4306	.4319
1.5	.4332	.4345	.4357	.4370	.4382	.4394	.4406	.4418	.4429	.4441
1.6	.4452	.4463	.4474	.4484	.4495	.4505	.4515	.4525	.4535	.4545
1.7	.4554	.4564	.4573	.4582	.4591	.4599	.4608	.4616	.4625	.4633
1.8	.4641	.4649	.4656	.4664	.4671	.4678	.4686	.4693	.4699	.4706
1.9	.4713	.4719	.4726	.4732	.4738	.4744	.4750	.4756	.4761	.4767
2.0	.4772	.4778	.4783	.4788	.4793	.4798	.4803	.4808	.4812	.4817
2.1	.4821	.4826	.4830	.4834	.4838	.4842	.4846	.4850	.4854	.4857
2.2	.4861	.4864	.4868	.4871	.4875	.4878	.4881	.4884	.4887	.4890
2.3	.4893	.4896	.4898	.4901	.4904	.4906	.4909	.4911	.4913	.4916
2.4	.4918	.4920	.4922	.4925	.4927	.4929	.4931	.4932	.4934	.4936
2.5	.4938	.4940	.4941	.4943	.4945	.4946	.4948	.4949	.4951	.4952
2.6	.4953	.4955	.4956	.4957	.4959	.4960	.4961	.4962	.4963	.4964
2.7	.4965	.4966	.4967	.4968	.4969	.4970	.4971	.4972	.4973	.4974
2.8	.4974	.4975	.4976	.4977	.4977	.4978	.4979	.4979	.4980	.4981
2.9	.4981	.4982	.4983	.4983	.4984	.4984	.4985	.4985	.4986	.4986
3.0	.4987									
3.5	.4997									
4.0	.4999									

*Example: For z = 1.96, shaded area is 0.4750 out of the total area of 1.0000.

577

CHI-SQUARE TEST

Assume the following data for corn, Zea mays, where the kernels are scored for aleurone color: 2,187 colored and 1,813 colorless. Determine, by using chi-square analysis, whether the data best fits the hypothesis of testcross progeny for a single gene pair with complete dominance (i.e., 1:1), or the hypothesis of F_2 progeny for two gene pairs showing epistasis (i.e., 9:7). The smallest value of χ^2 calculated will determine to which hypothesis the data best fits. Then, take the lowest χ^2 value and determine its validity using the χ^2 table shown in problem 15-34.

Solution: We use the following formula to solve this problem:

$$\chi^2 = \Sigma(d^2/e)$$

d = observed - expected

Σ = sum

We now present the calculations for each hypothesis in tabular form:

a) Hypothesis of 1:1

Phenotype	Observed	Expected(e)	Deviation(d)	d^2	d^2/e
colored	2,187	2,000	187	34969	17.484
colorless	1,813	2,000	-187	34969	17.484

$$\chi^2 = 17.484 + 17.484 = 34.968$$

b) Hypothesis of 9:7

Phenotype	Observed	Expected(e)	Deviation(d)	d^2	d^2/e
colored	2,187	2,250	-63	3969	1.764
colorless	1,813	1,750	63	3969	2.268

$$\chi^2 = 1.764 + 2.268 = 4.032$$

578

Thus, because chi-square is smaller for our second hypothesis (9:7), we can say that it is a better fit than our first hypothesis (1:1).

Using the chi-square table in question 15-33, we can check to see if our hypothesis and the observed data are close enough for us to consider that our 9:7 hypothesis is valid.

First, we must find the degree of freedom (df) using this formula:

$$df = n - 1$$

n = # of different classes of outcome
(colored and non-colored)

so

$$df = 2 - 1 = 1$$

Now, using the table, we find that $x^2 = 4.032$ with df = 1 corresponds to an approximate probability value of 0.05. This means that a deviation as large or larger than that observed might occur by chance 5 percent of the time. Experimenters consider this value borderline and in this case additional experiments would be desirable.

● **PROBLEM 15-34**

You are given Mendel's original data on the inheritance of yellow versus green cotyledons. In his experiment, 8023 individuals were scored. Of the 8023, 6022 were yellow and 2001 were green. We expect that yellow and green will appear in a 3:1 ratio respectively. Using the chi-square test (x^2), how well does Mendel's data fit our proposed ratio?

Solution: The chi-square (x^2) test makes use of probability values in the determination of whether or not a given set of data fits a particular ratio. In this case our hypothesis is that yellow versus green appears in a 3:1 ratio.

The formula for the chi-square test is:

$$\chi^2 = \Sigma(d^2/e),$$

where Σ stands for "the sum of", and d represents the deviation from e, or the expected value. If all 8023 of the offspring conformed perfectly to the 3:1 ratio, the number of yellow would be 6017 and the number of green would be 2006, both these values being rounded to the nearest whole number. To find out if Mendel's values are close enough to the expected to be valid let us carry out the test:

Hypothesis	3 yellow	1 green
Observed	6022	2001
Expected (e)	6017	2006
Deviation (d)	5	-5
d^2	25	25
d^2/e	0.004	0.012

$$\chi^2 = 0.004 + 0.012 = 0.016$$

Now, we have obtained the χ^2 value. In order to continue our evaluation we must make use of a chi-square table to determine if Mendel's data will fit our ratio and if any deviations observed are due purely to chance.

Before we can make use of the chi-square table we must calculate one more measurement -- the degree of freedom (df). The formula for df is n - 1, where n is the number of different classes of outcome; in this case, green and yellow. Hence:

$$df = n - 1 = 2 - 1 = 1$$

one degree of freedom is available.

Looking at the table, we find that $\chi^2 = 0.016$ with df = 1 corresponding to an approximate probability value of 0.90. This means that 9 times out of 10, or 90 times out of 100, a deviation as great as the one observed would be due purely to chance. Since a value of P = 0.05 is considered borderline, a value of P = 0.90 indicates that Mendel's data fits the proposed ratio very closely.

TABLE OF CHI-SQUARE

			Probability			
n	.99	.98	.95	.90	.80	.70
1	0.000157	0.000628	0.00393	0.0158	0.0642	0.148
2	0.0201	0.0404	0.103	0.211	0.446	0.713
3	0.115	0.185	0.352	0.584	1.005	1.424
4	0.297	0.429	0.711	1.064	1.649	2.195
5	0.554	0.752	1.145	1.610	2.343	3.000
6	0.872	1.134	1.635	2.204	3.070	3.828
7	1.239	1.564	2.167	2.833	3.822	4.671
8	1.646	2.032	2.733	3.490	4.594	5.527
9	2.088	2.532	3.325	4.168	5.380	6.393
10	2.558	3.059	3.940	4.865	6.179	7.267

			Probability			
n	.50	.30	.20	.10	.05	.02	.01
1	0.455	1.074	1.642	2.706	3.841	5.412	6.635
2	1.386	2.408	3.219	4.605	5.991	7.824	9.210
3	2.366	3.665	4.642	6.251	7.815	9.837	11.345
4	3.357	4.878	5.989	7.779	9.488	11.668	13.227
5	4.351	6.064	7.289	9.236	11.070	13.388	15.086
6	5.348	7.231	8.558	10.645	12.529	15.033	16.812
7	6.346	8.383	9.803	12.017	14.067	16.622	18.475
8	7.344	9.524	11.030	13.362	15.507	18.168	20.090
9	8.343	10.656	12.242	14.684	16.919	19.679	21.666
10	9.342	11.781	13.442	15.987	18.307	21.161	23.209

● **PROBLEM** 15-35

In summer squash, spheroid fruit genes are dominant over genes for elongated fruit. A cross between two different homozygous spheroid-fruited varieties results in the following F_2:

> 89 disc
> 62 spheroid
> 11 elongated

Ascertain the fit of this data to a reasonable modified dihybrid ratio using chi-square analysis. Explain the pattern of inheritance, the F_1 genotype and phenotype, and the F_2 genotypes.

Solution: In a classical dihybrid cross the phenotypic ratio of F_2 should be 9:3:3:1.

In the present problem the F_2 generation consists of the following fruit shapes:

disc 89
spheroid 62
elongated 11

Inspection of these numbers yields an approximate ratio of 9:6:1. Using the chi-square test we can see how well the data fits to this ratio:

Observed	expected(e)	deviation(d)	d^2	d^2/e
89	91	-2	4	0.04
62	61	1	1	0.02
11	10	1	1	0.10
				0.16

$$\chi^2 = \Sigma(d^2/e) = 0.16$$

Now, finding the degree of freedom, number of classes - 1, and referring to the chi-square table in problem 15-34, we find P $\approx$ 0.90 or 90%. Therefore, we can say that the data fit our 9:6:1 hypothesis.

To explain the pattern of inheritance, we can illustrate the cross:

A = spheroid   a = elongated
B = spheroid   b = elongated

(spheroid) AAbb x aaBB (spheroid)

F_1: Aa Bb

F_2:
9 A - B - (disc)
3 A - bb (spheroid)
3 aaB - (spheroid)
1 aabb (elongated)

There is complete dominance at both gene loci. Interaction between 2 dominants produces a new disc phenotype.

In one month at a public health clinic, 70 patients were found to have the same inherited disorder: 55 were males and 15 were females. Assuming a 1:1 ratio for males versus females, use the chi-square (χ^2) test to determine if any association of the disease with the male sex is statistically significant.

Solution: In this case we will be implementing the chi-square test to determine if the amount of deviation from the 1:1 ratio is significant enough to make any assumption that the disorder is sex linked.

	Male	Female
Observed	55	15
Expected (e)	35	35
(Assuming 1:1 ratio)		
Deviation (d)	20	-20
d^2	400	400
d^2/e	11.43	11.43

$$\chi^2 = \Sigma(d^2/e) = 11.43 + 11.43 = 22.86$$

Now, we need to find the degree of freedom (df). There are only two classes of outcome (the afflicted person will be male or female). Thus, n = 2 and df = n - 1 = 1.

Now, we are ready to consult the χ^2 table in problem 15-34. The table shows that the probability value for $\chi^2 = 22.86$ at df = 1 is much less than 0.01. This indicates that a ratio of 1:1 is completely inapplicable to the data and that association of the condition with the male sex is highly significant.

SHORT ANSWER QUESTIONS FOR REVIEW

Choose the correct answer.

1. What is the mean of the following measured
    quantities? 10, 11, 12, 13, 20, 25, 27, 30, 35
    (a) 25.5 (b) 20.3 (c) 18.5 (d) 18.3   b

2. What is the median of the quantities in question
    1? (a) 10 (b) 13 (c) 20.3 (d) 25 (e) 20   e

3. The mode of the quantities 30, 31, 31, 33,
    50, 60, 65 is (a) 30 (b) 31 (c) 50 (d) 60

    b

4. The modal class in question 2 is (a) 50, 60, 65
    (b) 31, 50, 60 (c) 30, 31, 31 (d) 30, 31, 50   c

5. A population that is relatively heterozygous
    for a particular trait would show a (a) low
    heritability. (b) high heritability. (c) no
    heritability. (d) none of the above   b

6. The total genetic variance for a given trait in
    a population of swine is 250. The variance due
    to epistatic effects is 20 and the environmental
    variance is 350. What is the heritability of the
    trait? (a) .20 (b) .30 (c) .40 (d) .50   b

7. In guinea pigs, black coat color is dominant
    over white coat color. If a black hetero-
    zygous guinea pig (Bb) is crossed with a
    homozygous white (bb) guinea pig, what is
    the probability that the first offspring will
    be white? (a) ¼ (b) ½ (c) 3/4 (d) 0   a

8. If two heterozygous black guinea pigs (Bb)
    are crossed, what would be the probability
    that the first three offspring will be black,
    white and black, or white, black, and white
    respectively? (a) 2/20 (b) 3/16 (c) 4/14
    (d) 5/12   b

9. Which of the following numbers is representa-
    tive of a continuous variable? 65^2, 65.3, 65,
    .03 (a) 65^2 (b) 65.3 (c) 65 (d) .03 (e)
    both b and d   e

10. The normal distribution for a trait existing
    in a large population reveals that (a) all
    individuals are homozygous for that trait.

(b) more individuals are found closer to the average value. (c) fewer individuals possess the extreme genotype. (d) both b and c

d

11. When two garden inflated yellow peas were crossed, the observed offspring phenotypes were; 193 green inflated : 184 yellow constricted : 556 yellow inflated : 61 green constricted. What is the approximate phenotypic ratio? (a) 1:2:1 (b) 2:1:2:1 (c) 9:3:3:1 (d) none of the above

c

12. If we use the chi-square test to evaluate the ratio in question 11, we can conclude that the genes coding for the two traits (a) assort independently. (b) are linked. (c) are sex-linked. (d) are epistatic.

a

13. The degrees of freedom for a sample with four phenotypes is (a) 4 (b) 3 (c) 2 (d) 1

b

14. A cross between two creepers (chickens affected with a genetic condition) produces a progeny of 775 creepers and 388 normal chicks. What is the closest phenotypic ratio? (a) 3:1 (b) 2:1 (c) 1:1 (d) 2:2

b

15. What is the possible mode of inheritance of the creeper trait in question 14? (a) sex-linked (b) epistatic to the normal allele (c) autosomal recessive-lethal when homozygous (d) both a and b (e) none of the above

c

Fill in the blanks.

16. The mean of a sample is the _____ of all the quantities in the sample _____ by the number sampled.

sum
divided

17. _____ is simply the square root of the variance.

Standard
deviation

18. The different expressions of a particular trait are due to genetic differences, _____ differences or the combined interaction of both.

environ-
mental

19. _____ is the measure of the degree to which

SHORT ANSWER QUESTIONS FOR REVIEW

a phenotype is genetically determined and
environmentally influenced.

Heritability

20. The _____ distribution is a method for
determining the probability of occurrence of
all possible outcomes in a given problem.

binomial

21. The study of human inheritance is not always
possible because individual matings produce a
_____ number of offspring.

small

22. The probability that the first two children
born to a couple will be male is _____.

one
quarter

23. A _____ random variable is a variable that
can only take isolated values.

discrete

24. Time is a _____ variable.

continuous

25. The _____ curve is widely used to describe
continuous variables.

bell-shaped

26. When evaluating experimental data by the
chi-square test, only the actual _____ data
can be used, not derivations.

numerical

27. If two phenotypes appear in a ratio of 4:16,
the probability value is between _____
and _____.

.7, .5

28. The ratio 9:3:3:1 has _____ degrees of
freedom.

two

Decide whether the following statements are true
or false.

29. The mean of a sample is the number sampled
divided by the sum of all the quantities in the
sample.

False

30. In the set of numbers {1,19,27,18,6}, 27 is
the median.

True

31. In the set of numbers {1,19,27,18}, 27 is
the median.

False

32. It is impossible for one number to be the mean,
median and mode in a specific set of numbers.

False

|

33. The variance stands for the average squared deviation from the mean. | True

34. To ascertain the standard deviation in a set of numbers, simply square the variance. | False

35. The standard deviation is preferred over the variance as a method of measure because its units are more specific. | True

36. Heritability is not dependent upon the inheritance of certain traits. | False

37. The probability that a couple will give birth to a girl rises significantly if they have three boys first. | False

38. In a dark room with 18 containers, 3 of which contain Drosophila, the probability of picking one container filled with Drosophila is 0.167. | True

39. In humans, a 1:1 sex ratio exists. The probability that a couple who plan to have four children will have all four girls is 0.125. | False

40. A discrete variable may only take isolated values. | True

41. The number of offspring in a litter of kittens is an example of a continuous variable. | False

42. Any normal distribution will fit perfectly under a bell curve. | True

43. The chi-square (χ^2) test is used to determine whether a set of data fits into a particular ratio. | True

44. The chi-square (χ^2) test can determine the amount of deviation from a given ratio. | True

APPENDIX

Recombinant DNA: The Technique of Recombining Genes
From One Species With Those From Another

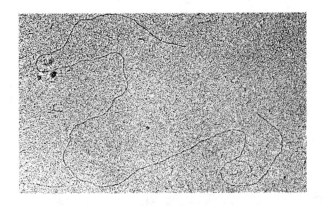

Electron micrograph of the DNA, which is the plasmid SP01
from *Bacillus subtilis.* This plasmid which has been
sliced open is used for recombinant DNA research
in this bacterial host

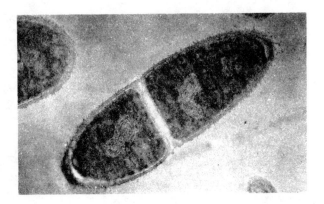

Electron micrograph of *Bacillus subtilis* in the process of
cell division. The twisted mass in the center of each
daughter cell is the genetic material, DNA

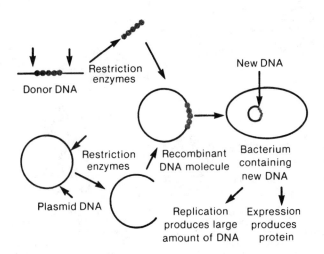

Restriction enzymes recognize certain sites along the DNA
and can chemically cut the DNA at those sites. This makes
it possible to remove selected genes from donor DNA molecules and insert them into plasmid DNA molecules to form
the recombinant DNA. This recombinant DNA can then be
cloned in its bacterial host and large amounts of a desired
protein can be produced.

The Product Development Process

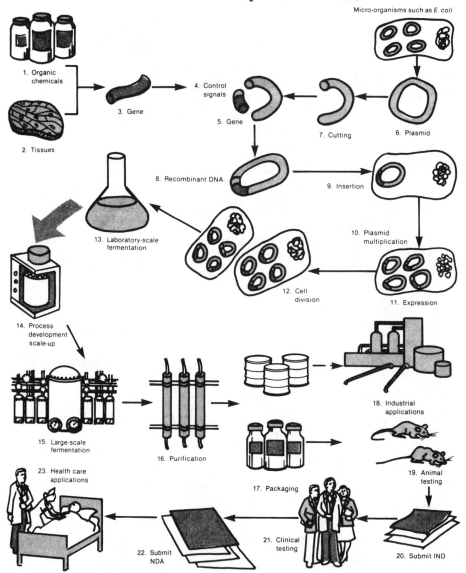

Micro-organisms such as *E. coli*

1. Organic chemicals
2. Tissues
3. Gene
4. Control signals
5. Gene
6. Plasmid
7. Cutting
8. Recombinant DNA
9. Insertion
10. Plasmid multiplication
11. Expression
12. Cell division
13. Laboratory-scale fermentation
14. Process development scale-up
15. Large-scale fermentation
16. Purification
17. Packaging
18. Industrial applications
19. Animal testing
20. Submit IND
21. Clinical testing
22. Submit NDA
23. Health care applications

The development process begins by obtaining DNA either through organic synthesis (1) or derived from biological sources such as tissues (2). The DNA obtained from one or both sources is tailored to form the basic "gene" (3) which contains the genetic information to "code" for a desired product, such as human inteferon or human insulin. Control signals (4) containing instructions are added to this gene (5). Circular DNA molecules called plasmids (6) are isolated from micro-organisms such as *E. coli*; cut open (7) and spliced back (8) together with genes and control signals to form "recombinant DNA" molecules. These molecules are then introduced into a host cell (9).

Each plasmid is copied many times in a cell (10). Each cell then translates the information contained in these plasmids into the desired product, a process called "expression" (11). Cells divide (12) and pass on to their offspring the same genetic information contained in the parent cell.

Fermentation of large populations of genetically engineered micro-organisms is first done in shaker flasks (13), and then in small fermenters (14) to determine growth conditions, and eventually in larger fermentation tanks (15). Cellular extract obtained from the fermentation process is then separated, purified (16), and packaged (17) either for industrial use (18) or health care applications.

Health care products are first tested in animal studies (19) to demonstrate a product's pharmacological activity and safety, in the United States, an investigational new drug application (20) is submitted to begin human clinical trials to establish safety and efficacy. Following clinical testing (21), a new drug application (NDA) (22) is filed with the Food and Drug Administration (FDA). When the NDA has been reviewed and approved by the FDA the product may be marketed in the United States (23).

Applications of Genetics

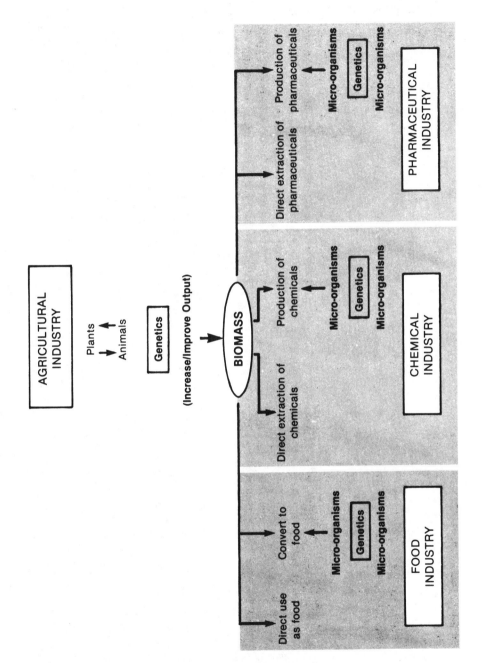

The Inheritance Pattern of Pea Color

Y = yellow gene   g = green gene

Homozygous yellow-seed peas have the genetic composition YY.
Homozygous green-seed peas have the genetic composition gg.

Each parent contributes only one seed-color gene to the offspring. When the two YY and gg homozygotes are crossed, the genetic composition of all offspring is Yg:

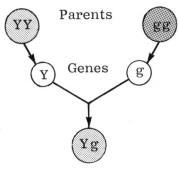

Offspring

All Yg offspring are heterozygous, and all have yellow seeds, indicating that the Y yellow gene is dominant over the g green gene.

When these Yg heterozygotes are crossed with each other:

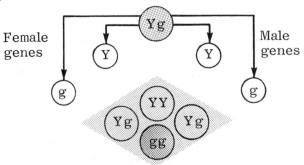

¼ of the total are homozygous YY, having yellow seeds
¼ of the total are homozygous gg, having green seeds
¼ of the total are heterozygous Yg, having yellow seeds

Thus, $\frac{3}{4}$ of these offspring will have yellow seeds, but their individual genetic composition, YY of Yg, may be different.

Chromosomes

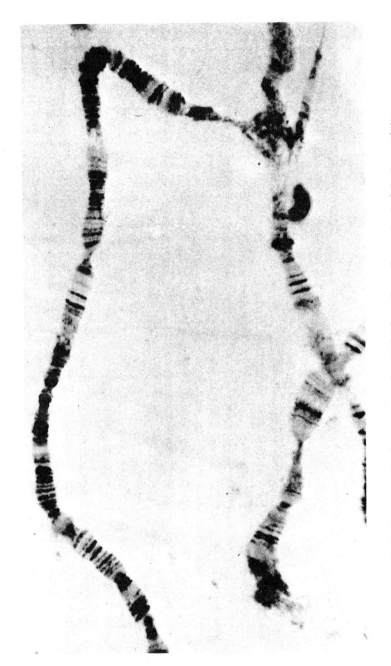

Optical micrograph of chromosomal material from the salivary gland of the larva of the common fruit fly, *Drosophila melanogaster*

The Structure of DNA

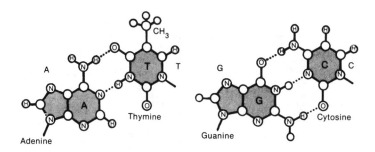

The pairing of the four nitrogenous bases of DNA:
Adenine (A) pairs with Thymine (T)
Guanine (G) pairs with Cytosine (C)

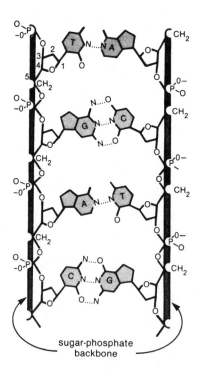

The four bases form the four letters in the alphabet of
the genetic code. The *sequence* of the bases along the
sugar-phosphate backbone encodes the genetic information.

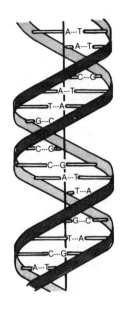

A schematic diagram of the DNA double helix.

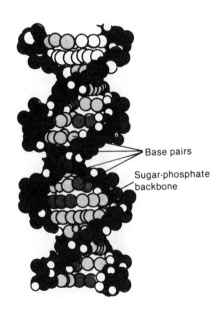

A three-dimensional representation of the DNA double helix.

The DNA molecule is a double helix composed of two chains. The sugar-phosphate backbones twist around the outside, with the paired bases on the inside serving to hold the chains together.

Replication of DNA

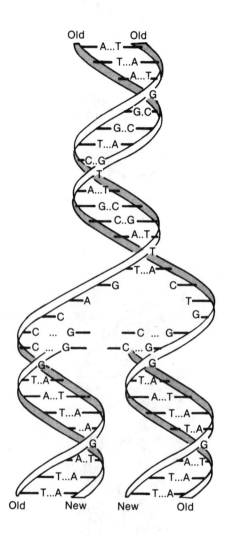

When DNA replicates, the original strands unwind and serve as templates for the building of new complementary strands. The daughter molecules are exact copies of the parent, with each having one of the parent strands.

The Genetic Code

SECOND BASE A — THIRD BASE

FIRST BASE	A	G	T	C
A	phe	phe	leu	leu
G	leu	leu	leu	leu
T	ileu	ileu	ileu	met
C	val	val	val	val

SECOND BASE G — THIRD BASE

FIRST BASE	A	G	T	C
A	ser	ser	ser	ser
G	pro	pro	pro	pro
T	thr	thr	thr	thr
C	ala	ala	ala	ala

SECOND BASE T — THIRD BASE

FIRST BASE	A	G	T	C
A	tyr	tyr	och*	amb*
G	his	his	gln	gln
T	asn	asn	lys	lys
C	asp	asp	glu	glu

SECOND BASE C — THIRD BASE

FIRST BASE	A	G	T	C
A	cys	cys	end*	trp
G	arg	arg	arg	arg
T	ser	ser	arg	arg
C	gly	gly	gly	gly

*och (ochre); amb (amber), and end are stop signal for translation, i.e., signal the end of synthesis of the protein chain.

Amino acid	Three-letter symbol
alanine	ala
arginine	arg
asparagine	asn
aspartic acid	asp
asn and/or asp	asx
cysteine	cys
glutamine	gln
glutamic acid	glu
gln and/or glu	glx
glycine	gly
histidine	his
isoleucine	ileu
leucine	leu
lysine	lys
methionine	met
phenylalanine	phe
proline	pro
serine	ser
threonine	thr
tryptophan	trp
tyrosine	tyr
valine	val

Each amino acid is determined by a three letter code (A, G, T, or C) along the DNA. If the first letter in the code is A, the second is T, and third is A, the amino acid will be tyrosine (or tyr) in the complete protein molecule. For leucine (or leu), the code is GAT, and so forth. The dictionary above gives the entire code.

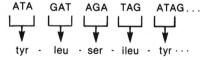

ATA   GAT   AGA   TAG   ATAG...

tyr - leu - ser - ileu - tyr ···

Transduction: The Transfer of Genetic Material in Bacteria by Means of Viruses

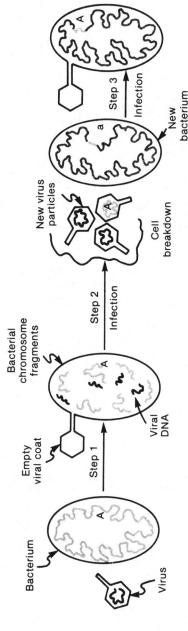

In step 1 of viral transduction, the infecting virus injects its DNA into the cell. In step 2 when the new viral particles are formed, some of the bacterial chromosomal fragments, such as gene A, may be accidently incorporated into these progeny viruses instead of the viral DNA. In step 3 when these particles infect a new cell, the genetic elements incorporated from the first bacterium can recombine with homologous segments in the second, thus exchanging gene A for gene a.

Conjunction: The Transfer of Genetic Material in Bacteria by Mating

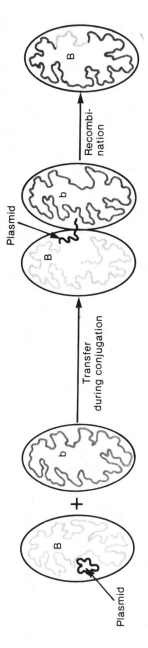

In conjugation, a plasmid inhabiting a bacterium can transfer the bacterial chromosome to a second cell where homologous segments of DNA can recombine, thus exchanging gene B from the first bacterium for gene b from the second.

An Example of How the Recombinant DNA Technique May Be Used To Insert New Genes Into Bacterial Cells

The first part of the technique involves the manipulations necessary to isolate and reconstruct the desired gene from the donor:
  a) The RNA that carries the message (mRNA) for the desired protein product is isolated.
  b) The double-stranded DNA is reconstructed from the mRNA.
  c) In the final step of this sequence, the enzyme terminal transferase acts to extend the ends of the DNA strands with short sequences of identical bases (in this case four guanines).

II. A bacterial plasmid, which is a small piece of circular DNA, serves as the vehicle for introducing the new gene (obtained in part I above) into the bacterium:
  a) The circular plasmid is cleaved by the appropriate restriction enzyme.
  b) The enzyme terminal transferase extends the DNA strands of the broken circle with identical bases (four cytosines in this case, to allow *complementary base pairing* with the guanines added to the gene obtained in part I).

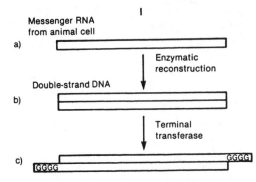

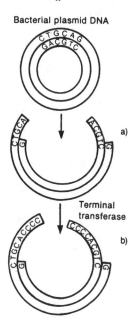

III. The final product, a bacterial plasmid containing the new gene, is obtained. This plasmid can then be inserted into a bacterium where it can be replicated and produce the desired protein product:
  a) The gene obtained in part I and the plasmid DNA from part II are mixed together and anneal because of the complementary base-pairing between them.
  b) Bacterial enzymes fill in any gaps in the circle, sealing the connection between the plasmid DNA and the inserted DNA to generate an intact circular plasmid now containing a new gene.

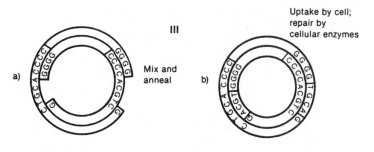

Recombinant DNA: The Technique of Recombining Genes From One Species With Those From Another

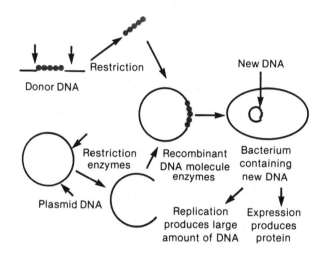

Donor DNA — Restriction

New DNA

Plasmid DNA

Restriction enzymes

Recombinant DNA molecule enzymes

Bacterium containing new DNA

Replication produces large amount of DNA

Expression produces protein

Diagram of Products Available From Cells

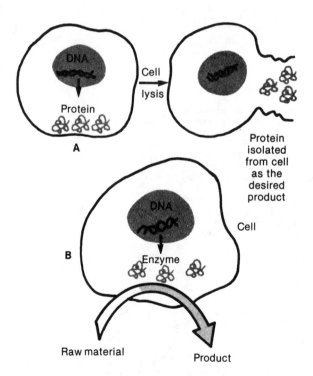

DNA

Cell lysis

Protein

A

Protein isolated from cell as the desired product

DNA

Cell

B

Enzyme

Raw material

Product

In (**A**) DNA directs the formation of a protein, such as insulin, which is itself the desired product. In (**B**), DNA directs the formation of an enzyme which, in turn, converts some raw material, such as sugar, to a product, such as ethanol.

GLOSSARY

Acridine dyes Chemical mutagens which cause frameshift mutations in the DNA.

Acrocentric chromosome A chromosome with its centromere towards one end of its length.

Adenine A purine base found in DNA and RNA.

Agouti Grizzled color of fur in animals resulting from light and dark banding on each hair.

Albinism In animals it is the absence of pigment in hair, eyes and skin. It is the absence of chlorophyll in plants.

Alkylating agents Chemical mutagens which add organic chemical groups to guanine (e.g., ethyl methansulfonate donates a methyl group to guanine).

Allele Any member of either a pair or a series of forms of a given gene.

Allopolyploid Polyploid in which the chromosome sets are non-homologous and arise from different species.

Allozymes The slightly different enzymes that arise from alleles at the same locus.

Amino acids These are the building blocks of proteins. Chemically, they contain a carboxyl (COOH) group and an amino (NH_2) group.

Anaphase The mitotic stage during which the single-stranded daughter chromosomes move apart. Late in this phase the chromosomes approach the poles of the spindle. This is also the stage that would be arrested following the administration of colchicine, a microtubule inhibitor.

Anemia Deficiency of hemoglobin or a reduced number of erythrocytes.

Aneuploidy The addition or deletion of parts of a chromosomal set.

Antibody A substance present in the body that helps to fight off foreign substances (antigens).

Anticodon Three bases in a tRNA molecule that are complementary to the three bases of a codon in mRNA.

Antigens A substance that stimulates the production of antibodies when introduced into an organism.

Anti-sense strand The strand of DNA not used as the template for mRNA. It is used to generate a complementary-sense strand during replication.

Astral fibers Fibers which radiate in other directions from each centriol but never run through the spindle.

ATP Adenosine triphosphate; an energy-providing compound in cells.

Autoimmune disease Characterized by production of antibodies against tissue components in the individual's own body.

Autopolyploid A sudden multiplication of the chromosomes in a normal individual due to nondisjunction of chromosomes during meiosis.

Autoradiography The imaging of a

radioactive-labeled substance produced over a period of time to allow for decay radiations to develop on the film.

Autosome Any chromosome which is not a sex chromosome.

Autotetraploid A nucleus which has four sets of chromosomes. This nucleus produces the recessive phenotype less frequently than the autodiploid.

Auxotroph A mutant organism which requires one or more nutritional supplements to grow.

B-cells Lymphocytes which are formed in the stem cells of bone marrow and are processed in the bursa. They are responsible for humoral immunity.

Bacteriophage A virus that attacks bacteria.

Barr Body Chromatin mass present in the nucleus of most female mammals. They result from the inactivation of all but one X chromosome.

Base analogs Chemical mutagens which cause substitutions of the naturally-occurring base pairs.

Binomial Distribution A method for determining the probability of occurrence of any of all the possible events for certain types of problems. It is expressed mathematically as

$$P(X) = \frac{N!}{X!(N-X)!} \; P^X \; Q^{N-X}$$

Bloom's Syndrome A chromosomal disorder (high frequency of chromosomal breakage) characterized by dwarfism.

Cancer cells A mass of clone cells which multiply and are unresponsive to the body's mechanism for controlling cell division.

Carrier An individual carrying a recessive gene that is not expressed.

Centriole Central granule of the centrosome that appears to be the most active area on the centrosome.

Centromere The area where two chromatids are bound to each other. It divides the arms of a chromosome into characteristic lengths. It also serves as a point of attachment to a spindle fiber during cell division for directional movement of chromosomes toward the poles.

Chemotaxis The behavior of an organism after the introduction of specific chemicals.

Chi-square test Allows for the determination of whether or not a given set of data fits a particular ratio. It is expressed mathematically as $X^2 = \Sigma \, (d^2/e)$.

Chiasma; pl. chiasmata The point of change or crossing over that occurs in two of a group of four chromosomes during prophase I of meiosis.

Chloroplast A green-colored structure in a plant cell's nucleus that contains chlorophyll which synthesizes starch.

Chromatid One of two identical strands resulting from the self-duplication of a chromosome while undergoing either meiosis or mitosis.

Chromatin Strands of DNA complexed with histone proteins and other organic compounds. The chromatin fiber can be considered as a basic structural unit of the chromosome.

Chromosomes Microscopic structures present in the nuclei of cells that carry the genes in a linear order. They are visible through a microscope during cell division.

Cistron The functional unit in a DNA system. One cistron in the DNA represents one polypeptide that will be synthesized.

Clones All individuals derived from a single individual by vegetative propagation.

Codominance When alleles produce different effects when heterozygous.

Codon Three adjacent nucleotides

that represent (code for) one specific amino acid.

Coefficient of Coincidence It is expressed mathematically as

$$C.C. = \frac{\text{observed frequency of double crossovers}}{\text{expected frequency of double crossovers}}$$

Colchicine An alkaloid that is added to cells to arrest spindle formation, thus interrupting mitosis by stopping movement of chromosomes to the poles.

Competence The degree to which a bacterial cell allows DNA to be incorporated and complete genetic transformation.

Complementary genes Genes which, if presented separately, give similar phenotypic traits but if given together interact to produce a different trait.

Complementary strand The strand of DNA which is matched to an original strand of DNA by base pairing.

Complementation The principle used to determine whether bacteriophage have mutations in separate genes or whether the mutations are allelic.

Concordant twins Twins which are alike with respect to a specific trait.

Conjugation The transmission of genetic material between bacteria through a specialized sex pilus.

Consanguineous marriage A marriage between two individuals that have a common-blood ancestor.

Continuous fibers Spindle fibers which run from pole to pole in a cell.

Continuous variable A variable which may fall into a range of values, depending on the accuracy of measurement.

Cotransformation A process that involves the ligation of a cloned gene to a cloned selectable marker in order to introduce the genes into mammalian cells.

Cri-du-chat Syndrome A deletion in the short arm of chromosome No. 5 in humans resulting in severe retarda-

tion and a cat-like cry in infants.

Cross breeding Mating between individuals who are from different races or species.

Crossing over An exchange of genes between chromosomes producing new combinations of genes not present in the parents.

Crystallized intelligence A component of intelligence which is a function of training and intelligence.

Cytosine A pyrimidine base found in DNA and RNA.

Deletion The absence of a segment of a chromosome consisting of one or more genes.

Desynapsis The separation of paired chromosomes with the sister chromatids remaining joined at the centromere occurring during diplotene.

Diakinesis Stage in meiosis when chromosomes are maximally condensed and chiasmata slide to the ends of the chromatids.

Deficiency See Deletion.

Dihybrid An individual that is heterozygous for two different pairs of alleles.

Dihybrid cross A cross in which two traits are being examined.

Dioecious A unisexual organism which is either a male or a female.

Diploid An organism or cell having 2 complete sets of chromosomes (2n).

Diplotene During this late meiotic prophase stage, the paired chromosomes separate in a process called desynapsis. Sister chromatids, however, continue to be held together by their centromeres.

Discordant twins Twins which are different with respect to a specific trait.

Discrete random variable A variable which can only take isolated values.

(e.g., the number of apples in a bushel).

DNA Deoxyribonucleic acid. The chemical material of which genes are made.

DNA B protein Enables primase to begin RNA synthesis during DNA replication.

DNA polymerase I Removes primer and fills in gaps during DNA replication.

DNA polymerase III holoenzyme Synthesizes DNA during DNA replication.

Dominance When one member of the allelic pair is seen more often phenotypically than the other which is usually suppressed.

Dosage compensation The elimination of genes that are present in two doses in the heterogametic sex.

Double crossover Two gene loci are exchanged during crossing over.

Down's syndrome Also called trisomy-21, it is a chromosomal disorder in which the affected individual has an extra chromosome, number 21. The syndrome results in mongolism and a low resistance to disease.

Duplications The occurrence of an extra copy of a piece of chromosomal material on the same chromosome or genome.

Electrophoresis The migration of particles that are suspended in an electric field.

Enzyme A protein that catalyzes (speeds up) certain chemical reactions.

Episome A bacterial genetic factor that can exist either as an autonomous circular element in the cytoplasm or integrated into the chromosome.

Epistasis The suppression of the activity of one or more genes by one or more genes that are not allelic to the first gene or genes.

Eukaryote An organism composed of cells with true nuclei.

Euploidy The addition or deletion of an entire chromosomal set.

Excision repair A method of repairing thymine dimers, utilizing enzymes to remove the dimer and then filling in the gap.

Expressivity The degree of effect or the extent to which a gene expresses itself in different individuals.

F_1 First filial generation.

F_2 Second filial generation.

F factor The fertility factor in bacteria. It is an episome.

Fanconi's Anemia Characterized by chromosomal structure instability. Victims also show an increased susceptibility to cancer.

Fertilization The union of a male gamete (sperm) and a female gamete (ovum) to form a zygote.

Flagellum; pl. flagella The whiplike locomotor structure in certain organisms.

Fluid intelligence A type of intelligence which is a function of brain development and is completed by age 14.

Frameshift mutations Result from the addition or subtraction of one or several base pairs in the DNA.

FSH (follicle-stimulating hormone) A gonadotropic hormone, secreted by the hypothalamus, which stimulates a few egg follicles to undergo maturation each month.

G-bands Band patterns which appear all along the chromosomes, except at the ends, when stained.

Galactosemia An inherited disorder which results in a buildup of dietary galactose because its metabolism is blocked.

Gamete A mature reproductive cell. In males it is the sperm, and in females it is the egg.

Gametogenesis The formation of gametes.

Gene The hereditary unit or factor present in a fixed location on a chromosome.

Gene frequency The representation of one allele as a proportion in a breeding population.

Gene pool Total of all genetic information in the breeding members of a population.

Genetic drift The purely random fluctuations in gene frequency mainly due to a small population size.

Genetic equilibrium A breeding population with a total absence of mutations, no gene exchange with the outside, and random reproduction. Gene frequencies remain constant.

Genetics The study of heredity and variance.

Genome A complete set of genes and chromosomes inherited as a group from one parent.

Genotype The genetic makeup of an organism.

Geotaxis Gravity-oriented locomotion.

Germ cells Reproductive cells which, when mature, are capable of fertilization to keep the species going.

Giemsa (G) stain Chemical reagent used to make visible the G-bands on the chromosomes.

Globulins Proteins commonly found in blood that are insoluble in water. Alpha, beta, and gamma globulins are present in human blood.

Gonad Sexual organs that produce the gametes. In males it is the testis and in females it is the ovary.

Guanine A purine base found in DNA

and RNA.

Gyrase 1) Helps to supertwist DNA molecules along with ATP.
2) Helps to unwind DNA helix during DNA replication.

Haploid An organism or cell having only one complete set of chromosomes (n).

Hardy-Weinberg Law States that in a population at equilibrium both gene and genotype frequencies remain constant from generation to generation. It is expressed mathematically as

$$p^2(AA)+2pq(Aa)+q^2(aa) = 1$$

Helix A structure that is spiral in shape.

Hemizygous A nucleus which can only possess one set of the homologous gene pair. An (XY) male is considered hemizygous for a given trait rather than hetero- or homozygous because its Y chromosome does not have a locus for that genetic trait.

Hemoglobin A conjugated protein located in the erythrocytes in vertebrates. It plays an important role in carrying oxygen to all cells of an organism.

Heredity The transmission of traits from parental organisms to their progeny.

Heritability A measure of the degree to which a certain trait is controlled by inheritance.

Heteromorphic homologous chromosomes Easily-distinguished homologous chromosomes.

Heterosis The superiority of the heterozygous genotypes with respect to one or more traits when compared to the corresponding homozygotes.

Heterozygote An organism possessing different alleles on homologous chromosomes for one or all given characteristics.

Hfr High frequency recombination strain of Escherichia coli.

Histocompatibility Complex A locus
present on chromosome No. 6, of
humans, that allows for the differentiation between self and non-self.

Histones A major protein component
of the chromosomes having a high
content of basic amino acids arginine
and lysine.

Homologous chromosomes Chromosomes
bearing genes for the same character.

Homozygote An organism possessing
an identical pair of alleles on homologous chromosomes for one or all given
characteristics.

Hormone A chemical produced by
certain glands in plants and animals
which influences the activity of another
part of the organism.

Hybrid The offspring of homozygous
parents that differ in at least one
gene.

Hybridization The crossbreeding of
different strains of plants or animals
in which a hybrid may be formed.

Hyperploid nucleus A nucleus which
possesses more genetic information
than a normal nucleus.

Hypoploid nucleus A nucleus which
contains less genetic information
than a normal nucleus.

Immunity The resistance of the body
to foreign substances.

Immunization The induction of
resistance to a foreign substance
by producing antigen specific antibodies.

Immunoglobulins See Globulins.

Inbreeding Mating among individuals
who are common-blood relatives.

Incomplete dominance Heterozygous
alleles are expressed that are
different from those of the parents,
producing noticeable hybrids.

Independent assortment The random
distribution of genes into gametes

when the genes are present on
different chromosomes.

Inducer Substance that increases
the amount synthesized of the
enzyme(s) needed to metabolize it.

Intelligence The ability to learn or
understand.

Interferon A protein that is synthesized by the body upon virus
infection that helps rid the body of
the infecting organisms by inhibiting
virus formation.

Interphase This is the stage between
mitotic divisions, during which the
cell performs all necessary metabolic
processes.

Inversion A rearrangement of genes
in a chromosome in such a way that
their order becomes reversed in the
chromosome.

Ionizing radiation Radiation used to
knock out electrons in order to ionize
an atom in a chromosome molecule.

Isochromosomes Chromosomes in
which one arm has been deleted and
replaced by a piece identical to the
remaining arm.

Karyotype The way the chromosomes
of an individual appear at metaphase.

Karyotype analysis The technique
of fixing, staining, and photographing
cells at the metaphase stage for complete
study of the individual chromosomes.

Kinetochore Same as centromere.
Point of attachment to a spindle fiber
of a chromosome during cell division.

Kinetochore fibers Spindle fibers
which run from one pole to a
kinetochore on a chromosome.

Klinefelter's Syndrome Phenotypical
males who have two X chromosomes
plus a Y chromosome.

Leptotene The stage in meiosis which
has chromosomes identical to those in

the prophase of mitosis. They appear as slender threadlike fibers.

L.H. (luteinizing hormone) A gonadotropic hormone which stimulates the egg to be released and the follicle to become the corpus luteum.

Ligase An enzyme that joins the ends of DNA during DNA replication.

Linkage Genes on the same chromosome tend to stay together during the formation of gametes. Linked genes do not sort independently.

Linkage group A group of linked genes.

Linkage map A linear representation of how genes actually lie on their specific chromosomes.

Locus; pl. loci A known position on a chromosome that is always filled by a specific gene or one of its alleles.

Lymphocytes White blood cells.

Lymphokines Produced by T-cells to assist with cell-mediated immunity.

Lysis The infection of a bacteria by a bacteriophage and the subsequent destruction of the cell membrane with cell explosion as the final result.

Lysogenesis The incorporation of viral DNA into bacterial chromosomes and subsequent division of the newly-affected cell.

Map unit One unit on a linkage map. It represents one percent of crossing over.

Maternal Having to do with the mother.

Mean The sum of all measurements divided by the total number of measurements.

Median The middle value in a group of numbers arranged in order of size.

Meiosis The process by which the chromosome number of a reproductive cell becomes haploid, forming gametes in animals and spores in plants. This helps in variability through recombination. Four daughter cells result, each with half the number of chromosomes that were present in the original cell.

Merozygote Partial zygote formed through transformation in bacteria.

Metacentric chromosome A chromosome with its centromere equidistant from either end of the chromosome.

Metaphase The mitotic stage during which the chromosomes are arranged on the equatorial plane of the spindle and between the centrioles. The end of this phase is triggered by the separation of the chromatids of each chromosome, thus doubling the number of total chromosomes.

Microtubules Hollow filaments in the cytoplasm that serve many purposes, including formation of locomotor apparatus in motile cells and also formation of the spindle during mitosis.

Mitosis The process by which all somatic cells duplicate. Two daughter cells result from the splitting of the original cell that are identical to the original cell in all characteristics. It is broken down into five stages: Interphase, Prophase, Metaphase, Anaphase, and Telophase.

Mode The number that occurs with the greatest frequency among a given group of numbers.

Modifier A gene that affects the final expression of another gene.

Monoecious An organism with male and female gametes - mainly plants with both staminate and pistillate flowers.

Monohybrid The offspring resulting from a cross between parents that differ from one another by alleles at one locus only.

Monohybrid Cross A cross in which only one trait is being examined.

Morphology The study of the shapes and structures of an organism compared to similar structures in other organisms.

Multigene cross A cross in which more than three traits are being examined.

Multiple alleles Three or more alleles representing one locus on a given pair of chromosomes that control a single trait.

Mutagen An agent found in the external environment that is capable of causing mutation.

Mutant A cell or organism showing the change brought about by a mutation.

Mutation A change in the DNA at a specific locus in an organism.

Mutation rate Can be solved mathematically as

$$\text{Mutation rate} = \frac{\text{number of mutants}}{\text{total number of cells}}$$

Muton The smallest unit which, if altered, gives rise to a mutant phenotype.

Natural selection The survival of individuals that have better adapted to their natural environments.

Negative control This form of control utilizes repressors and inducers to turn off a genetic system that would otherwise be turned on.

Neocentric fibers Spindle fibers that attach to any part of the chromosome except at the kinetochore.

Non-consanguinous marriage A marriage between two individuals that do not have a common-blood ancestor.

Nondisjunction Homologous chromosomes fail to separate in meiosis, resulting in too many chromosomes being present in some of the daughter cells and not enough chromosomes present in the others.

Nucleolus Storage area for ribosomal RNA, present in some metabolic cells.

Nucleotide One unit in the DNA molecule containing a phosphate, a sugar, and a nitrogenous base.

Nucleus Part of the cell which carries the genetic information that directs activities of the cell. It is completely surrounded by nuclear membrane.

Nullisomics Organisms having a (2n-2) number of chromosomes. They have completely lost a pair of chromosomes.

Oncogenes Genes which may cause cells to become cancerous.

Oocyte The cell that undergoes meiosis to form the egg cell.

Oogenesis The formation of the ovum in animals.

Operon A group of genes that form a control unit.

Ovum The egg; the mature female germ cell.

P The symbol used to represent the parental generation or the parents of a specific individual.

Pachytene The stage in meiotic midprophase in which the actual physical exchange of genetic material is believed to occur.

Paracentric inversions Chromosomal inversions which do not include the area of the centromere.

Parthenogenesis The development of an individual from an unfertilized egg.

Paternal Having to do with the father.

Pathogen A disease-causing organism or virus.

Pedigree A graphic representation of the familial history of an individual. It can be done in chart, table, or diagrammatic form.

Penetrance The percentage of individuals in a population who carry a gene in the correct combination for its expression and who express the gene phenotypically.

Percent recombination This is

expressed mathematically as

$$\% \text{ recombination} = \frac{\text{total number of recombinant progeny}}{\text{total number of test cross progeny}} \times 100$$

Pericentric inversions Chromosomal inversions which include the centromere.

Phenocopy A phenotype produced by the environment stimulating the effects of a known mutation.

Phenotype Those characteristics which are either observed on an individual or are discernible by other means.

Phenyketonuria (PKU) An inborn error of metabolism resulting in severe mental retardation.

Pheromones Chemicals produced by one sex of an organism to attract a member of the opposite sex. Most organisms use their sense of smell to detect these chemicals.

Photoreactivation A method of repairing thymine dimers using visible light.

Plaque A clear area on an opaque culture plate of bacteria that is where a virus has killed the bacteria.

Plasmids Self-replicating, extra-chromosomal circular pieces of bacterial DNA.

Pleiotropy When a single gene locus has more than one phenotypic effect.

Polar bodies In female animals, these are the smaller cells produced during meiosis that do not develop into egg cells.

Polydactyly The appearance of more than the normal five digits on the hands or feet.

Polygene One gene that is part of a group of genes that deal with quantitative inheritance.

Polygenic inheritance In this type of inheritance the whole range of variation is covered in a graded series.

Polygenic traits Traits which show a continuous variation in phenotypes instead of distinct classifications (e.g., not only red and white, but pink also).

Polymorphism The maintenance of two or more kinds of individuals in a breeding population.

Polypeptide A compound containing more than two peptide groups held by peptide bonds.

Polyploidy An organism having two or more complete sets of chromosomes due to aberrant meiosis.

Polytene chromosome A giant bundled chromosome resulting from continuous duplication without separation. The chromosomes of the salivary gland of the Drosophila are good examples of this.

Positive control This form of control utilizes components to enhance gene activity.

Postadaptive resistance The presence of a substance induces the resistance to that substance.

Preadaptive resistance The resistance to a substance is present in an organism before the substance is introduced into the organism.

Primase An enzyme that synthesizes RNA primers during DNA replication.

Probability The likelihood that an event will occur.

Progeny The offspring resulting from a particular mating.

Prokaryote An organism which does not contain true nuclei in its cell(s).

Prophase The mitotic stage during which the chromosomes shorten and thicken, and the nuclear membrane disintegrates. An intricate system of microtubules aggregate at either end of the cell forming the spindle.

Prototroph An organism which can grow on a minimal medium containing basic materials such as glucose and inorganic salts.

Pseudoalleles Genes that are closely linked and behave as if they were alleles but have been separated by crossing over.

Purines The two-ringed bases in DNA and RNA, adenine and guanine.

Pyrimidines The one-ringed bases in DNA, cytosine and thymine, and in RNA, cytosine and uracil.

Q-bands Chromosome band pattern resulting from quinacridine staining. This type of banding does not form at the ends of the chromosome.

Quinacridine Chemical reagent used in chromosome staining. It inserts itself into the DNA complex and produces fluorescent bands when excited by ultraviolet light.

R - and T - banding technique Technique used to detect terminal deletions on abnormal chromosomes.

Random reproduction The indiscriminate selection of a mate and of many other requirements contributing to success in producing viable offspring.

Recessive The member of the allelic pair that cannot be expressed phenotypically when the dominant member is present.

Reciprocal cross A second cross involving the same strains as the first cross but carried out by sexes opposite to those in the original cross.

Recombination New combinations of traits observed in an organism that are different from the parental combinations exhibited.

Recombination frequency Represented mathematically as

R.F. $\dfrac{\text{number of recombinants}}{\text{total number of offspring in that generation containing the recombinants}}$

R.F. x 100 = number of map units between the two genes.

Recon The smallest unit that is interchangeable, but not divisible, by recombination.

Replication A reproduction or duplication process that involves copying from a template.

Rep protein Unwinds the helix during DNA replication.

Repressor A molecule which interacts with DNA to inhibit the synthesis of the gene products.

Resistance The ability of an organism to fight off harmful foreign substances.

Restriction enzymes Enzymes that cut double stranded DNA molecules at very specific DNA sequences that these enzymes recognize.

Restriction map A map which locates the relative sites on DNA that are attacked by specific restriction enzymes.

Reverse transcriptase A viral enzyme that can catalyze the synthesis of DNA from RNA.

Ribosomes Structures in the cytoplasm of cells which are responsible for protein synthesis.

RNA Ribonucleic acid, the information-carrying chemical of plant viruses.
1) **mRNA** transcribes genetic information from DNA by the process of transcription.
2) **tRNA** transfers amino acids to the ribosomes for incorporation into proteins by the process of translation.
3) **rRNA** makes up the ribosomes.

Sense strand The strand of DNA used as the template for mRNA.

Segregation When paternal and maternal chromosomes are separated at meiosis, phenotypic differences can be observed in the offspring. This was Mendel's first principle of inheritance.

Sexduction An F factor-mediated form of transduction.

Sex-influenced trait Genes governing this trait may reside on any of the autosomes or on the homologous portions of the sex chromosomes. Dominant or recessive expression of these traits is determined mainly by the sex of the bearer, and by the presence of sex hormones.

Sex-linked trait A trait produced by a gene present only on the X chromosome.

Shuttle vectors Contain sequences that signal DNA replication in both E. coli and yeast.

Single crossover Only one gene locus is exchanged during the crossing over.

Somatic cells Those cells in body tissues containing two sets of chromosomes, one donated by the male parent and the other by the female parent.

Sperm; pl. spermatozoa Mature male germ cells.

Spermatids The four cells formed after two meiotic divisions of a primary spermatocyte. They will form four spermatazoa after differentiation.

Spermatocyte The cell that after two meiotic divisions forms four spermatids.

Spermatogenesis The process by which mature sperm cells are formed.

Spindle An aggregate of microtubules that forms in the cell to facilitate mitosis.

Spore 1) A protoplasmic unit that can, under certain conditions, develop asexually into a new individual.
2) In higher plants it is the haploid meiotic product that will eventually give rise to male or female gametes.

SSB protein Protects single-stranded regions during DNA replication.

Standard deviation The measure of variability in a population.

Standard error A measure of variability of a population of means.

Statistic A value based on a sample of a population from which estimates of a population value can be obtained.

Sticky ends Free ends of a chromosome resulting from radiation breakage which are capable of rejoining.

Synapsis Pairing of homologous chromosomes in meiotic prophase.

Tay-Sachs Disease A recessive disease resulting in the degeneration of the nervous system.

T-cells Lymphocytes which are formed in the stem cells of bone marrow, processed in the thymus, and are responsible for cell-mediated immunity with the production of lymphokines.
1) **Killer T-cells** Responsible for skin graft rejection, killing tumors, and killing virus-infected cells.
2) **Helper T-cells** Interact with B-lymphocytes and microphages to produce antibodies.
3) **Supressor T-cells** Mediate the activities of killer and helper T-cells.

Telocentric chromosome A chromosome with its centromere at the very end of its length.

Telophase This is the last mitotic stage during which the spindle fibers disappear and nuclear membranes form around both new sets of chromosomes. The end of this stage is signified by the separation of the original cell into two daughter cells.

Template A mold or model. DNA is the template for mRNA.

Test cross 1) A cross between an individual with an unknown genotype and one that is fully recessive to determine if the individual is homozygous or heterozygous for a certain allele.
2) A backcross to the recessive parental type.
3) A test to determine linkage.

Tetrad The group of four chromatids formed by the association of split homologous chromosomes during meiosis.

Thymine A pyrimidine base found in DNA but not in RNA.

Thymine dimers Chemical bonds between adjacent thymine residues on DNA caused by irradiation with ultraviolet light.

Thymus A gland in the chest that helps process T-cells.

Transcription The reading of the template DNA strand and subsequent formation of mRNA.

Transduction Bacteriophage-mediated recombination in bacteria.
1) Abortive transduction Bacterial DNA is injected into a bacterium by a phage, but no replication occurs.
2) Generalized transduction Any transfer of a bacterial gene from a phage to a bacterium.
3) Restricted transduction Transfer of bacterial DNA restricted to only one site on the bacterial chromosome.

Transformation 1) The addition of foreign DNA to a culture bringing about genetic recombination.
2) The donation of fragments of genes from one bacterium to another.

Transforming agent The foreign DNA added to a culture during transformation.

Transgressive segregation Segregation in which the variability of an F_2 generation is so great that some individuals show more extreme development than either parental type.

Transition The type of mutation caused by the substitution of one purine for another purine or one pyrimidine for another pyrimidine in DNA or RNA.

Translation The manufacture of proteins from mRNA strands.

Translocation The movement of a part of a chromosome to either a different region on the same chromosome or to a different chromosome.

Transposons Short segments of DNA which are incapable of self-replication.

Transversion A mutation in which a purine replaces a pyrimidine or vice-versa on DNA or RNA.

Trihybrid An organism produced by homozygous parents differing in three traits.

Trihybrid cross A cross in which three traits are being examined.

Turner's Syndrome Phenotypical females who only have one X chromosome and no Y chromosome.

Ultraviolet light Electromagnetic waves of very high frequency used to induce chromosomal breakage.

Uracil A pyrimidine base found in RNA but not in DNA.

Variance The square of the standard deviation. It is the degree of dispersion in a sample.

Variation Differences occurring among members of the same species.

Viral interference An initial viral infection prevents a secondary infection of the same cell by a different virus.

Wahlund's principle State that when mating occurs between populations the frequency of homozygous genotypes is reduced.

Wild type The phenotype that is used as the standard for comparison.

X-chromosome The chromosome associated with sex determination. The female usually has two and the male has one.

Xeroderma pigmentosum A disease in which the mechanism that repairs ultraviolet-induced damage in DNA is defective.

Y-chromosome   The chromosome that
is paired with an X chromosome in
males. They usually carry only a
few genes.

Zygote   1) The cell formed by the

union of two gametes.

2) The organism growing from the
original zygote formed.

Zygotene   Stage in meiotic prophase
when synapsis occurs.

INDEX

Numbers on this page refer to <u>PROBLEM NUMBERS</u>, not page numbers

Numbers on this page refer to __PROBLEM NUMBERS__, not page numbers

Ultraviolet (UV) light, 2-6,
   2-7, 5-4, 5-5
Unicorn, 7-17
Uracil, 9-2, 9-4, 9-14, 9-26

Vaccination, 10-27, 14-14
Valine, 9-33, 9-34
Variability, 1-5, 1-6
Variable:
   continuous, 15-23, 15-30
   discrete, 15-23
   random, 15-24, 15-25
Variance, 15-1 to 15-3, 15-6,
   15-25, 15-31
   dominant, 15-5, 15-6
   environmental, 15-5, 15-6
   environmental/genetic, 15-5
   epistatic, 15-5, 15-6
   genetic, 15-5, 15-6
   of a population, 8-30
   phenotypic, 15-5, 15-6
Viral interference, 10-27
Virus, 10-19
   Epstein-Barr, 10-26
   foot-and mouth disease
   (FMDV), 14-14
   herpes, 10-26
   influenza, 10-19
   poliomyelitis, 10-19
   retrovirus, 14-5
   RNA tumor, 10-25
   Rous sarcoma (RSV), 10-28
   smallpox, 10-19
   SV40, 10-19, 14-1
   tobacco mosaic (TMV), 10-19

Wahlund's principle, 8-15
Whatmore, P., 12-12
Wheat, kernel color, 6-10
Widow's peak, 8-7
Wobble hypothesis, 9-35, 9-36
Woodyard, E.R., 12-11
Wright, 15-6

Xanthine dehydrogenase, 14-7
X chromosome, 4-1, 4-9
Xeroderma pigmentosum, 2-7,
   5-4
X-ray diffraction, 2-1
X-rays, 2-6

Y chromosome, 4-1, 4-24
   and behavior, 12-12
Yeast, 14-8

Zea mays (corn), 1-8, 15-33
   height, 6-15
   kernel type, 7-10, 7-16
   leaf type, 7-16
Zinkernagel, Rolf, 13-13
Z-score, 15-24, 15-25, 15-28
Zygote, 1-9
   bacterial, 10-8
Zygotene, 1-5, 1-8